Chinese Medicine for Maximum Immunity

CHINESE

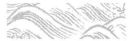

Understanding the

MEDICINE

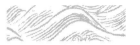

Five Elemental Types for

FOR MAXIMUM

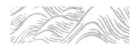

Health and Well-Being

IMMUNITY

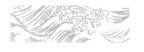

Previously published as *The Five Elements of Self-Healing*

Jason Elias, L.Ac., and

K̶ Ketcham

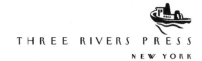

THREE RIVERS PRESS

NEW YORK

Published by Three Rivers Press, New York, New York.
Member of the Crown Publishing Group.
Originally published as *The Five Elements of Self-Healing: Using Chinese Medicine for Maximum Immunity, Wellness, and Health* in hardcover by Harmony Books in 1998.
First paperback edition printed in 1999.

Random House, Inc. New York, Toronto, London, Sydney, Auckland
www.randomhouse.com

THREE RIVERS PRESS is a registered trademark and the Three Rivers Press colophon is a trademark of Random House, Inc.
Printed in the United States of America

Library of Congress Cataloging-in-Publication Data
Elias, Jason.
    [Five elements of self-healing]
    Chinese medicine for maximum immunity : understanding the
five elemental types for health and well-being / by Jason Elias and
Katherine Ketcham. — 1st pbk. ed.
    Previously published: The five elements of self-healing / Jason
Elias, Katherine Ketcham. New York : Harmony Books, 1998.
    1. Medicine, Chinese. 2. Health. I. Ketcham, Katherine, 19
    R602.E46   1999
    610'.951—dc21

ISBN 0-609-80273-9
Book design by Susan Hood
Illustrations of the five elements by Jeanne McMene

10   9   8   7   6   5   4

To our children:

Adam Elias
Robyn, Alison, and Benjamin Spencer

CONTENTS

Acknowledgments   ix

Introduction by Jason Elias: The Journey of a Thousand Miles   xi

Part One. Understanding the Powers Within   1

Introduction to Part One   3

1. Who Am I? A Questionnaire   9
2. Wood: The Commander   21
3. Fire: The Lover   49
4. Earth: The Peacemaker   71
5. Metal: The Artist   93
6. Water: The Philosopher   117
7. A Delicate Balance   141

Part Two. The Healing Zones   167

Introduction to Part Two   169

8. Level One: The *Wei Chi*   171
   Recurrent Colds and Flus • Allergies and Food
   Sensitivities
9. Level Two: The *Chi*   209
   Chronic Sinusitis • Asthma • Irritable Bowel
   Syndrome • Inflammatory Bowel Disease (Crohn's
   Disease and Colitis) • Chronic Skin Disorders
   (Eczema and Psoriasis)

10. Level Three: The Blood   277
    Arthritis (Rheumatoid Arthritis and Osteoarthritis) •
    Lupus (Systemic Lupus Erythematosis) • Chronic
    Fatigue Syndrome • Type II Diabetes (Adult Onset
    Diabetes Mellitus)

11. Level Four: The Organs   339
    Cancer • HIV / AIDS (Human Immunodeficiency
    Virus, Acquired Immune Deficiency Syndrome)

Appendix I: Resources   391
Appendix II: Making Your Own Herbal Formulas   401
Appendix III: Acupressure Points   405
Index   409

ACKNOWLEDGMENTS

Every book is a journey, full of winding roads and countless adventures. The pathway to this book was paved thousands of years ago by ancient Chinese sages such as Lao-tzu, Confucius, Huang Di, and Qi Bo, who helped create the philosophical and practical system we now call traditional Chinese medicine. Many modern healers have followed their bright lights to illuminate the way. Those who have made our journey easier by offering expert advice and insights from their own experience include Leon Hammer, Bob Duggan, Mark Seem, Ted Kaptchuck, Simon Mills, Frank Lipman, M.D., Doug Heller, M.D., Richard Nagle, M.D., and Perle Besserman.

I give special thanks to those who have combed the manuscript and offered valuable suggestions: Steve Cowen, M.D., and Larry Baskind, M.D., for their encouragement and critical review of the medical data; Fara Kelsey for her insight and critique of the herbal sections; Bob Lesnow and Ellen Marshall for their expertise on clinical nutrition and the use of supplements; Amarish James Caruso for his insights into the "yogic" connection to the five elements; and Marc Grossman for his general support and critical support. And an extra-special thanks to Berkana Gervais for her unending support through this process.

For their support, camaraderie, and professional guidance we owe a deep debt of gratitude to our friends and colleagues at Integral Health Associates: Bob Lesnow, David Lester, Ellen Marshall, Kady Bray, Lynn Walcott, and Marc Grossman, with special thanks to Marc for his insights on vision.

We are deeply indebted to our literary agents, Janis Vallely and Jane Dystel, who have advised and encouraged us countless times in the three years spent researching and writing this book.

At Harmony Books our sincere thanks go to all who have played a part in the creation of this book, especially Leslie Meredith for her commitment to the idea from the very beginning, and Andrew Stuart, who shepherded us through the final stages.

Our greatest debt, as always, is to our families: Jason's mother, Betty Elias; his wife, Brigit; and his son, Adam; and Kathy's mother, Joan Ketcham; her husband, Patrick Spencer; and her children, Robyn, Alison, and Benjamin Spencer. Their love has guided our steps from beginning to end.

Introduction by Jason Elias
THE JOURNEY OF A THOUSAND MILES

> Prevent trouble before it arises.
> Put things in order before they exist.
> The giant pine tree
> grows from a tiny sprout.
> The journey of a thousand miles
> starts from beneath your feet.
>
> —Tao Te Ching

I will never forget the first time I read *The Yellow Emperor's Classic of Medicine,* a five-thousand-year-old book that describes the philosophical foundation and practical techniques of traditional Chinese medicine. It was the summer of 1968, the first of several summers I spent at Esalen Institute in Big Sur, California, studying with such luminaries as Joseph Campbell, Alan Watts, and Ilana Rubenfeld and investigating the healing powers of the body, mind, and spirit.

That particular summer marked the beginning of my adventures into the world of Eastern philosophy and ancient healing techniques. In the late afternoon after class and discussion group, I'd walk to the cliffs overlooking the beach, sit down in the shade of the wind-bowed cedars, and read the *The I Ching,* the *Tao Te Ching,* and *The Yellow Emperor's Classic of Medicine.* Losing myself in the gentle wisdom of the ancient sages, I felt as if I understood for the first time the exquisite harmony and continuity of life, where night always follows day, the rising moon shadows the setting sun, and the present rests on the enduring foundation of the past. The same sun rose and set on Confucius, Lao-tzu, Huang Di, and Qi Bo, and the same ocean lapped at the edges of their country as they searched for answers to the questions that disturbed my own peace of mind.

One of my favorite passages in *The Yellow Emperor's Classic of Medicine* occurs on the very first page, when Huang Di, the Yellow Emperor, asks his minister Qi Bo why people in the days of old enjoyed longer, happier lives. Does the world itself change from one generation to the next, he asks, or have people forgotten how to live in harmony with the enduring laws of nature? Qi Bo gently answers the young emperor's questions, speaking at length about the many dramatic changes in lifestyle and philosophy that have contributed to the present predicament of chronic disease, premature aging, and a general state of disharmony.

"In the past," Qi Bo observes, "people practiced the Tao, the Way of Life . . .

> They understood the principle of balance, of yin and yang, as represented by the transformation of the energies of the universe. Thus, they formulated practices such as Dao-in, an exercise combining stretching, massaging, and breathing to promote energy flow, and meditation to help maintain and harmonize themselves with the universe. They ate a balanced diet at regular times, arose and retired at regular hours, avoided overstressing their bodies and minds, and refrained from overindulgence of all kinds. They maintained well-being of body and mind; thus, it is not surprising that they lived over one hundred years.
>
> These days, people have changed their way of life. They drink wine as though it were water, indulge excessively in destructive activities, drain their jing—the body's essence that is stored in the kidneys—and deplete their qi [vital energy]. They do not know the secret of conserving their energy and vitality. Seeking emotional excitement and momentary pleasures, people disregard the natural rhythm and order of the universe. They fail to regulate their lifestyle and diet, and sleep improperly. So it is not surprising that they look old at fifty and die soon after.

This conversation took place nearly five thousand years ago, yet I heard the same concerns being raised at Esalen that summer, and I hear them repeated with even more urgency today. Health care practitioners, philosophers, environmentalists, and concerned citizens are still pondering the connections between the rise in chronic illnesses and changing lifestyle patterns. Why, we wonder, is our health declining? In what ways does our modern lifestyle contribute to premature aging and chronic, degenerative illness? What can we do to restore the natural order and live in peace and harmony as people did in the days of old?

As a thoroughly modern healer trained in both Eastern and Western techniques, I know too well that the problems we face today are infinitely more complicated and life-threatening than they were in the days of Huang Di and Qi Bo. Unlike our ancient ancestors, we live in a world that is slowly but surely being poisoned by technology, industry, and human encroachment on the natural world. A few statistics aptly illustrate the magnitude of today's American environmental dilemmas: Over sixty percent of the population—150 million Americans—live in areas where carbon monoxide levels and ozone pollution are considered "unsafe"; every year industry releases more than 2.4 billion pounds of hazardous chemicals into our atmosphere; air pollution is responsible for an estimated 50,000 premature deaths every year; according to a study by the Environmental Protection Agency, up to 1,700 cancer deaths each year can be attributed to toxic air pollution. The risk of health problems due to air pollution is six times greater for children. Every year more than 250,000 children suffer from serious respiratory problems due to air pollution. In a recent EPA survey of large public water systems served by groundwater, forty-five percent were found to be contaminated with industrial solvents, agricultural fertilizers or pesticides, or other toxic synthetic chemicals.

Our drinking water is polluted with more than 2,100 toxic chemicals, many of them toxic to the kidneys, liver, brain, and cardiovascular system, and some are known carcinogens. Only a handful of our nation's six thousand public water systems, which were established decades ago to disinfect water rather than to purify it, are capable of removing these chemicals.

The foods we eat are heavily processed and highly refined, and they contain staggering amounts of synthetic chemicals. In 1966 the average American ingested three pounds of chemical food additives every year; by 1974 the figure had risen to five pounds. Today we consume an average of nine pounds of food additives every year.

Of the six billion animals raised each year in the United States for human consumption, the vast majority receive antibiotics in their feed every day, for a total of twenty million pounds of antibiotics each year. Antibiotic-resistant bacteria develop routinely in these animals and are passed along to humans when they eat meat. As a result of these practices and the widespread use of antibiotics in standard medical practice (more than 240 million prescriptions for antibiotics are written every year), viral and bacterial infections rarely seen before the antibiotic era are now becoming commonplace, and drug-resistant bacterial strains (dubbed "killer microbes" and "superbugs") are multiplying.

As industry and technology systematically destroy the air we breathe, the water we drink, and the food we eat, our health problems have increased dramatically. While modern medical science has virtually eliminated the virulent diseases that threatened the lives of our ancestors (smallpox, diphtheria, polio, typhoid fever), a different kind of disease process is gradually destroying the body's ability to protect and heal itself.

Twenty-five years ago when I first began practicing what is now called "complementary medicine"—a combination of Western psychology, Eastern philosophy, nutritional science, massage therapy, and stress reduction techniques—most of the people walking through my door sought relief for such problems as generalized arthritic complaints, digestive upsets (chronic gas, bloating, indigestion, "nervous" stomach, heartburn), high blood pressure, lower back pain, chronic anxiety, panic attacks, and insomnia. After several months of treatment, the great majority of these patients experienced significant relief from their problems.

Today many of my patients have difficulty articulating the precise nature of their problems. They talk about feeling off balance, out of sorts, or out of sync. Chronic depression and apathy are common symptoms, as are migrating aches and pains, lethargy, and a crushing sense of fatigue. I often hear comments like these:

"I just don't have any energy."

"I can't seem to get up in the morning."

"I have no spark."

"I want to feel like my old self again."

Furthermore, the nature of the diseases is changing. In my first twenty years of practice, I saw perhaps ten patients with lupus; in the last year alone, I've added five new lupus patients to my caseload. Patients with chronic allergies and/or sinus infections have more than quadrupled. Fully one fifth of my caseload are cancer patients, a figure that has doubled in the last twenty years. Every week I see patients with diseases and disorders that were unknown or unnamed twenty or thirty years ago—irritable bowel syndrome, chronic fatigue immune deficiency syndrome, fibromyalgia, environmental illness, and HIV/AIDS.

What is happening in our world to increase our susceptibility to chronic immune disorders? The answer to this troubling question seems self-evident: Our immune systems—our innate ability to defend ourselves against disorder and disease—are slowly but surely being weakened by the ongoing devastation of our planet's delicate ecosystems and by the tens of thousands of chemical pollutants contaminating our air, food, and water, as well as lifestyle changes that are affecting our emotional and psychic well-being.

Consider:

• Forty to fifty million Americans—approximately one in five—suffer from *chronic allergies;* every year the number increases.

• The percentage of American children diagnosed with *allergic dermatitis* has increased from three percent in the 1960s to ten percent in the 1990s.

• Thirty-five million Americans—approximately one in seven—suffer from *chronic sinus infections;* every year the number rises.

• 14.6 million Americans, including five million children, suffer from asthma—an increase of 61 percent since the early 1980s. The death toll has nearly doubled in the last two decades, to 5,000 a year.

• Twenty to thirty percent of U.S. citizens have been diagnosed with *irritable bowel syndrome* (IBS), a disease that wasn't even listed in medical texts and nursing dictionaries twenty-five years ago; more than one third of the people in the Western world have experienced, at least temporarily, the full collection of symptoms known as IBS.

• More than two million Americans have been diagnosed with *inflammatory bowel disease* (Crohn's disease or colitis).

• Nearly 40 million Americans suffer from *arthritic conditions.*

• Between 1.4 and 2 million Americans have *lupus,* a chronic autoimmune disease that causes inflammation of various parts of the body, especially the skin, joints, blood, and kidneys; more people have lupus than have AIDS, multiple sclerosis, cerebral palsy, sickle-cell anemia, and cystic fibrosis combined.

• *Adult-onset diabetes* (type II diabetes mellitus) is the seventh leading cause of death in the United States; our refined-carbohydrate, high-fat, high-sugar, low-fiber diet is an uncontested factor in the rising incidence of this disease.

• Fifteen million Americans suffer from *eczema,* a chronic skin disease; ten percent of children under three have eczema.

• 6.4 million Americans have *psoriasis;* every year between 150,000 and 260,000 new cases are diagnosed.

• Since 1950 the incidence of *cancer* has increased by 44 percent. Although cancer mortality is now finally dropping, having fallen by almost three percent from 1991 to 1995, the American Cancer Society estimates that more than 75 million people alive today will eventually develop some form of cancer. By the year 2000, researchers believe, cancer will surpass heart disease as the number-one cause of death in the United States.

• Between 1973 and 1987 lung cancer increased by 32 percent, melanoma by 83 percent, and non-Hodgkin's lymphoma by 52 percent; breast, prostate, and kidney cancers have also increased significantly.

• A 1990 study by the World Health Organization found that between 1968 and 1987 cancers of the brain and central nervous system more than doubled in people between the ages of 75 and 84 and almost doubled among those aged 65 to 74; in American boys under 10, researchers note a 16 percent increase in these cancers.

• Over the last fifty years, researchers report a two- to fourfold increase in testicular cancer.

• Since 1983 the number of reported AIDS cases has grown by more than one thousand percent. More than one million Americans are infected with the HIV virus, while 22 million people worldwide are HIV positive and 7.7 million have full-blown AIDS. Expensive new drug treatments offer hope for stalling the progression of the disease, but preventive efforts remain controversial and basically ineffective—every minute five more people worldwide are infected with HIV. Experts estimate that by the year 2000, one in every hundred people worldwide will have AIDS. The fastest-growing group of HIV-infected Americans is heterosexuals, who now account for 15 percent of cases.

As I reflect upon the health crisis now facing us, I keep hearing Qi Bo's gentle, insistent voice: "In the past, people practiced the Tao, the Way of Life," he said. "They understood the principle of balance . . . they maintained well-being of body and mind." The words are thousands of years old, but the wisdom is timeless. If you understand the principles of balance and live in harmony with the natural laws of the universe, can you, too, discover the secret to health and well-being?

I believe you can, and I know from experience that the pathway to health and harmony is not as formidable as it may initially seem. "The brilliant gem is in your hands," advises a favorite Zen saying. We don't have the time to wait until the ozone hole is mended, the groundwater is purified, and the air is once again free from contaminants. To restore harmony, we must initiate the change ourselves, taking control of our bodies and accepting responsibility for our health. If we can restore balance within ourselves, we will have taken the necessary first step to restoring balance without.

Five thousand years ago Chinese physicians developed a philosophical yet eminently practical approach to healing called *Wu Hsing* or the Five Element System. This unique classification and diagnostic system was designed to help you understand who you are, why you behave and feel the way you do, and how the world inside you mirrors the energy and vitality of the natural world. Using this system you can learn to recognize imbalances in body, mind, and spirit and correct them before illness strikes.

The Chinese believe that the Five Elements—Wood, Fire, Earth, Metal, and Water—govern the physical, emotional, and spiritual existence of human beings just as they regulate the cycles of growth and change in the external world. An excess or deficiency in any one of these basic forces immediately and powerfully affects your physical health and emotional well-being. Once you learn how to balance these energies, regulate their flow, and adjust any excesses or deficiencies, you can create health and harmony in your life.

Each of the Five Elements has a unique nature and spirit, and every human being has a constitutional affinity to one or more of them. The aggressive, forceful energy of *Wood* is most obvious in the season of spring, when the buds swell to bursting and the seeds sprout into tender shoots that, against all odds, push their way through the earth to burst into vigorous life. If Wood is your predominant energy, you are like the greening stem of spring, driven by the need to stay in motion and reach to new heights, yet firmly grounded by a sense of self and "home"—the place where you fit and belong. Your roots are driven deep; your potential is unlimited.

The radiant energy of the sun, which is the power of *Fire,* is felt most intensely during the season of summer. Fire is the force that generates passion, compassion, and creativity. If you are energized by Fire, you are filled with enthusiasm and a blazing love of life. You draw others to you as the flame draws the moth, and you thrive on drama and excitement. Your intense craving for affection and close physical relationships will prove to be either your greatest strength or your most notable weakness.

The power of *Earth* is captured in the image of a garden: fertile, nourishing, solid, yet forgiving, the power of Earth is strongest in late summer and early fall—harvest time. If you are energized by the power of Earth, you are a natural mediator who thrives on harmonious relationships; discord and dissension throw you off balance. A sense of kinship and connectedness to others is essential to your health and happiness. Earth energy helps you find a center between opposing forces, teaching you how to resolve your differences and find sensible solutions to even the most difficult problems.

The power of *Metal* is symbolized by a majestic, snow-capped mountain. Reaching toward the heavens, yet firmly grounded in the earth, the mountain stands as a symbol of inner strength, endurance, and tranquillity. If you are energized by Metal, you are disciplined and precise, strong-willed yet willing and able to adapt to changing circumstances. Drawn to the core issues of life and the higher truths of art and philosophy, you seek to develop your character by devoting your attention to ethics, morality, and the acquisition of knowledge. Your season is autumn, the time of year when you begin to compress and contract your energy, pruning back and pulling inward in preparation for winter.

The power of *Water,* which is most evident in winter, can be seen in the raindrops that freeze overnight into icicles and melt in the morning, falling softly to the ground to dissolve into mist when warmed by the sun. Water changes shape effortlessly and yet never loses its essential character. If Water energizes you, you are dependable, infinitely resourceful, and single-minded in pursuit of your goals. Difficult or demanding situations do not cause you to hesitate or retreat, for you have a firm, unshakable sense of self, and you follow the path before you with strength, purpose, and determination.

Each of the Five Elements interacts in unique patterns and cycles to create your individual personality, emotional responses, spiritual desires, and physical strengths or weaknesses. When one power is excessively strong or weak, specific physical, emotional, and spiritual imbalances may occur. Excess Wood energy, for example, can lead to aggressive behavior, impatience, explosive anger, arrogance, or greed, while deficient Wood energy is often associated with anxiety, restlessness, insomnia, fatigue, and lethargy. Physical manifestations of excess Wood energy might include high blood pressure, muscle cramps, heartburn, and migraine headaches, while deficient Wood energy can lead to insomnia, allergies, visual disturbances, low blood pressure, and digestive problems.

When I introduce my patients to this ancient system, I am always amazed to see how quickly they grasp its underlying philosophical concepts. Even more astonishing are their emotional reactions—their hunger to better understand themselves, their immediate response to the beauty and integrity of the Five Elements, their intuitive understanding of their intimate relationship with the natural world. The enchanting metaphors become realities, windows through which you can see and feel the energy forces within your own body, mind, and spirit. When you begin to feel that kinship with the natural world, you also gain a sense of your innate capabilities and potential.

In this book you will journey into this ancient system, learning how to use the Five Elements to maintain balance and restore harmony to body, mind, and spirit. In Part I you will explore the many intricacies and complexities of Wood, Fire, Earth, Metal, and Water and learn how imbalances can lead to physical, emotional, and spiritual disorders. In each chapter you will find detailed suggestions for restoring harmony, along with specific advice on stress-reduction techniques, dietary changes, exercise regimens, Chinese and Western herbs, nutritional supplements, and acupoints. Once you learn how to keep the Five Elements in harmonious balance, you will know how to prevent disease and quickly restore health and harmony when illness threatens.

In Part II you will journey beyond prevention to explore the causes, symptoms, and treatments—both conventional and complementary—of the most common immune system disorders. You will learn how underlying imbalances in Wood, Fire, Earth, Metal, and Water create an internal environment conducive to the development of disease—from the relatively benign colds and flus to the more chronic and distressing problems of allergies, asthma, sinus infections, arthritis, chronic fatigue syndrome, eczema, and psoriasis and the life-threatening diseases of lupus, diabetes, cancer, and HIV/AIDS. And you will discover many ways to use the Five Elements of Healing to restore health and harmony.

Hundreds of gentle remedies and time-tested strategies are offered to help you:

- Identify the symptoms of imbalance in Wood, Fire, Earth, Metal, and Water energies
- Reduce physical and emotional stress, which can drain the energy of the immune system and increase your vulnerability to disease
- Choose foods that will complement your natural energy and invigorate your immune system
- Avoid the excessive use of powerful drugs, particularly antibiotics, which can modify or suppress the activities of your immune system, leaving you susceptible to renewed infection
- Select specific exercises that will support your vital energy
- Detail the most effective combination of vitamin and mineral supplements for prevention and treatment of various diseases and disorders
- Decide which herbs and herbal formulas—Western and Chinese—can be used most effectively to strengthen your individual system
- Stimulate specific acupoints to relieve anxiety, combat depression, improve memory, restore energy, lift your spirits, and relieve pain
- Create the space and time for solitude and silence
- Express your emotions clearly and with gentle force
- Work with your doctor or other health care professional to create comprehensive solutions to your health problems
- Regard illness as a time to reevaluate your life and reassess your basic needs

Your immune system is truly an astonishment of wonders. The healing forces that ebb and flow within your body, mind, and spirit are powerful beyond your imagining. You are not a passive victim, helplessly waiting for the next microorganism to penetrate your defenses and lay you low. Your body deals with these bugs all the time, knocking them silly and then sweeping away the debris while you eat, sleep, and go on with your life, completely unaware that anything unusual has taken place.

The West conceives of the immune system as a great military machine, replete with grenades, machine guns, and Stealth bombers capable of annihilating hordes of invading enemies. The Chinese, on the other hand, choose more peaceful, pastoral metaphors based on the philosophy that the immune system's most important responsibility is to prevent war rather than engage in bloody battles to restore the peace. As Qi Bo said:

> In the old days the sages treated disease by preventing illness before
> it began, just as a good government or emperor was able to take the
> necessary steps to avert war. Treating an illness after it has begun is
> like suppressing revolt after it has broken out. If someone digs a well
> when thirsty, or forges weapons after becoming engaged in battle,
> one cannot help but ask: Are not these actions too late?

In ancient Chinese medical texts, the human body is compared to a garden
filled with lush vegetation, brightly petaled flowers, and magical healing herbs.
Streams and pools of vital energy flow in, through, and underneath the vegetation to cleanse and invigorate even the most remote corners of the body's kingdom. This vital, invisible, ever-flowing source of healing energy is called *chi*.

One form of *chi*—the *wei chi*—is roughly analogous to the Western concept
of the immune system. In the Chinese metaphor the *wei chi* is imagined as a massive assemblage (more than a trillion strong) of gardeners and groundskeepers
who work around the clock hoeing, weeding, irrigating, and fertilizing to assure
the integrity and vitality of our internal ecosystem. Some gardeners carry only
trowels, rakes, and hoes, while others are equipped with sophisticated communication equipment and detection devices, and still others (an elite group) have
access to potent chemical weapons.

When danger threatens, diligent laborers dig up weeds and exterminate unwelcome pests. If stronger measures are needed to repel a particularly noxious
weed or tenacious bug, master landscapers know precisely which plants to spray
with their potent chemicals, leaving the healthy vegetation untouched.

The groundskeepers and landscapers who weed and tend every molecule of
space within the garden that is your human body maintain physical and emotional
balance, assuring your long-term health and happiness. They don't ask for much
in return: nutritious food, pure water, clean air, and plenty of room to move
around and do their work, and most important, your belief in the healing capabilities of your own body.

Modern researchers are discovering that the immune system responds immediately and decisively to hormones and neurotransmitters flowing out of the
brain. The immune system, it appears, actually "talks" to the brain, and it's more
than a long-distance relationship. Bill Moyers's groundbreaking book, *Healing
and the Mind,* quotes Dr. David Felten, M.D., Ph.D., a professor of neurobiology

and anatomy at the University of Rochester School of Medicine, telling the story of how he first discovered the intimate connection between body and mind:

> One day I was looking through a microscope at tissue sections of liver in order to identify nerves that travel alongside blood vessels. I was having trouble seeing what the cells really looked like, so I said, "Let's go to the spleen. Everybody knows what the spleen looks like." So I started looking at blood vessels and some of the surrounding areas in the spleen. And there, sitting in the middle of these vast fields of cells of the immune system, was a bunch of nerve fibers. I looked at them and thought, What is this? Nerve fibers aren't supposed to talk to cells of the immune system. What are they doing here?
>
> So we cut some more sections, and looked—and there they were again. We tried other blocks of tissue, and there they were again. They kept showing up again and again. We and others eventually discovered nerve fibers going into virtually every organ of the immune system and forming direct contacts with the immune system cells.

In later experiments Felten and his colleagues discovered that when they removed the nerve cells from the spleen or lymph nodes, the immune response was suddenly severed, as if a wind storm snapped a cable and the lines went dead.

Modern research is confirming what the Chinese have always understood: "So much of all illness begins in the mind," said Huang Di, the Yellow Emperor. In the final years of the twentieth century, we are finally beginning to accept the long-held truth that body and mind are not only connected, they literally "talk" to each other all the time, in an ongoing dialogue that dramatically influences your health and well-being.

What can modern medicine learn from ancient wisdom? How can physicians improve their success in treating chronic illness? As chronic diseases and disorders escalate, affecting the health and well-being of tens of millions of Americans, many physicians are beginning to consult healers trained in such "unorthodox" practices as acupuncture, herbal medicine, bodywork, and meditative techniques, asking for their help with cases considered "incurable" by Western standards. In the past several years I've been approached by dozens of physicians from virtually every specialty. Here are just a few examples of the ways we worked together to solve patients' problems:

• Jared, a seven-year-old asthma patient, was referred to me by his pediatrician, who was concerned about the long-term effects of steroid drugs on his young patient. The pediatrician had been discussing the case with another doctor in his practice, who suggested that acupuncture and herbal medicine might help control the symptoms and prevent future asthma attacks. After five months of acupuncture sessions and herbal remedies, Jared was completely weaned off prescription medications. He continues to carry his inhaler with him in case of an emergency.

• When her gynecologist suggested surgery to remove a dermoid (solid) cyst on her right ovary, thirty-seven-year-old Rebecca decided to give acupuncture and herbal medicine a try. Although her doctor was openly skeptical, he agreed that delaying surgery for several months would do no harm. After three months of treatment, the doctor ordered an ultrasound, which showed no evidence of the cyst. Not quite believing his eyes—dermoid cysts are solid, and surgical removal is considered standard procedure—the doctor ordered another sonogram, which confirmed the findings. Four years later Rebecca remains cyst-free.

• Bill came to me at the recommendation of his rheumatologist, who for years had referred his patients with chronic, intractable pain to acupuncturists. Two years earlier Bill was seriously injured in an auto accident; his back and shoulder muscles were in constant spasm, and the muscles on either side of his spine were chronically inflamed. Because he was in constant pain, Bill had been unable to return to work. Pain-killers, anti-inflammatory drugs, and cortisone injections offered only temporary relief, so at the prodding of his physician, Bill reluctantly agreed to try acupuncture. Over a period of several months Bill began to notice that the pain was subsiding; six months after treatments began, he pronounced himself "completely cured" and returned to work full time.

• For three years Robert had been taking prescription medications for high blood pressure and elevated cholesterol levels. Concerned about the side effects associated with the drugs, Robert's wife spoke to his cardiologist, who agreed to work with me in an attempt to wean Robert off the drugs. With daily exercise, simple dietary changes, nutritional supplements, and herbal therapy, Robert's blood pressure and cholesterol levels lowered dramatically.

I continue to work with Robert's doctor, who routinely asks his patients if they would be willing to complement standard medical care with alternative healing techniques to control their symptoms and reduce the risk of coronary artery disease. "Unfortunately," he recently told me, "the vast majority of my patients would rather take pills than make significant changes in their lifestyle."

• Several years ago an internist called to ask for my help with a difficult case. For more than two years his six-year-old daughter Carolyn had been suffering from chronic sinus infections; repeated doses of antibiotics, prescription nasal sprays, and antihistamines had not been able to cure the problem or alleviate her symptoms. After major surgery she experienced temporary relief, but within a few months the sinus infections returned. Herbs and acupuncture (with magnets rather than needles, which she feared) worked almost immediately to offer Carolyn significant relief; within a few months she was using only herbs to control her symptoms, and today, nine years old, she only rarely succumbs to a sinus infection.

After witnessing Carolyn's amazing recovery, her father enrolled in acupuncture and herbal medicine courses designed specifically for practicing physicians. He routinely advises his patients to investigate the healing wonders of these ancient medical techniques.

In my ongoing association with dozens of highly skilled physicians, I've become convinced that traditional Chinese medicine and modern medical science can be joined together to create a system of healing that offers the best of both worlds. Chinese medicine, with its emphasis on preventive strategies and gentle, supportive remedies, offers a perfect complement to Western medicine, with its powerful arsenal of diagnostic, surgical, and pharmaceutical tools designed specifically to treat and cure established diseases.

Each system has its own strengths and weaknesses, which are offset by the strengths and weaknesses of the other. If you have a heart attack, stroke, ruptured appendix, brain hemorrhage, broken bone, head injury, bacterial or fungal infection, or any other acute medical or surgical emergency, the choice is clear: Western medicine can diagnose your problem in record time, offer fast, effective relief for your symptoms, and possibly save your life. If, on the other hand, you have an acute viral illness or a chronic degenerative disease—or if you simply want to stay healthy and prevent disease before it occurs—traditional Chinese medicine offers you five thousand years of accumulated wisdom and gentle yet remarkably effective healing and immune-supportive remedies.

The two systems of medicine are also complementary in the way they focus their energy and attention. While Western medicine tends to concentrate on the disease rather than the patient, Eastern medicine focuses on the impact of the disease or disorder on the patient's emotional and spiritual health. For if we fail to take care of the mind and spirit, counsel the ancient sages, we will do great damage to the patient's ability to recover.

In a remarkable section of *The Yellow Emperor's Classic* Huang Di discusses "the Five Failings of Physicians." Each failing is based on a lack of compassion or an inaccurate assessment of the patient's lifestyle and emotional state of mind. When people today speak of "mind-body" medicine, they are repeating the concerns expressed by the Yellow Emperor thousands of years ago. There can be no question that these ancient principles still apply today and that by combining these ethical standards with the brilliant diagnostic and treatment skills of modern medicine, the patient, the doctor, and the world itself will benefit.

> The first failing occurs in diagnosis. When a physician overlooks factors such as a patient's social and material status that could contribute to the development of disease, that physician ends up making an incorrect assessment. . . . Lack of such observation is a loss to the physician of a valuable link that is essential in the accuracy of the diagnosis.
>
> The second failing occurs in treatment. When a physician neglects a patient's emotional experiences, which can affect the patient's health greatly . . . the consequence is further injury to the patient. It is significant to know the patient's lifestyle and emotional state because emotions such as anger damage the yin, while overexcitement scatters the yang. Treatment without understanding . . . may cause further exacerbation to a patient's condition.
>
> The third failing occurs when the physician lacks deductive reasoning. Much information about a patient's condition is gathered, in addition to careful observation of the body signs and inquiry of patient's symptoms, from lifestyle, occupation, social and family cir-

cumstances, emotional stress, and immediate environment. After gathering the pieces of information, it is the physician's task to utilize his knowledge and analyze through deduction the entire picture of the patient's illness. Inability to do this limits the physician's effectiveness.

The fourth failing occurs in counseling. When a physician lacks compassion and sincerity, when a physician is hasty in counseling and does not make the effort to guide the patient's mind and moods in a positive way, that physician has robbed the opportunity to achieve a cure. So much of all illness begins in the mind, and the ability to persuade the patient to change the course of perception and feeling to aid in the healing process is a requirement of a good physician.

The fifth failing occurs when a physician is simply inept and careless when administering medical care. A physician who is incompetent in medical skills fails to stem the patient's disease from deteriorating. Consequently, when the condition becomes grave, the physician gives a prognosis of death or incurable when the disease actually could have been reversed earlier.

"The Five Failings of Physicians" reminds us of how much we have to gain if ancient wisdom and modern science were to join hands, working together to reclaim the gifts of caring and compassion in this age of chronic, "incurable" disease. *Chinese Medicine for Maximum Immunity* strives to build a bridge between Eastern and Western medicine, offering detailed, step-by-step instructions for working together to create a system of medicine that honors the whole person: body *and* mind *and* spirit. With the light of ancient wisdom illuminating the shadows of modern disease, the reader is guided toward a broader understanding of the art of healing and the untapped power of the mind and spirit.

Part One

UNDERSTANDING
THE POWERS WITHIN

Introduction to Part One

Nature's richness lies in its power to nourish all living things; its
greatness lies in its power to give them beauty and splendor.

—*The I Ching*

You are a unique individual, unlike any other human being on this planet. Just as your fingerprints are yours and yours alone, so are your ideas, opinions, and behaviors completely distinctive. Your eyes behold a different world from the one that others perceive. The sound, smell, taste, and touch of your surroundings fires your senses in unique patterns and intensities. No one else feels your impulses, thinks your thoughts, or dreams your dreams.

What makes you unique? Why does a Beethoven sonata move you to tears, while a Bach concerto leaves you cold? Stricken by fear or grief, why do you seek the solace of solitude, while others crave the comfort of loving arms? Why do you eat nonstop when you're feeling blue, while your sister goes shopping and your brother jogs for two hours? Why is spring—or summer, fall, or winter—your favorite season? Why do you crave sweet—or salty, sour, bitter, or spicy—foods? Why do you love the color blue—or green, red, yellow, white, or black? Why would you rather sit by a river—or a mountain, forest, meadow, or sun-drenched beach—than anywhere else on earth?

The Chinese believe your unique responses to the world are determined by your affinity to certain basic energy forces that flow through you in distinctive ways. The balance and interaction between these natural forces determine the risks you take or avoid, the goals you set, the fears and doubts that assail you, the situations that cause you stress or conflict, the talents you have or have neglected, the values that motivate you, and the dreams that inspire you. Just as you can't change the color of your eyes or the shape of your hands and feet, your nature is part of you—you are born with it, and every aspect of your life will be shaped by it.

Thousands of years ago Chinese philosophers created the *Wu Hsing* (the Five Element System) to explain how the primary powers of nature—Wood, Fire, Earth, Metal, and Water—ebb and flow within human beings. Wood is the restless, aggressive energy that gives a tiny seed the power to develop into a firmly rooted tree. Fire's passionate, radiant energy is symbolized by the sun, which provides life-giving warmth to the world. Earth is the stable, balancing force that keeps us grounded and centered within ourselves. Metal's strong inspirational energy is symbolized by the precious gems and essential minerals that give form and structure to the world. Water's adaptable, infinitely resourceful energy can be seen in the rivers that flow to the sea, cleansing and invigorating everything that they touch.

Each of the Five Elements depends upon the others, and life itself depends upon their intricate balance and interdependence. Water irrigates the fields and forests so that Wood can grow. Wood feeds Fire, which burns to ash, nourishing the Earth. Earth provides a firm foundation and stable support for the mountains of Metal that rise upward toward the heavens. Metallic ores and rocks underlie the river channels that give Water its direction, while minerals and trace elements give Water its nourishing richness. Each element nourishes and is nourished by the others.

Just as the elements feed and sustain each other, so do they restrain and inhibit each other. Water controls Fire by quenching it. Fire restrains Metal by melting it, allowing it to be shaped and molded. Metal inhibits Wood by cutting it (symbolized by the ax chopping the tree). Wood restrains Earth by covering it, literally rooting it in place and preventing erosion. Earth controls Water by absorbing it and forming natural dams and riverbanks to prevent it from overflowing its channels.

The Five Element System is ancient and exotic, yet it is eminently practical and immediately accessible. If you are energized by Wood, you can recognize the similarities between the force that drives the sap in the tree and the energy that pushes you to seek out challenges and adventures. If you have an affinity to Fire, the power literally burns within you, a steady pilot light that infuses your life

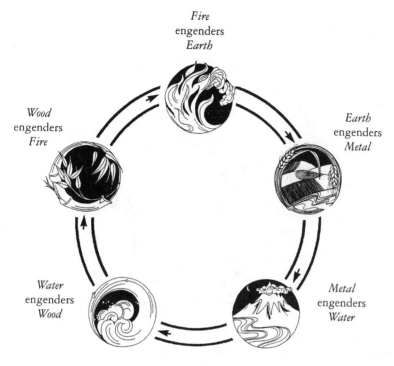

*Fire
engenders
Earth*

*Earth
engenders
Metal*

*Wood
engenders
Fire*

*Metal
engenders
Water*

*Water
engenders
Wood*

THE GENERATION CYCLE
Supporting Sequence: *Sheng*

with passion and joy. Earth types need only look out their window at their green, growing gardens to understand the nourishing, stabilizing nature of their energy. Metal types feel a powerful connection to the core issues and underlying structures of life, intuitively understanding that its most meaningful moments occur when movement stills and silence reigns. Water types know from observing the behavior of rivers that their power resides in remaining flexible and adaptable, always yielding to current conditions.

As you learn about the Five Elements, you will learn a great deal about yourself and your relationship to the natural world, but equally as important, you will learn tolerance for others. The differences between us are not flaws indicating that one of us has strayed from the norm, but symbols of the wondrous complexity of life. What would our world be like without rivers and oceans, without mountains, woodlands, and fertile fields, without the radiance of the sun or the reflected light of the moon?

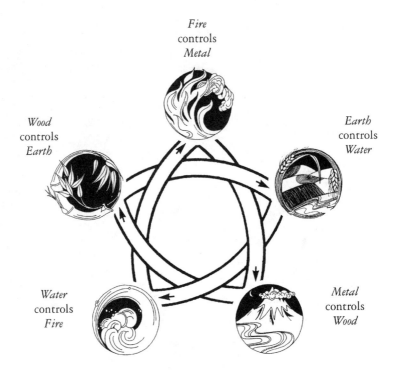

Fire
controls
Metal

Wood
controls
Earth

Earth
controls
Water

Water
controls
Fire

Metal
controls
Wood

THE CONTROL CYCLE
Restraining Sequence: *Ke*

The beauty and integrity of our world depend on all the elements, and each element expresses its basic nature in unique ways. The tree can no more melt like the icicle than the river can stay rooted in one place. The sun can't shine cold, the earth can't spin square, the mountain can't rise forever. The nature of things determines the way they grow, mature, change, and erode away.

Just as the natural world must follow its own inner laws of being, so is human behavior shaped by forces beyond our control. Recognizing that all living things are guided by "an inner light" that they "must involuntarily obey," as *The I Ching* advises, we learn to be more tolerant and forgiving. A tendency to make quick judgments is replaced by thoughtful consideration of the underlying forces that directly influence our thoughts, feelings, and behaviors. When a friend seems excessively needy or meddlesome, you recognize her affinity to Earth, the energy that needs to be in the center, surrounded by activity. If your husband chooses to seclude himself rather than join in a group activity, you understand his strong affinity to Water, which is reflective and directed inward. When a colleague becomes aggressive and forceful when things don't go her way, you appreciate the power and force of her Wood energy.

The Five Element System gives you a deeper understanding of the invisible energy patterns that influence you and the people you know and love. As you embark on this journey to discover who you are and how you can best fulfill your individual destiny, you will learn how to assess your strengths and weaknesses and set reasonable goals through a knowledge of your limitations. Instead of living at the whim of fate or blindly following the advice of the experts, you will learn to take responsibility for your life and develop self-mastery through constant self-examination. You will discover that your health and well-being depend on living in harmony with the natural world, you will learn tolerance and compassion for others, and you will gain a deeper appreciation for the complex interplay of forces that determine your basic nature.

Most important of all, you will learn who you are and how to be true to yourself. So many of our problems—physical, emotional, and spiritual—come from trying to be something or someone that we are not. We find ourselves in situations or relationships where we struggle to fit into someone else's conception of who we should be. That sense of not fitting, of not belonging, creates significant stress that, over time, increases our vulnerability to disease and disorder.

The Five Element System will guide you to a deeper understanding of who you are and how you can be true to your own nature. Remember, there is no one right way to be. As the ancient philosophers who wrote *The I Ching* reassure us: "If the individual acts consistently and is true to himself, he will find the way that is appropriate for him. This way is right for him and without blame."

The following story shows how the search for the "true" self leads us back home to the place where we fit and belong.

> There once was a child made all of salt who yearned to know who she was and where she had come from. One day she embarked on a long journey, traveling to many foreign lands to seek the answer to her questions. Eventually she came to the coastline of a vast ocean.
>
> "How wonderful!" she exclaimed, putting one foot in the water.

"Don't be afraid," the ocean whispered to her, "for if you continue, you will find what you seek."

The salt child put her other foot in the water and waded deeper and deeper, her body dissolving with each step. When she was fully immersed and her body had become one with the ocean, she cried out in a voice filled with wonder, "Ah, now I know who I am."

1. WHO AM I? A QUESTIONNAIRE

Everything becomes spontaneously what it should rightly be, for in the law of heaven life has an inner light that it must involuntarily obey.

—The I Ching

Which of the Five Elements—Wood, Fire, Earth, Metal, or Water—surges most strongly within you? Are you most like the supple birch tree bending in the wind, the sun setting crimson behind a bank of clouds, the fertile fields that nourish and provide for all living things, the snow-capped mountain reaching toward the heavens, or the rushing river flowing to the sea?

The following questionnaire will help you determine the relative strengths and weaknesses of your affinities to the Five Elements. In Section One you'll find a list of physical characteristics and symptoms, while Section Two describes psychological inclinations and behavioral tendencies.

Put a check mark next to each statement that accurately describes your present-day condition or a predictable pattern you have experienced in the past. Because an affinity to a particular element or an imbalance within that element may be expressed in a wide range of sometimes opposing symptoms, some of the statements in Section Two contain contradictory phrases, as in "I enjoy (or dread) public speaking." If either alternative accurately describes you, place a check next to the statement. After finishing the questionnaire, you'll learn what your responses indicate about your affinities to Wood, Fire, Earth, Metal, or Water.

Section One

PHYSICAL CHARACTERISTICS

____ Muscular, athletic physique with well-proportioned hands, arms, legs, and head. Thick, somewhat coarse skin. Jaw and chin dominate the face (1)

____ Fingernails and toenails tend to split, peel, and crack easily (1)

____ Oily skin, especially around the face, nose, and scalp (1)

____ A subtle greenish hue around the eyes and mouth (1)

____ High-pitched ringing in the ears (1)

____ Blurred vision (1)

____ Dry, red, itchy, or teary eyes (1)

____ Chronic headaches, particularly around the temples; migraine headaches (1)

____ Difficulty swallowing, especially when tense (1)

____ Sudden, sharp, migrating pains in the eyes, ears, nose, throat, genitals, armpits, or between the ribs (1)

____ Chronic tension in the neck and/or shoulders (1)

____ Menstrual problems: strong painful cramps, erratic cycles, PMS with irritability and mood swings (1)

____ Cramps or twitches in the muscles of the eyes, face, calves, or feet (1)

____ Abdominal pains (1)

____ Spinal aches or pains (1)

____ Sciatica (radiating pain from the lower back down the leg) (1)

____ Tendency to develop muscle and tendon injuries (1)

____ Digestive disturbances: heartburn, constipation, or ulcers (1)

____ High blood pressure (1)

____ Cysts and lumps (sebaceous cysts, breast lumps, endometrial cysts) (1)

____ Graceful, willowy physique. Soft, warm skin. Long neck, hands, and fingers. Delicate features. Eyes tend to dominate the face (2)

____ Bright red, often blotchy complexion; or noticeable lack of color (ashen complexion) (2)

____ Tendency to blush, particularly when nervous or upset (2)

____ Feelings of being cold and chilled; hands and feet feel chronically cold (2)

____ Spontaneous sweating, hot flashes, tendency to overheat (2)

___ Difficulties with perspiration: a tendency either to perspire too easily or to have difficulty perspiring (2)

___ Shallow breathing; a tendency to hold the breath (2)

___ Dizziness and fainting spells (2)

___ Skin eruptions—acne, pimples, boils, rashes—that feel "hot" or inflamed (2)

___ Varicose veins, hemorrhoids, thrombosis, or phlebitis (problems involving the veins and arteries) (2)

___ Heartburn (2)

___ Diverticulitis (inflammation of the colon) (2)

___ Rapid or irregular heartbeat; erratic pulse (2)

___ Heart palpitations, especially when excited or stressed (2)

___ Frequent urinary infections (2)

___ Sleep disturbances: insomnia, often intensified by excitement or anxiety; vivid or disturbing dreams; restless sleep (2)

___ Problems with the tongue: sores, inflammation, redness, or swelling (2)

___ Speech problems, especially stammering or stuttering; also slurring words or habitually speaking too quickly (2)

___ Seizures (2)

___ Strokes (2)

___ Rounded physique with broad hips and shoulders. Soft, smooth skin. Short, stubby hands and feet. Mouth and lips predominate the face (3)

___ Yellowish hue around mouth or temples (3)

___ Thick mucus in mouth, nose, and throat (3)

___ Swollen, sore, or bleeding gums (3)

___ Frontal headaches, usually connected with worrying (3)

___ Tendency to water retention; skin feels soft and puffy to the touch (3)

___ Nails and cuticles easily inflamed, misshapen, and tear easily (3)

___ Excessive belching or burping (3)

___ Gain weight easily; find it difficult to lose weight (3)

___ Craving (or intense dislike of) sweets and starchy foods (refined carbohydrates) (3)

___ Anorexia or bulimia (3)

___ Obesity (3)

___ Digestive problems: indigestion, abdominal pain, excess stomach acid (3)

____ Ulcers (3)

____ Blood sugar disturbances: hypoglycemia, diabetes (3)

____ Thyroid problems (especially hypothyroidism or deficient thyroid) (3)

____ Menstrual problems: irregular periods, lethargic with periods, bloating (3)

____ Fibroid tumors (3)

____ Hemmorhoids (3)

____ Varicose veins (3)

____ Symmetrical physique with long arms and legs and narrow shoulders. Small bones. Chiseled or delicate features. Nose predominates the face (4)

____ Dry, itchy skin with tendency to wrinkle prematurely (4)

____ Dry hair: ends split easily, hair lacks luster (4)

____ Dry, irritated throat and nasal passages (4)

____ Dry, scaly pimples, especially on the cheeks, beside the nose, or on the upper back (4)

____ Difficulty perspiring even when hot (4)

____ Nasal polyps (4)

____ Sinus problems: congested nose or sinuses, sinus headaches, chronic sinus infections (4)

____ Hay fever and other allergies, including food allergies or sensitivities (4)

____ Rashes or hives (4)

____ Chronic bronchitis (4)

____ Asthma, especially allergy-induced asthma (4)

____ Enlarged or hard lymph nodes, especially along the sides of the neck or under the jaw (4)

____ Numerous moles or warts (4)

____ Frequent sneezing or coughing due to changes in air temperature or pressure (4)

____ Bowel disturbances: diarrhea, constipation, or alternating diarrhea and constipation (4)

____ Spine and joint problems: inflexibility, stiff posture, chronic joint pain (4)

____ Sensitivity to climate changes, particularly to humid and excessively dry climates (4)

____ Eczema (4)

____ Psoriasis (4)

___ Lean physique with narrow shoulders and wider hips. Long fingers and toes. Sculptured features. Deep-set eyes. Ears tend to predominate the face (5)

___ Darkish hue around or under the eyes (5)

___ Hearing problems: loss of hearing, tinnitus (ringing in ears) (5)

___ Ear aches and pains; tendency to get ear infections (5)

___ Teeth problems such as multiple cavities or bone loss, weakening teeth (5)

___ Hair falls out easily, thinning hair, loss of head or pubic hair (5)

___ Sore aching feet (especially the soles of the feet) (5)

___ Excessive thirst, often feel parched or dry (5)

___ Urinary problems: frequent need to urinate, difficulty urinating, urinary tract infections (5)

___ Tendency to vaginitis or yeast infections (5)

___ Swelling and bloating due to water retention (5)

___ Aching and pain in lower back region (5)

___ Aching in lower part of the abdomen; lower abdomen often feels cold to the touch (5)

___ Pain and stiffness in the joints, particularly in the knees; pain tends to get worse in winter (5)

___ Brittle joints (5)

___ Instability of the spinal column; a tendency to "throw your back out" (5)

___ Osteoporosis or other problems involving degeneration of bone (5)

___ Prostatic problems: benign prostatic hypertrophy (enlargement or swelling of the prostate gland), prostate infections (5)

___ High blood pressure (hypertension) (5)

___ Illness or symptoms worse in winter or in very cold climates (5)

Section Two

PSYCHOLOGICAL/BEHAVIORAL CHARACTERISTICS

___ I tend to feel confident about my abilities (1)

___ I tend to do what I feel is right, regardless of what others might think (1)

___ I enjoy competition; my friends often describe me as competitive (1)

___ I feel compelled to win, sometimes at any cost (1)

_____ I am comfortable in conflict situations or under pressure (1)

_____ I can be bullheaded and stubborn (1)

_____ I like to take the lead and direct others in activities or work (1)

_____ I like to think of creative solutions to difficult problems (1)

_____ I tend to make hasty, irrational decisions (or I find it difficult to make decisions) (1)

_____ I am willing to stick with a plan of action even if the odds are not in my favor (1)

_____ I can be impulsive and feel a strong need to satisfy my impulses (1)

_____ I am typically direct and straightforward in my dealings with others (1)

_____ I can be insensitive, plowing ahead without paying attention to other people's needs (1)

_____ I tend to be critical of others and find it difficult to understand why they don't accomplish as much as I do (1)

_____ I enjoy public recognition of my talents and achievements (1)

_____ I tend to act boldly and decisively, even when I may not have all the expertise or information I need (1)

_____ I tend to speak forcefully and at times shout my words (1)

_____ I like to take risks (1)

_____ I am a workaholic (1)

_____ I am a procrastinator (1)

_____ I enjoy public speaking (1)

_____ When things don't go my way, I often feel off balance, uprooted, stuck, or unable to move (1)

_____ My characteristic response to difficult situations is to get angry; I sometimes have trouble controlling my anger (1)

_____ My greatest fears involve loss of control: being helpless, being confined, being stuck or unable to move (1)

_____ I have a strong preference (or distaste) for sour foods (vinegar, lemons, limes) (1)

_____ I have a strong preference (or distaste) for the color green (1)

_____ I have a strong preference (or distaste) for very windy conditions (1)

_____ I have a strong preference (or distaste) for the season of spring (1)

_____ My dreams often involve images of forests, growing plants, competition, trying to reach a goal (1)

____ I often feel restless or have difficulty sleeping between the hours of 11 P.M. and 3 A.M. (1)

____ I am empathic and can easily identify with other people's pleasure or pain (2)

____ I intuitively know what other people are thinking or feeling (2)

____ I am easily affected by other people's responses or opinions of me (2)

____ I tend to be animated, enthusiastic, and full of excitement about life (2)

____ I enjoy all my senses and love sensual pleasures (2)

____ I sometimes laugh too loud, too much, or at inappropriate times (2)

____ I enjoy physical contact and emotional intimacy (2)

____ I tend to thrive (or fall apart) in a stimulating environment: a big city, noisy office, etc. (2)

____ I like to live in the moment, letting bygones be bygones (2)

____ I am often thought of as eternally optimistic, even when others try to dampen my enthusiasm (2)

____ I'm considered magnetic or charismatic; other people seem to be drawn to me (2)

____ I would find it difficult to live without laughter or joy in my life (2)

____ I enjoy (or dread) public speaking and public recognition (2)

____ I have difficulty containing my emotions and tend to wear them on my sleeve (2)

____ I am uncomfortable with conflicting emotions or desires (2)

____ I often feel anxious and afraid for no apparent reason (2)

____ I can be scatterbrained and absentminded (2)

____ I find it difficult to say no (2)

____ I dread rejection, which makes me feel cut off from others (2)

____ I need a lot of support or praise; I tend to doubt myself (2)

____ I tend to be vulnerable, especially in relationships (2)

____ Communication is very important to me, and I work hard to communicate honestly and directly with people (2)

____ My characteristic response to difficult situations is to get overly excited, flustered, and emotional (2)

____ My greatest fears involve being alone or abandoned (2)

____ I have a strong preference (or distaste) for bitter foods (bitter greens, coffee without sugar) (2)

____ I have a strong preference (or distaste) for the color red (2)

____ I have a strong preference (or distaste) for very hot climates (2)

____ I have a strong preference (or distaste) for the season of summer (2)

____ My dreams often involve images of romantic relationships, sexual encounters (2)

____ My energy is either extremely high or totally depleted between the hours of 11 A.M. and 3 P.M. (2)

____ I tend to be nurturing; I enjoy taking care of others (3)

____ I tend to be a mediator and peacemaker; I like to solve problems and help others reconcile theirs (3)

____ I become easily upset or unsettled with conflict or discord (3)

____ I value loyalty and commitment and expect my friends and family to do the same (3)

____ I am extremely adaptable and easily mold myself to different situations (3)

____ When I am with different people, I can be a different person (3)

____ I find it easy to be with people I don't know well (3)

____ I don't need a lot of stimulation to be happy; just being with my family and friends is enough (3)

____ I thrive on peaceful settings, tranquil surroundings, and natural beauty (3)

____ I often feel too needy; I particularly need to know that I am needed (3)

____ I often feel left out, as if people were making plans without me (3)

____ I often have difficulty asking for what I need (3)

____ I have difficulty being alone (3)

____ I need stability in my life (3)

____ I tend to put the needs of others before my own (3)

____ I easily get overly involved in other people's problems (3)

____ I like being the center of my social network (3)

____ I tend to eat when I feel lonely or uncomfortable (3)

____ I like the feeling of being "full" with food, friends, social engagements, and work, but I sometimes feel weighted down or overstuffed (3)

____ I tend to set unrealistic expectations and often feel disappointed in the way things turn out (3)

____ I tend to worry or obsess about problems (3)

____ I have obsessive/compulsive tendencies (3)

____ My characteristic response to difficult situations is to worry about the outcome or to interfere, hoping to change the outcome (3)

____ My greatest fears involve being lost, alone, or far from home (3)

____ I have a strong preference (or distaste) for sweets (3)

____ I have a strong preference (or distaste) for the color yellow (3)

____ I have a strong preference (or distaste) for very damp climates (3)

____ I have a strong preference (or distaste) for late summer (Indian summer) (3)

____ My dreams often involve images of houses, backyards, and grassy fields (3)

____ My energy is either extremely high or totally depleted between the hours of 7 P.M. and 11 P.M. (3)

____ I tend to be neat and orderly in my personal appearance (4)

____ I take pride in being efficient and methodical (4)

____ I like making lists to create order in my life (4)

____ At times I become obsessed with the need for order and organization (4)

____ I am content with just a few close friends or relationships (4)

____ I am bored with superficiality; I like to concentrate on quality and substance (4)

____ I am immediately and powerfully affected by my environment; junk and clutter make me extremely uncomfortable (4)

____ I dislike crowds, waiting in line, traffic lights, and the like (4)

____ In social situations I tend to be stiff and somewhat formal (4)

____ I like to be in control; spontaneity frightens me (4)

____ I sometimes fear contamination: drinking from another person's glass, using restaurant utensils, sitting on public toilet seats (4)

____ I tend to be a perfectionist and can be excessively critical of myself (4)

____ I restrain myself from expressing my feelings; others sometimes describe me as unemotional or unfeeling (4)

____ I value organization in myself and others (4)

____ I am interested in spiritual disciplines and approaches to life (4)

____ I love to collect rare or beautiful objects: artwork, jewelry, books, and so on (4)

____ I tend to accept what authority dictates (4)

____ I feel strongly committed to certain moral principles and standards of conduct (4)

____ I enjoy tasks that require logical and analytical approaches to problem solving (4)

____ I enjoy doing puzzles, solving riddles, and reading good mysteries (4)

____ I don't like to get caught up in other people's dramas (4)

____ I feel proud of the fact that I am able to resist temptation (4)

____ My characteristic response to difficult situations is to feel overwhelmed with sorrow or grief (4)

____ My greatest fears involve crowds, chaos, and corruption (4)

____ I have a strong preference (or distaste) for pungent and spicy foods (4)

____ I have a strong preference (or distaste) for the color white (4)

____ I have a strong preference (or distaste) for very dry climates (4)

____ I have a strong preference (or distaste) for the season of autumn (4)

____ My dreams often involve mountain peaks, snow, or the interiors of boats, cars, or trains (4)

____ I often feel restless, agitated, or full of energy between the hours of 3 A.M. and 7 A.M. (4)

____ I tend to be introverted and keep my thoughts to myself (5)

____ I value my solitude and need time to be alone (5)

____ I deeply resent attempts to intrude on my privacy (5)

____ I have few friends and avoid most social situations; as a result I often feel lonely (5)

____ I tend to avoid intimate relationships (5)

____ I prefer to work alone (5)

____ Because I have my own thoughts and opinions, others sometimes find me eccentric (5)

____ I have a tendency to be paranoid (5)

____ I am patient and persevering, even when the odds are against me (5)

____ I am known for my ability to be objective and impartial in most situations (5)

____ I tend to be skeptical, even cynical (5)

____ I find it difficult to adapt to new situations (5)

____ I sometimes get deeply depressed for no apparent reason (5)

____ I often wake up with feelings of dread or foreboding (5)

____ I am insatiably curious and have a vivid imagination (5)

____ I like to know how mechanical objects work, and I enjoy taking them apart and putting them back together again (5)

____ I like to figure things out for myself; I don't like to be given the answer or solution (5)

_____ I am very attentive and am constantly taking things in that others don't seem to notice (5)

_____ I value reason, logic, and intelligence, and I enjoy all intellectual pursuits (5)

_____ When I'm in conflict with others, I tend to feel a sense of underlying anxiety or dread (5)

_____ I can be incredibly stubborn; when I know I'm right, I won't bend or compromise (5)

_____ I have a strong will; I stand up for myself and my beliefs, even when I'm at odds with everyone around me (5)

_____ My characteristic response to difficult situations is to feel a sense of dread or foreboding, imagining the worst that could happen (5)

_____ My greatest fears include a fear of heights, fear of water, fear of people, fear of the dark, and fear of death (5)

_____ I have a strong preference (or distaste) for salty foods (5)

_____ I have a strong preference (or distaste) for the color blue and/or black (5)

_____ I have a strong preference (or distaste) for very cold climates (5)

_____ I have a strong preference (or distaste) for the season of winter (5)

_____ My dreams often involve images of lakes, rivers, oceans, or dark, mysterious places (such as caves) (5)

_____ My energy is either extremely high or totally depleted between the hours of 3 P.M. and 7 P.M. (5)

SCORING THE QUESTIONNAIRE

The questions are numbered—1, 2, 3, 4, or 5—and grouped accordingly. Total the number of check marks you placed in each section, and enter them in the chart below.

	1 (Wood)	2 (Fire)	3 (Earth)	4 (Metal)	5 (Water)
Physical	_____	_____	_____	_____	_____
Psychological/ Behavioral	_____	_____	_____	_____	_____
Totals	_____	_____	_____	_____	_____

The totals indicate which element or elements most strongly influence your physical health, emotional responses, and behavioral inclinations. Some people fall clearly into one type or another, while many others have a clear affinity to two or more elements; certain individuals (a rare minority) are strongly influenced by all five.

In Chapters 2 to 6 we will explore each of the Five Elements in detail, describing balanced energy patterns and characteristic symptoms of excessive or deficient energy. If your symptoms indicate an imbalance of energy, you'll learn what you can do to restore harmony, including lifestyle changes, stress-reduction strategies, dietary adjustments, nutritional supplements, exercise routines, Western herbs, Chinese herbal formulas, acupressure points, ways to invigorate your senses, and questions you can ask yourself to help pinpoint the underlying meaning of your illness.

In Chapter 7, "A Delicate Balance," you will meet six combination types, men and women who have strong, natural affinities to two or more elements. Through their experiences you will learn how the Five Elements combine and interact, and you will discover how various healing strategies can be adapted to individual needs.

2. WOOD: THE COMMANDER

Adapting itself to obstacles and bending around them, wood in the earth grows upward without haste and without rest. Thus too the superior man is devoted in character and never pauses in his progress.

—*The I Ching*

David had always taken his good health for granted. He worked hard, played hard, ate hard, and drank hard, and his body had always bounced back, ready for more. Now, in his mid-thirties, he was beginning to show signs of wear and tear, and he didn't like it at all. Marching into my office, grabbing my hand, and giving it a forceful shake, he immediately launched into a description of his problems and requested a cure.

"I've had a bad stomach for as long as I can remember," David began, speaking in a loud, forceful tone of voice. Although he initially sat down opposite me, he was soon pacing back and forth, gesturing with his hands, his brow furrowed, his back and shoulder muscles tensed. "Whenever I'm under stress—and I'm always under stress—I get acid reflux and intense gas pains. I've learned to live with these problems by taking Tagamet and antacids with me everywhere I go, but lately the pain and discomfort have increased to the point where over-the-counter drugs don't work anymore. I'm a trial lawyer, and I've got a mountain of work piled up on my desk. To make matters worse, I'm a partner in my firm, so I have to take part in all the socializing and drinking and late-night meetings."

At this point in his soliloquy, David threw his hands up into the air. "I know, I know, I need to change my ways," he said. "Believe me, I'm motivated—I just met with a surgeon who wants to take out my gallbladder. I don't trust doctors, I don't want anyone cutting me open, and I don't have time for surgery. So just tell me what I need to do, and I'll do it. Promise."

"How about taking a seat?" I said, pointing to the chair. David laughed heartily and sat down, but within a few minutes he was shifting around, clearing his throat, and drumming his fingers on the desk. His forceful personality, impatient manner, loud, exclamatory voice, and jittery, pent-up energy all shouted out: *Wood.* In acupuncture school we would have described him as a relatively "pure" type, for everything about him, including the slightly oily texture of his skin, the greenish tinge around his mouth, and his muscular, well-proportioned body, fit neatly into the Wood category.

After conducting the standard examinations, I carefully outlined the steps David needed to take to restore balance. First, he had to eliminate or greatly reduce his alcohol intake and cigarette smoking. His liver and gallbladder were obviously rebelling against the toxic effects of these drugs as well as his standard diet of pastries for breakfast, fast foods for lunch, and calorie-rich, high-fat meals for dinner. I suggested a liver-healthy diet with plenty of fresh fruits, vegetables, and whole grains. Regular exercise, liver-supporting herbs such as dandelion and milk thistle, and therapeutic doses of vitamin C, vitamin A, vitamin E, selenium, and the herb pycnogenol would also help restore balance and harmony, I said.

I also learned that David had few outlets for his creative energy. During college and law school he had relaxed by taking photographs and working in a darkroom, but he hadn't picked up a camera in years. Once I pointed out the inherently creative nature of his Wood energy, which needs to express itself boldly and decisively (and particularly enjoys fast results), David agreed that spending some time in a darkroom might release some of his built-up tension.

Within a few weeks of our session David began to experience relief from his digestive upsets. He had no difficulty sticking to "the program," as he called it, for like most Wood types, he tackled any challenge with energy and enthusiasm. And whenever he lapsed and ate, drank, or worked too much, his stomach rebelled— a potent reminder of his vulnerability to stress.

An aggressive, dominant, and often domineering personality is characteristic of Wood types, whose energies can best be described as bold, ambitious, and fiercely competitive. If you are a Wood type, you are driven by invisible forces that compel you to stay in motion and constantly seek out new challenges and exciting adventures. It is your nature to be direct and forceful and to express your feelings to the world clearly and effectively, using your abundant energy to remove any obstacles that might be blocking your way.

The power of Wood can be compared to the tenacious energy of a sapling sinking its roots deep in the earth while simultaneously shooting upward at an astonishing rate of growth. "Adapting itself to obstacles and bending around them, wood in the earth grows upward without haste and without rest," notes the ancient Chinese text known as the *The I Ching*. Adaptable and pliable, the plant draws its power from the roots, which depend on the earth for sustenance. Rising slowly but surely, the seedling pushes upward with strength and purpose while always remaining supple and yielding.

If you are a Wood type, you are like the greening stem of spring, driven by the need to stay in motion and reach new heights, yet be grounded by a firm sense of self and "home"—the place where you fit and belong. While your roots are driven deep, your potential is unlimited. Blessed with vision, insight, and the ability to plan ahead, you are determined to find your way in the world and are prepared for any situation or obstacle that might present itself.

The predominant emotion associated with Wood energy is anger, which the Chinese consider healthy as long as it is balanced and clearly expressed. Viewed as a natural reaction to stress, frustration, or injustice, anger helps to release pent-up emotions, much as thunder helps to clear the air. When anger builds up and is not released, the internal skies grow dark and stormy, fierce winds blow, and the thunderheads stack up in preparation for a mighty explosion.

Imbalances in Wood Energy

Problems arise for Wood types when they rely on unhealthy (high-fat, fried, greasy) foods, drink too much, take too many prescription or over-the-counter drugs, neglect exercise, or live for long periods of time with chronic, unrelieved stress. When the Liver is overburdened, Wood energy becomes constrained (what the Chinese call "constrained Liver *chi*"), and no matter how hard you push, you don't seem to get anywhere.* As a result, you feel frustrated and stunted in your growth, like a tree whose roots can't penetrate a thick layer of rock.

Psychological and emotional pressures can also lead to energy blockages. When you don't get your way, when your natural desire to move ahead and take charge is thwarted, when your creative energies are blocked, or when physical ailments or emotional problems contribute to boredom and inactivity, you will experience an uncomfortable buildup of internal pressure.

A healthy Wood type needs to be able to keep moving; when you encounter obstructions, you need to remove them quickly so that you can continue on your way. If for any reason you get stuck and your forward movement is impeded, your energy will build up and eventually stagnate, further weakening the Liver.

Imbalances in Wood energy arise from, and in turn are affected by, the organ systems associated with Wood: the Liver and the Gallbladder. Western medicine describes organs as strictly anatomical structures responsible for specific physiological activities, but in traditional Chinese medicine organs are discussed in both concrete and metaphorical terms that extend their influence into emotional and spiritual realms. The "Western" liver is perceived as a kind of chemical refinery responsible for storing, metabolizing, and distributing nutrients, removing dead cells and toxins from the blood, and transforming carbohydrates, fats, and proteins into glucose, which is used by the cells for energy.

The Chinese Liver is imagined as a brilliant military strategist that performs all the duties assigned to it by Western medical science and many others as well. Primarily responsible for the smooth flow of energy and blood to every cell in the body, the Liver is said to "command the blood." Its duties are described by the Yellow Emperor Huang Di in *The Yellow Emperor's Classic:*

> The liver stores blood. During the day the liver provides the blood
> for movement and activities, so that the blood can circulate through
> the channels and collaterals. At night, when one sleeps, the blood re-

---

*Whenever we refer to the Chinese organ, we will capitalize the first letter of the organ, such as Liver, Kidney, Lung, Heart, Spleen, Stomach.

turns to the liver. When the liver is nourished by the blood one can see. When the feet are perfused with blood, one can walk. When the hands are nourished by blood, they can grasp. When the fingers are provided with blood, one can carry.

As "Commander of the Blood," the Liver is also responsible for making sure that physical, emotional, and spiritual needs are kept in balance, just as a great military leader would consider the morale of his troops as being as essential to their strength and vitality as getting enough food and water. A healthy Liver keeps the blood, energy, and emotions in a perpetual state of flow, which in turn helps to create an openness to new ideas and experiences. If your energy is blocked or impeded for any reason, you will find it difficult to express and release your emotions, which will, in turn, affect your physical health and well-being.

The spirit of the Liver, the *hun,* is called "the creative spirit"; when the Liver energy is constrained, your ability to communicate with others and express yourself creatively is thwarted. Because creative expression is essential to healthy Wood energy, long-term obstructions will contribute to physical and emotional illnesses.

In Western medicine the pear-shaped organ known as the gallbladder is held responsible for concentrating and storing the bile produced by the liver. When bile is needed for digestion (especially the digestion of fats), the gallbladder sends it through the common bile duct into the duodenum of the small intestines. In Chinese medicine the Gallbladder is invested with additional duties that directly affect our emotional and spiritual well-being. Viewed as a wise and prudent judge, the Gallbladder rules over the body's kingdom with careful decision making and impeccable judgment. In emotional and spiritual terms, the Gallbladder moderates impulsive or reckless behavior. Rash decision making and indecisive behavior suggest an imbalance of energy in this organ sphere.

EXCESS WOOD

While Wood types tend to push themselves to the limit and perform admirably under pressure, excess Wood energy—what the Chinese call "overly *yang*" behavior—affects both the Liver and the Gallbladder, spawning a tendency to push ahead without adequate planning or thought. You become overly aggressive and try to push your way past any obstacles blocking your way. When you are frustrated in your efforts, you tend to behave like the proverbial bull in the china shop, crashing ahead without thinking, oblivious to the damage you are causing. When friends or family members disagree with you or object to your pushy, inconsiderate behavior, you respond with anger and denunciations. Excess Wood types are often described as having "a chip on their shoulders."

Not surprisingly, your inner tension is manifested in physical symptoms such as tight, bunched, or cramped muscles, migraine headaches, and digestive disturbances. Because it is part of your nature to be independent and self-reliant, you refuse to acknowledge your increasingly distressing physical and emotional problems. Only when your symptoms become too painful or too obvious to ignore will you turn to an expert for help, and even then excess Wood energy rules your behavior. Abrupt and forceful in your demands for a cure, you want fast relief and have little patience with long-term methods that require a commitment of time and energy.

Excess Wood: Physical Symptoms
- Hard, ridged, or cracked fingernails and toenails
- Oily skin with tendency to acne
- Muscular tension with cramps and spasms, usually in the head, neck, and shoulders but also in the hips, legs, hands, and feet
- Tendon injuries
- Sciatica (radiating pain following the course of the sciatic nerve from the lower back through the buttock and down the leg)
- Pain or tension in the temple area
- Headaches, especially migraines
- Visual disturbances: severe eyestrain, sharp eye pain, extreme headaches related to visual problems, conjunctivitis, glaucoma
- Dizziness, usually accompanied by nausea
- Ringing in the ears
- Menstrual irregularities, including heavy bleeding and abnormally frequent periods
- "Excess" PMS (premenstrual) symptoms, such as cramping, abdominal distention, severe headaches, severe emotional swings featuring anger, intense irritability, and acute anxiety

- Digestive disturbances such as heartburn, excessive, foul-smelling gas, or ulcers
- Cysts, lumps, and growths of all kinds (breast lumps, endometrial cysts, sebaceous cysts)
- Cancer of all kinds, but particularly liver and breast cancers
- High blood pressure, with tendencies toward atherosclerosis (hardening of the arteries)
- Chinese Wind Syndrome: The Chinese call the wind "the Chariot of One Hundred and One Diseases," ranging from tingling and numbness in the extremities to muscle twitches, eye twitches, migrating aches and pains, chills, seizures, and strokes

Excess Wood: Psychological and Behavioral Symptoms

- Tendency to be overly serious
- Difficulty relaxing
- Obsession with movement, action, and arousal
- Overpowering desire to win or accomplish a particular goal
- Lack of respect for authority
- Aggressive tendencies
- Insensitivity to other people's feelings or needs
- Agitation and irritability
- Violent outbursts of anger
- Tendency to make life difficult for others, particularly those who disagree with you
- Tendency to blame others when things don't go as planned
- Inflexible behavior patterns
- Workaholic tendencies
- Self-destructive tendencies
- Fears of being confined, restrained, or controlled by others

DEFICIENT WOOD

While excess Wood energy creates problems with rigidity, recklessness, and insensitivity to the needs of others, deficient Wood energy contributes to an internal weakening and eventual collapse. With Wood, as with Fire, Earth, Metal, and

Water, deficient energy patterns tend to follow a prolonged period of excess energy surging erratically through the system. Eventually your energy reserves are depleted, your power begins to spurt and sputter, and symptoms of distress become obvious to everyone.

Anger is focused inward, and feelings of shame and humiliation begin to invade your body, mind, and spirit. A danger of stagnation exists, for you don't have the energy to pull yourself out of the rut you find yourself in. You feel stuck in the mud, no longer capable of sending your roots deep into the soil to nourish and sustain your vital organs. Exhausted and despondent, you find it difficult to concentrate on anything for very long. As time goes by, your power dwindles and collapses.

Deficient Wood: Physical Symptoms

- Chronic tension in neck and shoulders
- Sleep disturbances: insomnia, difficulty falling asleep, fitful sleep
- Allergies of all kinds from hay fever to food sensitivities to dermatological allergies
- Itchy eyes, urethra, or anus
- Visual disturbances, including blurry vision, chronic eye strain, dry eyes, underconvergence (difficulty reading for long periods of time), and extreme sensitivity to light (photophobia)
- Muscle spasms and tics, such as eye twitches and restless leg syndrome
- Menstrual irregularities such as irregular menses, missed periods, light and/or short flows
- PMS (premenstrual syndrome) symptoms such as depression, bloating, chronic weeping, feelings of vulnerability, and low-grade or dull, chronic headaches
- Digestive problems including bloating, difficulty digesting foods such as dairy or wheat products, and food sensitivities or intolerances
- Unstable blood pressure (fluctuating between high and low)
- Lethargy, lack of energy

Deficient Wood: Psychological and Behavioral Symptoms

- General feelings of anxiety, unrelated to any particular situation or experience

- Restless, nervous energy
- Indecisive behavior
- Feelings of shame, embarrassment, and humiliation
- Fear of ridicule, often leading to suppressed emotions (anger, fear, shame)
- Tendency to blame yourself when things don't go as planned
- Blocked creative energy
- Feelings of being stuck and unable to move, as if caught in a trap
- Dependence on external sources of stimulation or sedation (coffee, soda, sugar, alcohol, cigarettes, tranquilizers)
- Withdrawal from others
- Frustration
- Depression, often accompanied by anger or resentment
- Feelings of helplessness and hopelessness

Restoring Harmony

If you recognize yourself as a Wood type with excess or deficient reserves of energy, numerous strategies are available to you to restore health and harmony. Because imbalances in the Five Elements directly affect your body, mind, and spirit, the process of restoring harmony necessarily involves changing your lifestyle, adjusting your diet, reducing your stress, strengthening your interpersonal relationships, and using various nutritional supplements, herbs, and acupoints to restore balance.

LIFESTYLE

Time of Day: If you intend to make drastic or long-term changes in your lifestyle, you might consider the Chinese "clock," which designates the hours between 11:00 P.M. and 3:00 A.M. as the time when Wood's power is most intensely concentrated. If your Wood energy is strong and balanced, you are probably a "night person." Take advantage of the late night/early morning hours to work, think, write letters, rearrange your schedule, plan the week ahead, and make important decisions.

If you are not a night person or if you need to sleep during these hours, rest assured that your Wood energy will be replenished as you sleep. Some people with imbalances in Wood energy wake up between 11 P.M. and 3 A.M. feeling agitated or disturbed; rather than trying to force yourself back to sleep, turn on the light and read or write until you feel tired again.

Season: Wood's season is spring, the time of year when all of nature comes alive again. If Wood is your predominant energy, you will learn a great deal about your own nature by paying careful attention to the changes occurring in the natural world in March and April. The swelling, bursting energy that moves the sap and forces the buds to open is the same powerful, directed energy that surges through your body, mind, and spirit. Become a careful observer of the unique energy of spring, always keeping in mind the words of the ancient Chinese philosopher Lao-tzu: "The hard and stiff will be broken, the soft and supple will prevail."

The Yellow Emperor's thoughts on the spring season are eminently useful for Wood types:

> The three months of the spring season bring about the revitalization of all things in nature. It is the time of birth. This is when heaven and earth are reborn. During this season it is advisable to retire early. Arise early also and go walking in order to absorb the fresh, invigorating energy. Since this is the season in which the universal energy begins anew and rejuvenates, one should attempt to correspond to it directly by being open and unsuppressed, both physically and emotionally.
>
> On the physical level it is good to exercise more frequently and wear loose-fitting clothing. This is the time to do stretching exercises to loosen up the tendons and muscles. Emotionally, it is good to develop equanimity. This is because spring is the season of the liver, and indulgence in anger, frustration, depression, sadness, or any excess emotion can injure the liver.

How to Reduce Stress: Of all the Five Elements, Wood is the most vulnerable to stress because the Liver—the organ system that replenishes and directs Wood energy—is burdened with the responsibility of eliminating stress from the body, mind, and spirit. If you are constantly under stress, the Liver has to work overtime, resulting in the rapid depletion of Wood energy.

The *The I Ching* uses the image of a roof-supporting pole bent to the breaking point to symbolize Wood energy when it is under extreme pressure:

> The load is too heavy for the strength of the supports. The ridgepole,
> on which the whole roof rests, sags to the breaking point.

The problem is that Wood types *like* the feeling of being pushed to the breaking point. You enjoy setting difficult goals for yourself and then pushing yourself to the limit to achieve those goals. A risk-taker and adventurer, you seek out challenge and thrive on competition. If your energies are out of balance, you set goals and take on projects that cannot be completed in the time appropriated. Inevitably, you end up banging your head against the wall, refusing to give up or give in even when it's clear the wall won't move. Wood types don't know the meaning of defeat; they keep pushing and shoving, draining their vital energy reserves and becoming increasingly frustrated, angry, and emotionally unstable.

As the stress level builds, you tend to become more dogmatic, digging your heels in when faced with opposition. Your muscles become tense, tight, and increasingly vulnerable to spasm and injury. Migraine headaches, digestive disturbances, hernias, ulcers, and cysts reflect the unyielding nature of the Wood energy, which can no longer flex and bend under pressure.

If the Wood energy becomes so dried and brittle from chronic stress that even a small spark can set it on fire, the Heart can become inflamed, leading to high blood pressure and atherosclerosis. The Gallbladder can also become irritated, leading to the buildup of gallstones, infections, ulcers, and hepatitis. As the heat builds up in the blood, the blood begins to congeal; in traditional Chinese medicine "congealed blood" is considered a precursor to cancer.

Flexibility is the key to restoring health and balance. As the graceful birches bend and sway with the wind, so do Wood types need to learn how to be flexible and adaptable. Goals can be set, but they should be reasonable and reachable. If a deadline cannot be met or a project completed in a specific period of time, Wood types need to learn how to change direction and "go with the flow."

To increase your flexibility and adaptability, try the following strategies:

Relaxation techniques: When you're stressed out, your muscles contract and create tension; but intentionally tightening those muscles will help you relax. When you tense your muscles, you become painfully aware of the discomfort associated with tension and the overall relief of relaxation. While there are many progressive relaxation techniques, you might start with this simple exercise developed by Edmund Jacobson, M.D., in the early part of this century. Jacobson's techniques, described in his book *You Must Relax,* have been improvised and expanded by many recent writers, most notably Herbert Benson, M.D., of Harvard Medical School in his book *The Relaxation Response.*

TENSE AND RELEASE EXERCISE

Begin by finding a quiet space where you will not be disturbed for ten minutes.

Clench your fists as tight as you can for ten seconds, then release, paying careful attention to the tension draining out of your body. Continue this tension-release exercise with your arms, shoulders neck, forehead, eyebrows, eyes, jaw, stomach, lower back, buttocks, thighs, calves, and feet.

Meditation: Meditation is a simple, easy-to-learn (but difficult-to-master) art that asks you only to live in the moment, clearing your mind of all thoughts about the past and the future and focusing on the here and now. Numerous scientific studies have shown that meditation soothes anger, alleviates anxiety, eases chronic pain, and reduces the symptoms of asthma, migraine headaches, and PMS (premenstrual syndrome).

You don't have to take a class or become a spiritual master to learn the art of meditation. We all meditate, although we may call it "daydreaming" or "being lost in space." Think about those times when you've been completely lost in the moment, enraptured by a winter sunset, entranced by a campfire, immersed in the haunting call of the loons on a faraway lake, or captivated by the luminous energy of lightning bugs on a moonless night. For just a moment your mind is happily imprisoned, and thoughts of deadlines, exams, meetings, and phone calls fade away to nothingness. That's meditation.

Wood types are often so busy doing things that they forget how to "be" and miss those meditative moments when time seems to stop and stand still. If you need help learning how to slow down and pay attention to the world that is passing you by, you might consider taking a meditation class. Because Wood types often have difficulty staying still for prolonged periods of time, it might be best to avoid meditative practices such as Zen or Vipassana that require prolonged "sitting." An "active" meditative practice like tai chi, which combines slow, gentle movements with deep breathing exercises, is well suited to Wood's driving energy. Painting or drawing, writing in a journal, and losing yourself in a good book are all meditative exercises when done in quiet and without distractions. Taking photographs and working in a darkroom, as David did in this chapter's opening case, is another example of a creative way to keep Wood energy focused and directed.

ANGER EXERCISE

San Diego psychiatrist Dennis Gersten suggests an exercise that will put a smile back on your face. Imagine that you're locked in a room with someone who has offended or provoked you. You are free to move around and talk as much as you want, but the object of your anger cannot move or speak. Say all the things you'd like to say, screaming and shouting if that makes you feel better. Don't hold back.

Now imagine that three buckets are placed before you. The first is filled with water, the second with honey, and the third with confetti. Dump the buckets in any order that you like on the person's head until you feel your anger drain away. Then give yourself the pleasure of a good laugh.

DIET

Wood types tend to keep themselves so busy and involved in the endless details of life that they claim they don't have time to eat. For them, skipping meals is common, as is eating on the run—grabbing a Coke and a bag of chips for lunch or pulling into a fast-food drive-through and eating in the car on the way to the next activity. If you have a natural affinity to Wood, try to take a few minutes to relax before eating, then sit down at the table, light some candles, and take the time to enjoy a good, nourishing meal. *Sitting down* is essential, because eating on the run strains your digestive system and contributes to stress, which overburdens the Liver. Your body needs fifteen to twenty minutes of rest several times a day in order to keep your energy flowing steady and strong.

If you suffer from an excess or deficiency of Wood energy, you will need to pay careful attention to the foods you eat. Doctors trained in both Eastern and Western medicine recognize that modern life is particularly injurious to the Liver. Toxins from the fatty, fried, processed, and refined foods we eat, chemicals in our water, toxins in the air (both outside and inside our homes or offices), and the numerous stresses and strains of life in the 1990s place an enormous burden on the Liver. You don't have to be a Wood type to have a stressed-out or over-burdened Liver, so these dietary suggestions apply to anyone whose life is periodically or constantly stressful.

One of the Liver's main duties is to store fats and, when necessary, convert them into glucose (blood sugar) to provide the body's cells with sufficient energy to perform their essential functions. Thus, when you eat lots of high-fat foods, you stress the Liver. Food additives, stimulants (coffee, soda pop, chocolate), cigarettes, alcohol, and other drugs can also damage the Liver, which is responsible for detoxifying the blood, filtering and destroying bacteria, neutralizing poisons, and disposing of worn-out blood cells.

To help your Liver create a smooth flow of blood and vital energy to every cell of your body, follow these general dietary guidelines:

• Restrict your fat intake. Pay special attention to reducing saturated fats, found in animal products (beef, pork, lamb, chicken, and duck), whole milk and whole milk products (cheese, butter, cream, ice cream, yogurt), and tropical oils (coconut and palm oil).

• Whenever possible, avoid "partially hydrogenated" oils, which are found in margarine, solid vegetable shortening, fried fast foods (McDonald's french fries, Kentucky Fried Chicken, deep-fried fish or chicken sandwiches), cookies, cakes, frostings, pies, pastries, doughnuts, crackers, frozen french fries, and packaged microwave popcorn. In addition to overburdening the Liver, these foods raise blood cholesterol levels and blood pressure, contributing to the rising incidence of heart attacks and strokes.

• Reduce your intake of the stimulant caffeine (found in coffee, teas, colas, and chocolate), which can trigger the fight-or-flight response, induce chronic or acute anxiety, and stress both the Liver and the adrenal glands.

• Reduce your consumption of soft drinks. These products are loaded with sugar and phosphorus, which leach calcium and magnesium from your body.

• Whenever possible, avoid processed and refined foods (white bread, refined flour products, refined sugar), which contain numerous chemicals and few essential nutrients.

• Buy organic (chemically untreated) meats, dairy products, fruits, and vegetables whenever possible.

• To remove toxic residues, soak store-bought fruits and vegetables in water treated with grapefruit-seed extract (available in most health food stores—follow the instructions on the package).

• Increase your intake of raw, whole foods: Vegetables and fruits are extremely low in fat, high in fiber, and chock full of vitamins, minerals, trace minerals, and phytochemicals that work to strengthen your immune system and counteract damage to the cells.

• Drink eight to ten 8-ounce glasses of fresh, filtered water every day. Ask your local health department to test your water for pollutants, have your water tested by an independent laboratory (look in the Yellow Pages under Laboratories–Analytical), or contact a mail-order water-quality testing service like National Testing Labs (1-800-458-3330) or Suburban Water Testing Laboratories (1-800-433-6595). If your water contains contaminants, you may want to purchase a water-filtering system through your plumber or by mail order. See Appendix I, Resources, for companies that sell high-quality water-filtering systems.

• Avoid alcohol completely (especially if you have a family history of alcoholism), or reduce your intake to one drink daily.

• If you smoke, stop.

• If you use illicit drugs—marijuana, cocaine, amphetamines—stop.

• Take prescription and over-the-counter drugs only when absolutely necessary.

If stress is a major problem in your life, and your diet is typical "American fare" with lots of fast, fried, canned, frozen, processed, and refined foods, you might want to try a periodic liver cleanse. We've adapted the following Seven Day Liver Cleanse from one offered by Elson Haas, M.D., in his book *Staying Healthy with the Seasons,* and we recommend that you try it in spring, the season of Wood. During the winter months most of us are forced to use canned or frozen fruits and vegetables, we don't exercise as much as we should, and we've gained a few pounds from overindulging during the holidays. Think of this liver cleanse as a spring cleaning that rids your body of the junk and clutter that have accumulated over the last year.

SEVEN-DAY LIVER CLEANSE

Every Day

• Drink *at least* two 8-ounce glasses of Special Lemonade (recipe on page 37) *and* eight 8-ounce glasses of fresh, filtered water daily.

• Take a bulking laxative; we recommend Yerba Prima's completely organic (nonchemically treated) Daily Fiber Powder. Twice daily mix a heaping teaspoon in water (or a combination of juice and water), and drink. Avoid commercial bulking laxatives such as Metamucil or Fiberall, which often contain artificial colors, flavors, and sweeteners, all of which you want to avoid during this liver cleanse. Always read the ingredients on the product label to make sure you are buying a natural form of the active ingredient (crushed psyllium seeds or husks). *Note:* Whenever you use dietary fiber, make sure that you drink plenty of water to keep the fiber soft and digestible.

• For twenty to thirty minutes every day, engage in some kind of gentle aerobic activity: Take a brisk walk, go on a bicycle ride, swim laps, or work out on your home fitness machine.

Days 1-7

• *Days 1 and 2:* Eat only raw, juiced, or steamed fruits and vegetables, spiced to taste. Quantity isn't an issue—you can eat as much as you want. Use cold-pressed, extra-virgin olive oil for salad dressing.

• *Day 3:* Drink only fruit juices and water (again, as much as you want), and at least *four* 8-ounce glasses of Special Lemonade.

• *Day 4, the liver cleanse day:* Drink a minimum of four glasses of Special Lemonade and as much filtered, spring, or distilled water as you want. Before bed take two tablespoons of olive oil followed by a glass of Special Lemonade.

• *Day 5:* Same as Day 3.

• *Days 6 and 7:* Same as Days 1 and 2.

SPECIAL LEMONADE

8 ounces water

Juice of one lemon or lime

⅒ teaspoon or less cayenne powder

1—2 tablespoons 100 percent maple syrup

NUTRITIONAL SUPPLEMENTS

To prevent illness and maintain general good health, take the following vitamins and minerals every day:

General Formula for Maximum Immunity

Vitamin A: 25,000 I.U. (in the form of beta-carotene or mixed carotenes)

Vitamin C: 2,000–3,000 mg.

Vitamin E: 400–800 I.U. (take the higher amount if you are over 50)

Magnesium: 500 mg. (chelated with amino acids)

Multivitamin and mineral supplement: Choose a formula with 100–200 percent of the RDA for various vitamins and minerals

For Extra Protection Add:

Selenium: 200 mcg. (take with vitamin E)

Coenzyme Q-10: 30 mg.

Pycnogenol (pine bark or grape-seed extract): 50 mg.

Zinc: 30 mg. (15 mg. of zinc is included in many multivitamin and mineral supplements)

EXERCISE

Wood types tend to be avid sports enthusiasts who thrive on watching competitive games *and* participating in vigorous exercise. Excess Wood types will often play in a sport until they're ready to drop from exhaustion; when they watch a sports event, they're the ones who follow the action by pacing up and down the sidelines or shout objections at the umpire from the stands. Deficient Wood types, on the other hand, often experience a fear of competition and suffer from feelings of being frozen or unable to move forward; without sufficient Wood energy available to them, they find it difficult to express themselves in appropriate or creative ways.

Regular exercise—for twenty to thirty minutes every day—is equally important for both excess and deficient Wood types. Because deficient Wood types often become inactive due to their low energy and motivation, they need to build up their strength and endurance before engaging in competitive sports or physically demanding exercise. Stretching exercises, swimming, brisk walking, gentle bicycling, treadmills, or cross-country ski machines help to limber up the muscles and tendons and prevent injuries.

Exercises that stretch and soften the muscles (tai chi, yoga, gentle aerobics, brisk walking) help to relieve pressure and circulate the energy evenly throughout the body, preventing muscle spasms and pulls. Once you're warmed up and in good physical shape, choose physically demanding exercises that allow you to express your aggressive energy: Running, mountain biking, backpacking, a competitive game of tennis or racquetball, or a solitary workout on a fitness machine all appeal to Wood's innate need to push hard and stay in constant motion.

Yoga exercise: This simple yoga *asana* (exercise) is specifically recommended for Wood types and will invigorate the Liver *chi* (energy).

Important note: Use this exercise as an adjunct to your regular yoga class. If you have never taken yoga, please find a certified instructor and attend classes to learn the proper techniques. Be sure to warm up with stretching and limbering exercises before trying this or any other yoga *asana.* Never force your body into any position or movement; if you feel pain, your body is telling you to back off. If you are not sure what you are doing, ask your yoga instructor for guidance.

THE BUTTERFLY

Sit on your mat with your legs out in front of you. Take three deep breaths. Now bring the soles of your feet together, and let your knees open out to the sides. Hold your feet as you sit tall. Breathe five slow, full breaths. Extend your legs out in front and bob your knees up and down. Lie on your back with knees up and feet flat. Take three deep breaths. Bring the soles of your feet together and let the knees gently open out—*do not force them open*. Breathe five full breaths. Extend your arms to the wall behind you, and press your palms and fingers together. Breathe five full breaths. Bring your knees into your chest for a gentle counter-stretch for the lower back, and hold for five breaths.

Repeat the entire sequence two times, then rest on your back for two minutes.

HERBS

Western

Many Western herbs work to support liver function, but the most effective and frequently prescribed are dandelion root and milk thistle.

Dandelion *(Taraxacum officinalis):* One of the richest of all plants in nutritive value and a cornerstone of traditional herbal treatments, dandelion is the archetypal liver tonic, helping this vital organ detoxify and cleanse the blood. Traditionally used for any condition involving the liver and gallbladder, including food sensitivities, hepatitis, cirrhosis, gallstones, and infections, dandelion also supports digestion and improves metabolism, gently cleanses the blood to help resolve acne, itchy or sensitive skin, and other skin conditions, and regulates blood sugar levels.

Milk thistle *(Caardus marianus, Silybum marianum):* Milk thistle's value as a liver tonic and cleanser was discovered by herbalists in the Middle Ages, and numerous modern-day studies confirm its effectiveness for Liver and Gallbladder disorders. The liver is overburdened by the stress of modern life and the ubiquitous presence of environmental toxins, and milk thistle offers general support, helping the liver eliminate toxins and regenerate dead and dying cells while relieving stress, fatigue, and overexertion.

Dosage: If you purchase your herbs in a health food store (either in tincture form or as dried herbs, in capsule or pill form), follow the dosage instructions on the label. Because herbs in dried form tend to lose their potency rather quickly, be sure to check the label for an expiration date.

For information on preparing your own herbs from the root, bark, leaves, flowers, or seeds of a plant, see Appendix II. In Appendix I, Resources, we offer a list of mail-order sources for high-quality herbs and herbal preparations.

Chinese

Chinese patent medicines are popular herbal formulas that are premixed in a factory in China in either pill or liquid form. Constitutional formulas work to support the immune system and gently correct imbalances in a particular area, such as deficient Earth or Water energy or constrained Liver *chi;* other remedies are formulated to combat the symptoms of specific diseases or disorders ranging from colds and flus to loss of sexual libido to arthritis and cancer. In Part I (Chapters 1–7) we offer constitutional remedies, while in Part II (Chapters 8–11) we often suggest stronger formulas specifically designed to treat or cure various illnesses.

Although certain patent formulas are extremely powerful and should be used only under the guidance of a qualified professional, most Chinese herbal preparations are completely safe and nontoxic. Throughout this book we suggest only those formulas that have been used for hundreds, even thousands of years, with great success and no potential for harm.

You can purchase formulas and other Chinese patent remedies in Chinese pharmacies (usually located in the Chinatown section of large cities), in larger health food stores, or through mail order; for information on buying or ordering individual herbs and herbal formulas, see Appendix I.

Hsiao Yao Wan ("Relaxed Wanderer Pills"): This is the standard remedy for "constrained Liver *chi,"* gently and effectively aiding the Liver in its job of flowing and spreading Wood energy (*chi*). The Emperor herb (the most powerful or most concentrated herb in the formula) is bupleurum, a Liver-supporting herb famous for its ability to break through obstructions and restore the free flow of energy and blood. Seven "attending" herbs—peony root, dong quai, poria fungus, atractylodes, ginger, licorice, and mint—support the Liver and digestive system, helping to relieve dampness, promote digestion, and move and disperse stuck energy.

You might want to keep this gentle remedy (said to be the most prescribed herbal tonic in Japan) in your medicine cabinet for use during stressful periods, especially when your digestive system is affected, or if you feel as if you have something stuck in your throat or in the pit of your stomach. The pills come in tiny pellet form; take eight pills three times a day or twelve pills twice daily.

ACUPOINTS

LIVER 3 ("Great Rushing"): This point can be imagined as a physical, emotional, and spiritual Roto-Rooter, breaking up blockages and obstructions and allowing energy and blood to flow through the system unimpeded. The "source point" for the Liver meridian, Liver 3 is used when the Liver energy is constrained or deficient. (There are twelve source points, one on each of the twelve main meridians; these points are said to have a powerful harmonizing effect on the vital organ associated with the meridian.)

Thousands of years ago the Chinese devised a map of the human body, identifying sixteen major meridians or invisible channels through which the life-giving energy of *chi* flows. Strategically located along the meridians, like cities on a highway map, are 365 primary acupuncture points (acupoints). By needling, massaging, or pressing these points, you can influence the vital energy flowing through the body, changing its direction, restoring its smooth and easy flow, and assisting it in its efforts to eliminate various pathogens from the body.

For the "Acupoint" sections of this book, we have selected only those points that are easy to locate and stimulate yourself. (See Appendix III for help locating the meridians and acupoints.) To find the point, read the general description of its location, and then let the point guide you to it by sliding your fingers along the general area until they stop in a natural depression or hollow, which tends to be slightly more sensitive to the touch than the surrounding area. When an imbalance or disharmony of energies exists, the acupoint is often extremely sensitive, even painful to the touch. Using your thumb or fingers, massage the point in small, circular movements, always moving in a clockwise direction. Continue for two or three minutes and repeat several times a day.

Common Uses
  • Supports the Liver, promoting the free flow of energy and blood
  • Expels "wind" conditions, which are thought to be caused by an imbalance in Liver energy, including tremors, muscle twitches, migrating pains, dizziness, and headaches

- Brightens the eyes, helping to resolve physical and psychological problems with vision
- Relieves migraine headaches
- Eases digestive problems associated with stress

Location: Liver 3 is located on the upper part of the foot, in the depression in the webbing between the big toe and the second toe. See illustration in Appendix III.

LIVER 14 ("Gate of Hope"): This acupoint supports Liver functions, stimulating the flow of blood and energy (*chi*) throughout the body, clearing clogged channels, and removing obstructions. The "alarm point" for the Liver orb, Liver 14 becomes extremely sensitive to the touch when the Liver is stressed or depleted of energy. (Alarm points are thought to connect directly to the vital organ associated with a particular meridian. They become spontaneously tender or hypersensitive to the touch when the organ's vital energy is out of balance.)

Common Uses

- Supports all Liver functions, stimulating the flow of energy and helping to remove blockages
- Breaks up "congealed blood," which can cause cystic breast disease, ovarian cysts, and uterine fibroids
- Relieves the stabbing pain associated with migraine headaches, chest pains, and gastric distress
- Promotes digestion, relieving constipation and bloating
- Restores hope and confidence in the future

Location: Liver 14 is located two ribs below the nipples on the mammillary line, in the space between the ribs. See illustration in Appendix III.

INVIGORATING THE SENSES

Vision: According to *The Yellow Emperor's Classic,* each of the Five Elements is directly linked with one of the five senses. The eyes are the sense organ invigorated and sustained by Wood energy; in acupuncture the originating point on the Gallbladder meridian is located directly next to the eye, and the Liver meridian has an internal branch that is said to nourish the eyes. Healing energy flows to and from the eyes through these invisible channels.

Although Western medicine makes no direct connection between a healthy liver and good vision, most practitioners would agree that stress contributes to dry eyes, blurry vision, and pain in and around the eyes. Prolonged, unrelieved tension and anxiety can actually injure the eyes and impair vision.

On an emotional and spiritual level, stress definitely affects your ability to form opinions, make decisions, and plan ahead. To think clearly, act instinctively, and rely on your powers of intuition, you need to be able to "see" with the inner eye of wisdom and experience. Abundant and free-flowing Wood energy generates keen insight, intuition, and foresight. No matter how difficult the challenges confronting you, you will be able to move forward with courage and faith, facing adversity with calm resolve and never doubting that good things lie just ahead. If, on the other hand, you tend to hesitate in difficult situations and are afraid to take risks, you might very well be suffering from an imbalance in Wood energy that affects your inner vision.

The color associated with Wood is green, the color of spring, and it signifies progress, creativity, and tranquillity. A natural attraction to the color green indicates your affinity with Wood, while a strong aversion to green may signal an imbalance in this energy. Practitioners of traditional Chinese medicine frequently use colors in diagnosing illnesses. A greenish hue around the eyes or mouth, for example, indicates an imbalance of Wood energy and suggests the need for various herbs and lifestyle changes to support the Liver and Gallbladder.

The color green is generally healing and soothing to Wood energies. "Green like jade" is regarded as the color of life, while "green as in a dying plant" is the color of death. A balanced shade of green is poetically described in *The Yellow Emperor's Classic:* "The color that produces liver *chi* is like white silk wrapping a green color." Certain shades of green may have a negative influence on Wood types, so be sensitive to your reactions, and avoid those tones that seem to irritate you or throw you off balance.

Placing healthy green plants in strategic places in your home, painting your office green, or wearing a green shirt or coat might help to inspire feelings of serenity and confidence in the future. Certain green vegetables—broccoli, peas, green beans, brussels sprouts, kale—are known to strengthen vision, so eat your fill!

In spring, the season of Wood, take a few moments every day to walk outside and look at the green growing plants in your garden, reassuring yourself that life constantly renews itself, year after year after year.

Sound: A strong, clear voice is a good sign that your Wood energy is abundant and well balanced. If there is a "shout" or "lack of shout" to your voice, an imbalance may be suspected. Excess Wood types tend to shout out their words in an aggressive, forceful way, while deficient Wood types exhibit a lack of strength or dynamic energy in the voice, resulting in a monotonous vocal tone with little or no inflection.

An effective healing sound for Wood is "Shhhhhhhhhhhhh," a quiet, relaxing tone that softens the shout associated with excess Wood energy. Find a comfortable, relaxed sitting position, keeping your spine erect, yet not stiff. Put your hands on either side of the lower end of the rib cage (the Liver is located on the right side), and take a deep, easy breath. As you breathe in, imagine that you are directing healing energy into your Liver. When you exhale, say, "Shhhhhhhhh," and imagine that you are releasing all your pent-up anger, hostility, and resentment. Continue this exercise for five or ten minutes every day.

Smell: For thousands of years men and women have been using perfumes, spices, and aromatic oils to alleviate fatigue, ease depression, restore energy, and invigorate the senses. Modern research has confirmed that they were on to something. Researchers at Yale University have discovered that certain smells (like lavender) work to increase alertness, decrease anxiety, and enhance the attention span, while the relatively un-exotic smell of spiced apples can lower blood pressure and alleviate panic attacks. At the University of Cincinnati, researchers report that certain fragrances increase work efficiency and typing speed. And in experiments conducted at International Flavors and Fragrances, women who smelled musk ovulated more often and found it easier to conceive. In another famous study, cats sniffed the herb lemon balm; after they died, when autopsies were performed, the inhaled molecules were discovered wedged into neurons in the hippocampus, providing clear evidence that certain smells directly affect the brain.

For Wood types, we recommend any of the following fragrances: *peppermint* to relieve tension headaches, restore energy, and lift the spirits (not to mention its ability to banish bad breath); *chamomile,* a sleep inducer, pain-killer, and mental relaxer; *lemon balm* for depression and melancholy; and *lavender* for anxiety, muscle cramps, and stress.

Taste: In traditional Chinese medicine the taste associated with Wood is sour, and a strong attraction or repulsion to acidic, tart, or tangy foods (vinegar, sour pickles, lemons, sorrel leaves, yogurt) is believed to indicate an affinity to Wood.

Foods with a sour taste are thought to stimulate and support Liver energy. As *The Yellow Emperor's Classic* explains it:

> With the arrival of spring the weather warms the earth. All plants begin to sprout and put forth green leaves, so the color associated with spring is green. Since most fruits and trees are immature and unripe at this time, their taste is sour. This sour taste can strengthen the liver.

High in vitamin C and potassium and rich in bioflavonoids, lemons stimulate gastric juices, aiding in digestion, and they assist the liver in metabolizing fat and detoxifying chemicals and waste products. In Western herbal traditions lemon juice and lemon water are frequently used to cleanse the liver and gallbladder, benefit the kidneys, lower high blood pressure, and reduce a fever.

To stimulate Wood energy, try foods with a sour taste. Put lemon slices in your drinking water, use vinegar and olive oil for your salad dressing, garnish your sandwich with a slice of dill pickle. Don't get carried away, however, for a craving for sour foods may indicate an imbalance in Wood energy, and overindulging could upset the delicate balance of energies within the body. As Qi Bo cautions: "Too much sour taste may cause overactivity of the liver and underactivity of the spleen."

Touch: The way you reach out and touch the world, and your response to being touched—by a lover, a child, the wind, a light rain, or the warming rays of the sun—is strongly influenced by your affinity to Wood, Fire, Earth, Metal, or Water. Wood types respond immediately and positively to strong pressure and a firm touch; in most cases they would choose a downpour over a gentle rain, a thunderstorm over stray wisps of clouds, a strong gust over a soft breeze.

Massage is a wonderful way to invigorate energy and stimulate healing. If your Wood energy is deficient, you might benefit from a gentler form of massage, but excess Wood types won't have much patience for soft massages that just barely touch their tense and tired muscles. Most Wood types prefer the "exquisite pain" of deep-connective-tissue massage, which is wonderful therapy for reducing muscle tension, improving circulation, soothing an overstimulated nervous system, easing headaches, and enhancing digestion. Shiatsu (vigorous finger pressure on selected acupressure points), Rolfing (a form of deep-connective-tissue massage designed to realign and strengthen the body to improve posture), and more vigorous forms of Swedish massage are favorite massage styles for Wood types.

You don't have to spend a lot of money on a professional massage to rub away your aches and pains—just find a quiet corner and spend ten or fifteen minutes massaging yourself. Here are a few suggestions for self-massage that are helpful for Wood types:

FOOT MASSAGE

Rub moisturizing lotion, massage oil (try peppermint-scented), or plain old vegetable oil on your fingers. Using both hands, lightly squeeze your right foot, moving from your ankle to your toe. Squeeze any sore spots for ten to twenty seconds. Press the sole of your foot, just beneath the ball, for twenty seconds. Gently pull the toes apart, and roll each toe back and forth several times. Repeat the massage with your left foot.

HEAD MASSAGE

Placing your thumbs just behind your ears, put the four other fingers of both hands on either side of the middle of the scalp with the pinkies at the hairline. Using firm, steady pressure, press your fingertips into the scalp. Slowly move your hands backward to the base of the skull, stopping every inch or so to apply firm pressure.

Return to the hairline, placing your fingers about an inch below the hairline, and repeat the massage, moving down to the base of the skull and back up again. Keep moving your fingers down your head until you've massaged your whole scalp. If you feel any sensitive spots, spend extra time massaging those areas. This entire exercise takes only three or four minutes.

QUESTIONS TO ASK YOURSELF

Fears and doubts assail us all, and Wood types are no exception. When Wood energy is out of balance, anxieties and uncertainties centering on direction, goals, and purpose in life tend to arise. The Wood type's greatest fear is being helpless and out of control.

If you feel off balance or out of sorts, use these questions to identify the source of your distress. Choose one or two questions that best describe your feeling. Write down your responses, and spend some time thinking about creative ways to overcome the obstacles confronting you.

- I tend to go off in a dozen directions at once: What is my purpose in life? What can I do to keep myself focused on the task at hand?
- I feel lost: What direction do I want to go in?
- I feel powerless: What can I do to take power back into my own hands?
- I feel confined, trapped, imprisoned: What can I do to break free?
- I am often frustrated: What obstacles confront me, and what can I do to break through them?
- I feel happiest and most energetic when I have a cause to believe in: Do I have a cause? Is it the right one?
- I love to compete, but I hate to lose: How can I learn to win gracefully and lose with dignity?
- I fear being out of control: What is the worst thing that could happen to me if I lost control?

A Story for Wood

Individuals with a strong affinity to Wood are driven by the need for action, movement, and fulfillment. The key to balancing Wood energy is the ability to control your emotions while clearly expressing your basic feelings and desires. A wonderful story shows us how to balance thought and action with gentle but effective force:

A young female disciple spent many hours trying to understand the spiritual concept of loving-kindness and treat others with respect and compassion. Sitting in her small room, she would fill her heart with loving-kindness for all living beings; yet each day as she went to the bazaar to buy her food, she would find her loving-kindness sorely tested by one shopkeeper who subjected her to unwelcome caresses.

One day she could stand no more and began to chase the shopkeeper down the road with her upraised umbrella. To her mortification, she passed her teacher standing on the side of the road observing the spectacle. Shame-faced, she went to stand before him, expecting to be rebuked for her anger.

"What you should do," her teacher gently advised her, "is to fill your heart with loving-kindness, and with as much mindfulness as you can muster, hit this unruly fellow over the head with your umbrella."

Famous Wood Types

John Wayne
Jane Fonda
Hillary Clinton
Bob Dole
Joan Rivers
Geraldo Rivera
Michael Jordan
Dorothy from *The Wizard of Oz*
Rabbit from *The House at Pooh Corner*

3. FIRE: THE LOVER

What is dark clings to what is light and so enhances the brightness of the latter. A luminous thing giving out light must have within itself something that perseveres; otherwise it will in time burn itself out. Everything that gives light is dependent on something to which it clings, in order that it may continue to shine.

—The I Ching

As my mother always used to say, 'Cold hands, warm heart,'" Jill said, laughing nervously, her graceful, long-fingered hands in constant motion as she described the symptoms that prompted her to try acupuncture and herbal medicine. "All day, no matter how warm it is outside, my hands and feet are cold, but at night I wake up drenched with sweat. Two minutes after I throw the covers off, I'm freezing to death. Then another hot flash blazes through me, and the whole thing starts over again." At this point Jill's voice began to tremble. "I also have panic attacks that make me feel like a deer caught in a car's headlights—I can't move, can't think, my heart pounds uncontrollably, and I want to die right there on the spot. I'm only forty-five, and I feel as if I'm being turned inside out, dozens of times a day. I just can't seem to get a grip on myself."

Jill pushed back her bright red hair in a gesture of impatience, then reached out to touch my hand as if I were the one who needed comforting. "I'm okay, really I am. Things aren't *that* bad. But maybe I can do something, make some changes in my life that will make me feel better in the long run—what do you think?"

Jill was a classic Fire type, full of energy and enthusiasm, vivacious, warm-hearted, and extremely emotional. When she spoke (her voice had a natural quaver, which worsened when she became upset or nervous), she seemed to hold her breath; after finishing a sentence, she would quickly take a deep breath and then plunge ahead. She explained that she had a phobia about public speaking that dated back to the eighth grade, when she had had a panic attack while giving a speech. Although naturally an extrovert, she pursued a writing career to avoid speaking in public; even answering the phone made her nervous.

After reassuring Jill that I knew of many gentle, supportive strategies that would diminish the severity and incidence of her panic attacks, hot flashes, and night sweats, reduce her anxiety, and restore her energy and enthusiasm for life, I began to tell her about the nature of Fire. "Fire types often find it difficult to separate themselves from the people they love," I explained, "and when feeling insecure or anxious, they can become clingy and overly emotional."

Jill nodded her head vigorously. "That's me," she said.

"Maintaining a separate identity is an important goal for Fire," I continued, "yet without close, loving relationships with friends, family, and the larger community, Fire types can lose their spark. Being disconnected from others, either literally or figuratively, is deeply disturbing to Fire types, so it is essential to keep the fires of passion and enthusiasm kindled. Think of a steady pilot light, and you'll have the right image for keeping your Fire energy in balance."

When I explained that excess Fire depletes the Kidney's reserves of water—just as the sun will evaporate a pool of water—Jill immediately grasped the need to contain her natural energy and set boundaries that would protect her from becoming overly excited or stimulated. Naturally creative, she treasured the metaphors and imagery associated with Fire because they helped her accept her limitations and celebrate her strengths.

If you are gifted with the radiant, passionate energy of Fire, you attract others to your light and warmth as the flame entices the moth. You love to be with people, and you work hard to create and sustain relationships. Highly intuitive, you often know what your friends are thinking or feeling before they do. You experience intense emotional pain when you are temporarily separated from your loved ones, for your desire to merge with others and "be one with everything" is consuming. With all your heart you believe that the fusion of two souls into one is the culminating experience of life.

The yearning to love another human being so deeply and intensely that you become one is both your greatest strength and your greatest weakness, for the potential exists to consume yourself with your own passion. Your thoughts and feelings may become so entangled with another's that you literally cannot tell where you end and the other begins. As Fire's flames leap out of control, this fusion threatens to become self-immolating. If Fire burns too hot for too long, its energy is gradually extinguished, the spark flickers and dies, and the flames turn to ashes.

Imbalances in Fire Energy

An imbalance of Fire energy causes a wide range of symptoms that affect many areas of the body, mind, and spirit. These disturbances inevitably derive from and, in turn, affect, one or more of the four organ systems associated with Fire: the Heart, the Pericardium (also called "Circulation Sex"), a solely functional (nonanatomical) system called the Triple Heater, and the Small Intestine.

The Heart: In Western medicine the small, hollow, muscular organ called "the heart" is considered the center of the circulatory system. Its primary responsibility is to serve as a pump that controls the flow of blood through the circulatory system. In fact, there are two "pumps" inside the heart: the pulmonary circulatory system, located in the right side of the heart, pumps blood through the lungs; the reoxygenated blood then flows back to the left side of the heart and is pumped out by systemic circulation to the rest of the body.

In Chinese medicine the responsibilities of the Heart are extended to the emotional and spiritual realms. In the ancient texts the Heart is compared to a supreme monarch responsible for maintaining internal peace and harmony. As Qi Bo explains to Huang Di in *The Yellow Emperor's Classic:* "The heart is the sovereign of all organs and represents the consciousness of one's being. It is responsible for intelligence, wisdom, and spiritual transformation."

Located at our core or center, the Heart is considered "the root of life" and "the seat of intelligence" that provides the inspiration for all the highly developed mental functions associated with being human: awareness, perception, intuition, inspiration, spiritual desires, and the ability to communicate thoughts, feelings, and emotions. The spirit of the Heart is known as *shen,* which governs intelligence and creativity.

The Pericardium: In Western medicine the pericardium is the sac that surrounds and protects the heart. To the Chinese this strictly structural definition misses the true spirit of the Pericardium, which is described in the ancient texts as "the court jester who makes the king [the heart] laugh, bringing forth joy." Just as the court jester offers the king relief from the heavy responsibilities involved with overseeing a vast kingdom, so does the Pericardium create an atmosphere of joy and good cheer, protecting the Heart by screening out unnecessary or undesirable ideas, thoughts, and images.

The Pericardium also provides the Heart with spiritual nourishment, overseeing all intimate relationships with lovers, friends, children, and parents. Numerous psychological disorders, including phobias, depression, anxiety, panic disorders, and speech problems, are viewed as imbalances within this vital organ.

The Triple Heater: The only organ within the Chinese classification system that is solely functional and has no structural counterpart (no corresponding organ exists in Western medicine), the Triple Heater is nevertheless considered an extremely powerful component of the body, mind, and spirit, responsible for heating and cooling the entire system. The Three Heaters include the Misting, the Factory, and the Swamp. The Misting rules the upper part of the body from the rib cage to the neck, housing the Heart and Lungs and ruling over the refinement and distribution of *chi* and blood. The Factory governs the middle part of the body, from the umbilicus to the rib cage; its duties of digestion and assimilation are carried out by the Stomach, Spleen/Pancreas, Liver, and Gallbladder. The lower heater, the Swamp, supervises the area from the belly button to the pubic bone and is responsible for the storage of wastes in the bowels and bladder and various gynecological functions.

Metaphorically, the Triple Heater rules over three different levels of consciousness. The Swamp is said to rule sensuality and sexual response; the Factory governs practical matters; and the Misting controls the spiritual domain. Working together to keep the body, mind, and spirit in harmonious balance, the Three

Heaters are responsible for maintaining peaceful, stable relationships both within the individual and between the individual and the larger society.

The Small Intestine: In Western medicine the small intestine is an organ consisting of three parts: the duodenum, through which pancreatic juices and bile flow, and the jejunum and ileum, where carbohydrates, proteins, and fats are broken down and absorbed into the body. Bulky and unusable portions of food pass through the small intestine and into the large intestine, where they are formed into wastes for eventual evacuation.

In Chinese medicine the Small Intestine is called "the Separator of the Pure from the Impure" and "the Minister of Information." After sorting out the "pure" nutrients from food and drink, the Small Intestine transports them to the Spleen, where they are transformed into energy (*chi*) and blood. The "impure" parts are passed on to the Large Intestine for elimination. A similar process takes place on the mental and spiritual level, where in order to stay healthy, we need to be able to filter out and absorb only the "nutritional" parts of our daily interactions with others and eliminate from consciousness the "undigestible" parts. When our emotional Small Intestine malfunctions, we have trouble discriminating between the healthy and harmful parts of our relationships, our psychological waters become clogged with debris, and confusion reigns throughout the body, mind, and spirit.

EXCESS FIRE

If an excess of Fire energy builds up within you, you will feel jittery and overexcited, as if you've had too much coffee or too little sleep. The comic Robin Williams is a perfect example of an excess Fire type. Spontaneous, unbridled joy bursts through the seams of his personality, and his energy seems to explode in a dozen places at once. Watching him perform, his hands circling like pinwheel firecrackers, his face red with exertion, his smile stretched to his ears, you can't help wondering when he is going to burn out. Yet he just keeps going and going and going.

Not all of us are so lucky, for if the excess energy continues to surge through our systems, the wires will burn out, just as a 110-volt electric line burdened with a 220-volt charge will snap, crackle, pop, and suddenly go *pfffffft*. The hyperexcitability associated with excess Fire energy leads to such physical symptoms as restlessness, manic behavior, generalized anxiety, panic attacks, palpitations, accelerated heart rate, cold and/or sweaty extremities, and painful, burning indigestion. The frenzied, frazzled nature of excess Fire energy also affects the emotions, often leading to irrational thoughts and to various phobias and fears. Excess Fire energy can also be exhausting to others, who feel smothered by the Fire type's unrelenting need for togetherness and intimacy.

Excess Fire: Physical Symptoms
- Excessive perspiration and a tendency to "overheat"
- Flushed complexion, ranging from rosy to bright red or purple
- Skin irritations or eruptions, including sores of the mouth, tongue, and lips
- Red and inflamed tongue, particularly on the tip
- Rashes or hives
- Speech disturbances: stuttering, choked or strained speech, constant tension in the throat, hoarseness
- Sleep disturbances: insomnia, vivid or disturbing dreams, restless sleep, waking up early
- Hot flashes
- Erratic pulse
- Irregular or rapid heartbeat
- Vertigo
- Fainting spells
- Palpitations
- Angina (pain in the chest or radiating down the left arm)

Excess Fire: Psychological and Behavioral Symptoms
- Restless, agitated, explosive energy
- Inappropriate, loud, and annoying laughter
- Extreme anxiety or restlessness, often bordering on mania
- Inability to concentrate or pay attention due to excessively manic energy
- Irrational thought patterns
- Fear of rejection

- Mood swings
- Fears of being overwhelmed
- Sudden irrational outbursts
- Rapid, pressured speech patterns
- Phobias about public speaking or any kind of public performance (stage fright)
- Hysteria, delirium, and various forms of depressive illness
- Lack of appetite, particularly when agitated or depressed
- Excessive desire for cold or iced drinks

DEFICIENT FIRE

In contrast to the manic excitability that marks excess Fire energy, a deficiency eventually leads to fatigue, lethargy, and disordered thought patterns. You have difficulty concentrating and paying attention, your thoughts are often chaotic and unfocused, your judgment is impaired, you wonder if you've lost direction in your life, and at times you feel overwhelmed by circumstances or swept along by events outside your control. You tend to be emotionally uncentered and unstable, experiencing difficulty expressing joy or generating warmth and affection. Your voice tends to drone on in monotony, and you find it difficult to smile or laugh. While your feelings may be intense, you just can't seem to summon up the energy or the confidence to express them in a healthy way. You've lost your spark and feel empty and chilled inside. Feelings of depression and hopelessness pervade your body, mind, and spirit.

Deficient Fire: Physical Symptoms
- Pale, ashen complexion
- Proclivity to blushing
- Shallow breathing; tendency to hold the breath
- Ringing in ears
- Rashes and/or eczema, especially on the elbows
- Insomnia: difficulty falling asleep or staying asleep
- Digestive problems, including constipation, gas, and heartburn
- Exhaustion

- Tendency to lightheadedness, especially when nervous or excited
- Excessive perspiration, especially when tired or nervous
- Difficulty maintaining sexual arousal
- Low blood pressure
- Heart irregularities and palpitations, including tachycardia (heart rhythm is too fast) and arrhythmia (irregular heartbeat or missed beats)
- Cardiac insufficiency or congestive heart failure

Deficient Fire: Psychological and Behavioral Symptoms

- Lack of originality and creativity
- Lack of spontaneity
- Eagerness to please
- Tendency to wear your heart on your sleeve
- Poor judgment in love relationships
- Intense need to be accepted
- Emotionally unstable
- Free-floating anxiety, reflecting restless (in contrast to excited) agitation
- Difficulty separating thoughts from feelings
- Tendency to go off in several directions at once
- Difficulty paying attention, thinking logically, and speaking clearly due to lack of energy and vitality
- Forgetfulness
- Muddled thought processes
- Monotonous, droning voice
- Conspicuous lack of humor
- Fear of rejection
- Fear of falling
- Loss of passion
- Exhaustion

Restoring Harmony

If you experience symptoms of excess or deficient Fire energy, the following strategies will help to restore balance and harmony.

LIFESTYLE

Time of day: Fire types thrive on excitement and stimulation, yet they also need moments of peace and quiet to simmer down and refocus their energies. Fire energy is most powerful between 11:00 A.M. and 3:00 P.M., so if you have important projects to complete or decisions to make, use these hours to your advantage. If you feel too revved up or, on the other hand, exhausted and drained of energy at this time of day, you may be expressing an imbalance in Fire.

Season: Because the power of Fire is felt most intensely in the summer, this may be the best time for you to concentrate on taking time off to relax and build up your energy. The summer months can also be your most vulnerable time; excessive heat and constant activity can overstimulate your system and stress your Heart. Always try to moderate your excitement and curb your tendency to burn the candle at both ends. Always keep in mind that the summer months can just as easily replenish your energy as exhaust it, in the same way as a half hour in the sunshine will rejuvenate you while an hour or two will drain you dry.

The Yellow Emperor has these instructive words about the season of summer:

> In the three months of summer there is an abundance of sunshine and rain. The heavenly energy descends, and the earthly energy rises. When these energies merge, there is intercourse between heaven and earth. As a result, plants mature and animals, flowers, and fruit appear abundantly.
>
> One may retire somewhat later at this time of year, while still arising early. One should refrain from anger and stay physically active, to prevent the pores from closing and the qi [*chi*] from stagnating. One should not overindulge in sex, although one can indulge a bit more than in other seasons. Emotionally, it is important to be happy and easygoing and not hold grudges, so that the energy can flow freely.

How to reduce stress: The Chinese believe that stress occurs when the gates to the Heart are stuck, either open or closed. When the gates are stuck open, Fire types have difficulty separating themselves from others around them; when the gates are stuck closed, their ability to open up emotionally is impaired. Because Fire types have trouble separating themselves from the people they love, their most stressful situations involve painful or disintegrating relationships: the breakup of a friendship, a divorce, or the death of a loved one. Being emotionally involved with someone who is anxious, tense, or unable to cope can also create serious emotional strain.

To reduce stress, *pay special attention to your relationships.* Be sure to spend a significant amount of time in the company of others, seeking out any and all situations that allow you to express yourself freely and openly. *Dancing* of any kind, for example, is a good way to create bonds of companionship, encourage laughter, and dissipate pent-up energy. Take a dance class, attend dance concerts, and go dancing whenever you have the opportunity. *Singing* and *listening to music* are also wonderful stress-relieving activities for Fire types. Crank up the stereo and sing along with your favorite musicians, or join a church or community choir. Opera and gospel music are often favorite choices for Fire types, who love the overflowing passion and sentiment. (Water types also love opera, but for different reasons; see page 126.)

Speech impairments are relatively common among Fire types and are another significant source of stress. Any disorder that affects your ability to communicate with others—stammering or stuttering, an illness that affects speech (stroke, minor brain damage), anxiety about public speaking, or panic attacks—will cause both acute and chronic stress. Since the Fire type's greatest talent is communication, their greatest fear is to be cut off from others. Anyone who has ever suffered from a speech disorder knows the deep, painful feelings of alienation and separation that occur when you cannot fully express your thoughts and feelings.

Because your ability to communicate with others is essential to your happiness, do everything you can to encourage and support relaxed, unpressured speech. *Breathing exercises* increase the oxygen available to your cells, which improves your physical energy, invigorates your thought processes, calms your emotions, and settles your spirit. Many spiritual traditions rely on special breathing techniques to bring "spirit" into the body, in the belief that the air we breathe contains, in addition to oxygen, a vital energizing force that animates and invigorates our bodies, minds, and spirits.

While people of all types can profit from daily breathing exercises, Fire types are the ones who can benefit the most from them. Because they get so excited about each and every event in their lives that they sometimes forget to breathe properly, Fire types are the most susceptible to constricted or chaotic breathing patterns. When Fire energy flares up and we become overexcited, breathing exercises help to ground our energy.

When you are anxious, tense, or need to relax, try this breathing technique:

THE CALMING BREATH

- Exhale completely, then close your mouth and inhale through your nose to a count of five. As you breathe in, imagine that pure, clean air is entering your lungs.
- Hold your breath for twenty counts, imagining that your cells are using this opportunity to empty their waste products into the bloodstream.
- Exhale to ten counts, visualizing the waste products exiting from your body.

This exercise follows a 1:4:2 ratio: 5 seconds, 20 seconds, 10 seconds. If this ratio is too easy for you, try 6:24:12 or 7:28:14. Experiment until you find the ratio that works best for you.

For extra energy try the Invigorating Breath (see page 126), and to open up your blood vessels, to relax constricted chest muscles, and for general relaxation, practice the Belly Breath (see page 80).

DIET

To keep your Fire energies strong and balanced, *increase your intake of "cooling"* (yin) *foods.* Raw fruits and vegetables, unsweetened fruit and vegetable juices, and tofu will help quench excess Fire energy, keeping you feeling cool and refreshed.

Red vegetables (tomatoes, red peppers, red chili peppers) tend to be more *yang* (heat-inducing) and can make you feel irritable and off-balance, so use them sparingly.

Bitter foods, beverages, and herbs are considered cooling in all herbal traditions because they support the liver (which the Chinese consider the mother of Fire) and calm the digestive system. Bitter vegetables include endive, escarole, kale, Swiss chard, raw spinach, and other dark green, leafy vegetables.

Green teas are usually bitter and offer the additional benefit of significant antioxidant actions; although green teas contain the stimulant caffeine, the benefits tend to outweigh the negative effects.

Coffee is definitely bitter, but the acids tend to produce heat in the system. If you feel you need the caffeine, *substitute green tea for coffee.*

If you feel agitated and overstimulated, or if your digestive system is upset, *try chamomile tea.* Chamomile is a soothing, stress-relieving herb that has been used for centuries to calm the nervous system of colicky babies and relieve numerous stress-related symptoms in adults. If you are extremely allergic to pollens, however, use chamomile with care: In rare cases, the chamomile flowers can induce an allergic reaction. (For information on preparing herbal teas, see Appendix II.)

As a general rule, but particularly if you suffer from excess Fire energy, *cut down on your intake of meat* (particularly red meat such as beef, pork, and lamb) *and dairy products* (milk, eggs, and cheese). These protein-rich foods are difficult to digest, causing the stomach to produce extra acid, which, in turn, can create stomachaches, cramps, gas, nausea, and heartburn. For deficient Fire types, warming foods like beef and chicken (use organic, nonchemically treated meat whenever possible), fish, beans, nuts, and seeds and moderate amounts of warming spices (cayenne, ginger, garlic) will gently turn up the internal heaters in your system, taking the chill away.

Reducing fats, particularly saturated and polyunsaturated fats, is good advice for anyone, but Fire has an additional reason to *beware of fats:* Fats contribute twice as many calories as proteins or carbohydrates, and the main function of calories is to produce heat. If you suffer from excess Fire symptoms, follow these basic rules for cutting back on fat:

• Reduce your consumption of saturated fats found in animal products (beef, pork, lamb, chicken, and duck); in whole milk and whole milk products (cheese, butter, cream, ice cream, yogurt); and in coconuts, coconut oil, and palm oil.

• Avoid all processed foods whose label or list of ingredients contains the words "partially hydrogenated oils"—margarine, solid vegetable shortening, fried foods, fast foods, cookies, frostings, pies, pastries, cakes, doughnuts, crackers, frozen french fries, and packaged microwave popcorn. These products have been subjected to the food-processing equivalent of a nuclear power reactor, getting their atoms bounced around and reconfigured by high heat and complicated chemistry. In this process the atoms realign themselves, changing from a natural ("cis") form to an unnatural ("trans") form, and trans-fatty acids (TFAs) are created. TFAs are devastating to the coronary artery system (Fire's most vulnerable area) and can increase the risk of heart attacks and strokes.

• Use extra-virgin, cold-pressed olive oil in all cooking and salad dressings. Brush or drizzle olive oil onto bread instead of using butter or margarine.

Last but definitely not least, be sure to *drink a minimum of eight to ten 8-ounce glasses of water daily.* Water will keep the Fire energies under control, aid the Kidneys in their work of filtering toxins from the body fluids, and assist the Liver in its detoxification duties.

NUTRITIONAL SUPPLEMENTS

To prevent illness and maintain general good health, take the following vitamins and minerals every day:

General Formula for Maximum Immunity

Vitamin A: 25,000 I.U. (in the form of beta-carotene or mixed carotenes)
Vitamin C: 2,000–3,000 mg.
Vitamin E: 400–800 I.U. (take the higher amount if you are over 50)
Magnesium: 500 mg. (chelated with amino acids)
Multivitamin and mineral supplement: Choose a formula with 100–200 percent of the RDA for various vitamins and minerals

For Extra Protection Add:

Selenium: 200 mcg. (take with vitamin E)
Coenzyme Q-10: 30 mg.
Pycnogenol (pine bark or grape-seed extract): 50 mg.
Zinc: 30 mg. (15 mg. of zinc is included in many multivitamin and mineral supplements)

EXERCISE

For Fire types the most important rule for exercising is to choose an activity you enjoy; if your exercise regime is boring or monotonous, you'll lose interest quickly. Competitive sports emphasizing team spirit (soccer, volleyball, softball, basketball) appeal to Fire's love of friendly competition, fast action, and companionship; if winning is the primary goal, however, you might want to try a congenial game of tennis or golf instead. Whenever there is a separation into winner and loser, Fire types and others who thrive on connection and intimacy can be thrown off balance. Another factor to consider is your competitor: Watch out for Wood types, who tend to be intensely competitive and can quickly turn friendly matches into fierce contests to determine a winner (and loser).

Competitive sports that require a lot of sitting and waiting for your turn to participate, such as swimming, diving, or gymnastics, can be difficult for Fire types, who thrive on constant activity and tend to get overly anxious when forced to wait and watch while others compete.

Swimming and water sports—water skiing, sailing, canoeing, kayaking—are ideal for excess Fire types. Winter sports like downhill skiing, cross-country skiing, and ice skating are also favorite Fire activities and will help you cool down an overheated system.

Although Fire types often enjoy exercising alone, you still prefer to have company close at hand. Riding a stationary bike or exercising on a home fitness machine in the TV room, surrounded by the family, would suit Fire's dual needs for action and companionship.

While Fire types enjoy short bursts of strenuous activity, you tend to burn out over extended periods of time or in long-distance events. Slow bike rides, gentle jogs, and short, moderate-paced walks are generally preferred to strenuous uphill biking, power walking, or marathon running.

Yoga exercise: This simple yoga *asana* (exercise) is specifically recommended for Fire types.

Important note: Use this exercise as an adjunct to your regular yoga class. If you have never taken yoga, please find a certified instructor and attend classes to learn the proper techniques. Be sure to warm up with stretching and limbering exercises before trying this or any other yoga *asana*. Never force your body into any position or movement. If you feel pain, your body is telling you to back off. If you are not sure what you are doing, ask your yoga instructor for guidance.

THE STAR SERIES

Stand on your mat in a wide stance. Press your feet lightly into the ground. Look straight ahead, and take a full breath. Extend your arms out to the sides to shoulder height with the palms facing down, fingers straight. Take five long, full breaths. (This position is particularly energizing for the Triple Heater.)

Bring arms down at the sides, and take five breaths. Look straight ahead, and raise your arms up to shoulder height with palms facing up. Hold for five breaths. (This variation opens the Heart meridian.)

Raise the arms straight up, and touch the palms together. Hold for five breaths. (This position opens the Conception Vessel and the Small Intestine.)

Now bring the arms out slowly, halfway between the head and shoulders, with the palms facing forward. Hold for five breaths. (This position opens and strengthens the Pericardium and the Small Intestine.)

Bring arms down at the sides and take ten slow, relaxed breaths.

This entire series can be repeated two times. If you are straining, you may need to shorten the holding times. To counterstretch, place your hands on your hips, bend your knees a bit, and fold yourself forward into a supported forward bend by placing your palms on the floor. Breathe into any tension in the lower back. Come up very slowly. Stand for five more breaths, then rest on your back for three minutes.

Exercise Cautions for Fire

◆ If you suffer from breathing difficulties, excessive perspiration, spontaneous perspiration unrelated to physical effort, tightness in your chest, or radiating pain down your arms, be sure to check with your physician before engaging in any strenuous exercise program.

◆ Because Fire types tend to perspire easily (or they may have the opposite problem and perspire too little, which contributes to a buildup of heat), be sure to drink plenty of water whenever you exercise.

HERBS

Western

Hawthorn berry (*Crataegus oxyacantha*): Hawthorn berry dilates peripheral and coronary blood vessels, improving the blood supply to the heart, lowering blood pressure, normalizing heart palpitations, easing the chest pains of angina, and generally stabilizing cardiac activity. One of the gentlest and most effective herbal tonics for the Heart and circulatory system, hawthorn is an "adaptogenic" herb that adjusts its actions to fit your needs, helping you adapt to physical, emotional, and environmental stress.

Motherwort (*Leonurus cardiaca*): Motherwort improves metabolism of the heart, reduces the heart rate, and relieves palpitations and tachycardia (abnormally rapid heart rate). Motherwort's gentle, tranquilizing qualities also help to ease nervous tension and induce sleep.

Dosage: If you purchase your herbs in a health food store (either in tincture form or as dried herbs, in capsule or pill form), follow the dosage instructions on the label. Because herbs in dried form tend to lose their potency rather quickly, be sure to check the label for the expiration date.

For information on preparing your own herbs from the root, bark, leaves, flowers, or seeds of a plant, see Appendix II.

Caution: If you have been diagnosed with heart problems or if you are using a heart medication, consult with a qualified professional before using any herbal remedy. If your cardiologist is not educated in the use of herbs—and most are not—ask if he or she would be willing to confer with your herbalist, acupuncturist, or naturopath.

Chinese

Tian Wang Bu Xin Wan ("Heavenly Emperor, Tonify the Heart Pill"): This famous Chinese patent remedy was formulated over a thousand years ago to nourish the Heart and support the functions of the Kidney *yin,* the invisible fluid energy that "mists" and nourishes the Heart with Water, keeping the Fire under control. The Emperor herbs are rehmannia root, which comprises over thirty percent of the formula and provides nourishing support to the Kidney *yin;* and zizyphus seeds (red jujube dates), used for thousands of years to improve stamina, increase longevity, and promote tranquillity. Nine attending herbs— biota seed, ophiopogon, dong quai, asparagus root, schisandra, scrophularia, polygala, ginseng, and sage—help to ease anxiety, calm restlessness, and allevi- ate insomnia.

Unless otherwise directed by a qualified herbalist, take eight pills three times daily or twelve pills twice daily.

In Appendix I we offer a list of mail-order sources for high-quality Chinese and Western herbs and herbal formulas.

ACUPOINTS

HEART 7 ("Spirit Gate"): The Heart is said to store spirit (*shen*), which the Chi- nese believe is reflected in the eyes. When the eyes sparkle and shine, the *shen* is considered strong, indicating a state of physical and emotional well-being; when the eyes appear dull or hazy, the *shen* is weak, indicating potentially serious un- derlying problems in the body, mind, and spirit. "Spirit Gate" can be imagined as the doorway to the palace where *shen* is stored.

Common Uses

 • Calms and pacifies the spirit, relieving generalized feelings of anxiety, ner- vousness, manic or obsessive-compulsive behaviors, agitation, and restlessness
 • Regulates and stabilizes the Heart, relieving palpitations and arrhythmias
 • Clears heat from the Heart, relieving menopausal symptoms such as night sweats and hot flashes
 • Lowers blood pressure

Location: Heart 7 is located on the inner crease of the wrist, in a depression lo- cated approximately half an inch in from the pinky side of the wrist.

CONCEPTION VESSEL 14 ("Great Palace Gate"): Called the front alarm (*mu*) point on the Conception Vessel, the meridian that runs down the center of the body, this point is thought to connect directly to the Heart. It becomes sponta- neously tender to the touch when Fire energy is out of balance. Famous for its ability to regulate the Heart, calm the spirit, and alleviate depression, "Great Palace Gate" is also used to relieve stomach and digestive upsets.

Common Uses
- Supports and protects the Heart
- Calms the spirit
- Eases emotional disturbances
- Reduces mental confusion
- Improves memory
- Eases stomachaches and pains, particularly in the upper abdominal region and chest

Location: Conception Vessel 14 is located in the hollow just below the breastbone, approximately six inches above the belly button.

INVIGORATING THE SENSES

Vision: Vibrant, contrasting, or clashing colors often appeal to Fire types, who will stop in their tracks to admire the deep purples, pinks, and reds of a summer flower garden. Beige has no place in Fire's wardrobe, except as a neutral backdrop to show off a beautiful necklace or bright silk scarf.

Red is the *color* associated with Fire, and a strong attraction or repulsion to red or orange may signify an imbalance in Fire. Because their complexion is typically rosy or ruddy, Fire types tend to avoid wearing red, which makes them feel, as one Fire type put it, "like an overripe tomato." Roses and dusky mauves are soothing colors for Fire.

Sound: A warm voice, joyous laughter, and robust sense of humor indicate balanced Fire energies. Inappropriate laughter or uncontrolled giggling often suggests an excess of Fire, while an inability to laugh or experience spontaneous feelings of joy points to a deficiency in Fire.

A healing sound for Fire is "Heeeeeeeeeeeee." Sit in a comfortable position with your back erect but not stiff. Place your hands over your heart, take a few deep breaths, and imagine that you can see the gates to your Heart open and close freely, without creaking. Breathe in slowly and deeply, letting the fresh, clean air enter through the gates and envelop your heart with healing energy. On exhalation say, "Heeeeeeeeee," and imagine the pent-up agitation, restlessness, anxiety, and irritability exiting through the gates of your heart.

Smell: Lavender will help calm frenzied Fire energy. A multipurpose first aid oil, lavender soothes both external burns and internal flare-ups of emotional and psychological distress. The healing powers of lavender were discovered in the 1920s by French chemist René-Maurice Gattefossé, the modern founder of aromatherapy, when he burned his hand in a laboratory accident, soaked the wound in a tub of pure lavender oil, and experienced immediate relief.

Modern scientific research confirms that lavender increases alpha waves in the brain, which help us relax. For frazzled nerves, anxiety, panic attacks, and general stress relief, inhale lavender directly from the bottle or add several drops of lavender oil to your bath water. You can also put two or three drops of lavender oil on a handkerchief or tissue and inhale deeply. If you find driving stressful, you might consider leaving the handkerchief on the dashboard of your car and letting the sun's heat diffuse the relaxing fragrance throughout the car.

Taste: The sense organ most strongly associated with Fire is the tongue, which makes sense when you consider its two basic duties: to help us speak clearly, and to give spice and flavor to life.

According to *The Yellow Emperor's Classic,* "the heart is benefited by the bitter taste." Bitter flavors are thought to have purging and eliminating qualities, helping the body rid itself of undesirable substances. In both Eastern and Western herbal traditions, bitter foods and beverages are used to cool down the system and eliminate excess heat. In addition to their cooling qualities, bitters offer general support to the Liver, promote the flow of bile, increase metabolism, aid digestion, and stimulate appetite.

The bitterness of coffee, tea, unsweetened chocolate, barbecued foods, and green, leafy vegetables (spinach, kale, endive, escarole, Swiss chard, dandelion greens) often appeals to Fire types; an extreme distaste or preference for these foods indicates an imbalance in Fire.

Make sure to use spicy foods in moderation, for they will increase the heat in your system and contribute to excessive flushing, perspiration, rapid heartbeat palpitations, and overall feelings of dryness and irritability.

Touch: Fire types need to be in touch, both literally and figuratively. You will touch your partner when you talk, rest your hand on an acquaintance's shoulder, freely offer hugs to both friends and strangers, and be delighted to receive them in return. When you are deprived of touch or are out of touch with those you love because of a disagreement or temporary separation, you will suffer physically, emotionally, and spiritually.

To keep your energy balanced and harmonious, make sure you are involved in relationships that allow you to be affectionate and physically expressive. Although at times you will need to curb your natural instincts to be demonstrative, do not attempt to deny or subvert them. If your spouse or friends have difficulty with your displays of affection, try to help them understand that your need for physical closeness is part of your basic nature.

Wear soft, luxurious materials like silk or rayon that feel sensuous to the touch. Work in the garden without gloves, digging your hands into the moist, warm soil. Take a pottery class just for the sensation of molding wet clay with your fingers. Give yourself a foot massage, or ask your partner for a backrub.

Better yet, splurge and have a professional massage. Swedish massage, which relies on five basic strokes to relieve muscle tension and soreness throughout the body, is particularly well suited to Fire types. You might want to ask your masseuse or masseur to concentrate on the soothing, rhythmic strokes (effleurage, petrissage, and vibration) rather than the friction technique (rolling and squeezing the muscles) or tapotement (chopping, beating, and tapping strokes). See what feels good to you, and don't be afraid to speak up if a particular technique feels uncomfortable or intrusive.

QUESTIONS TO ASK YOURSELF

If you feel off-balance or out of sorts with your family, friends, colleagues, or the world at large, these questions will help you discover the source of your distress and guide you to potential solutions. Focus on one or two questions that seem to relate most directly to your current problems or state of mind.

• I hate boredom and inactivity: What can I do to keep my mind and body occupied? Which activities nourish my enthusiasm for life while offering me adequate time to rest and regroup?

- I often feel tongue-tied, awkward, and incapable of expressing myself: What fears prevent me from speaking clearly?
- I am creative, but I often have difficulty transforming my ideas into reality: How can I focus my energies and give my creativity an outlet?
- I am always falling in and out of love: What do I want from love? How can I develop relationships that allow me to be myself?
- I fear being cut off from others: How can I stay connected to the people I love without losing myself in relationships?
- I can be hypersensitive to people and surroundings: How can I learn to keep my heart open without getting inundated?
- I crave intimacy with others, yet I also need time to be alone: What can I do to make sure that both needs are met?
- I am sometimes overwhelmed by intense sensations and feelings: What can I do to protect myself from overstimulation?
- I fear the future: How can I stay grounded in the present?

A Story for Fire

Your affinity to Fire gives you the capacity for great joy, which can be used to create strong, loving relationships. Intuitive and empathetic, you long to merge and fuse with others, and you suffer intensely when you are separated from those you love. A story from the Sufi tradition illustrates the pure, passionate heart of Fire:

> The great Sufi mystic Rumi, his heart filled with love and his body shaking with passion, knocked on the door of his beloved.
>
> "Who is there?" she asked.
>
> "It is your lover, Rumi," he answered.
>
> "Go away, for there is no room for the two of us here," the voice responded.
>
> Confused and distraught, Rumi went off to his meditations and prayers. Later he returned to the house of his beloved and knocked again.
>
> "Who is there?" she asked.
>
> "It is you," Rumi replied.

With a welcome, the door was thrown wide open, and the lovers passionately embraced.

Famous Fire Types
Robin Williams
Diane Keaton
Lucille Ball
Marilyn Monroe
Billy Graham
Elizabeth Taylor
Rosie O'Donnell
Santa Claus
Tigger from *The House at Pooh Corner*
Goofy, from the Disney cartoons

4. EARTH: THE PEACEMAKER

Just as the earth is boundlessly wide, sustaining and caring for all creatures on it, so the sage sustains and cares for all people and excludes no part of humanity.

—The I Ching

My best friend made the appointment for me," Diana said with a shy smile. "It's hard for me to admit I have a problem, and even harder to ask for help. I've always been that way. But lately my digestive system has really been acting up. I've been sick with the flu three times this winter, and I'm worried about my weight. Do you think you could help me?"

Wearing an ankle-length dress and Birkenstock sandals, her long hair pulled back in a ponytail, forty-seven-year-old Diana was the image of an "Earth Mother." ("I was a hippie in my youth," she laughed.) Her melodious voice, her short hands and fingers, the yellow tinge around her mouth and eyes, and her lifelong struggle to control her weight suggested a strong affinity to Earth. Like many Earth types, Diana was more comfortable giving attention to others than receiving it. As we talked, she kept looking at her watch. "You're certainly taking a lot of time with me," she said, a worried expression on her face. "I hope I'm not making you late for your next session."

Worrying was second nature to Diana. "I'm a worrywort," she admitted. "I worry about everything—violence in the schools, the ozone hole, pesticides in our foods, the Ebola virus, terrorism in the Middle East . . . you name it, I'll worry it to death." Keenly aware of the fact that fretting about events outside her control upset her digestive system, causing gas pains, bloating, and a tendency to constipation, Diana was hoping to find a way to worry less and enjoy life more.

Her weight was a major cause for concern. Now that her four children were off to college or living on their own, she ate continuously and had gained seven pounds in the last month. Sweets were her favorite food, and she often baked chocolate chip or peanut butter cookies. "I send boxes of cookies to my kids, but I always keep a few dozen for myself," she said.

Diana's affinity to Earth was also clear in her choice of careers. A social worker for the county, she helped men and women newly released from the state mental hospital find affordable housing. Although she enjoyed her work immensely and prided herself on helping people in need, she often had difficulty separating her own life from the lives of her clients. "Sometimes I don't know where they end and I begin," she admitted tearfully. "I spend most of my evenings and weekends on the phone, checking up on my clients. I don't even know how to take care of myself anymore—except," she sighed, "with those cookies I love so much."

In our sessions together we decided on many strategies to help Diana learn how to take better care of herself. She went on a low-fat diet, took daily walks, and set aside two hours every day (between 7 A.M. and 9 A.M.) to read, write in her journal, and walk Sadie, her golden retriever. Instead of baking cookies on Sundays, she made homemade soups and whole wheat breads. She loved to sing, and although initially reluctant ("Really, I'm tone deaf," she protested mildly), she joined her church choir, an activity she has come to enjoy immensely. Herbs and acupuncture helped to relieve her digestive symptoms, and she began to sleep better and feel more rested during the day.

Of all the changes in her life, however, the most essential to her peace of mind was her new garden. In the winter she seeded dozens of little pots and set them on her windowsills, watching over them tenderly. In the spring she transplanted the tender shoots, and throughout the summer she weeded and tended her plot. Then in late summer—her favorite season—she harvested her crop and gave overflowing boxes of fresh and canned vegetables to her friends and clients.

"As soon as I walk outside and smell the sweet soil, I feel grounded," she told me in a recent session. "How in the world did I live without my garden?"

If Earth is the primary power that molds and shapes your nature, you are naturally sympathetic and caring. You have great difficulty saying no, particularly to people who are in need. Blessed with a sunny disposition, patience, and a willingness to listen to other people's problems, you are a wonderful friend, a loving parent, and an eloquent spokesperson for peace and cooperation. Earth types are the volunteers who never say no, the friends who always offer a shoulder to cry on, the peacemakers who create harmony wherever they go.

Your tolerant and forgiving nature draws many different kinds of people to you. Friends, relatives, and complete strangers feel safe with you, for you accept life in all its glorious diversity and refrain from judging others. A sense of kinship with other human beings is essential to your health and happiness, and you have a gift for creating loving communities. While Fire types crave intense intimacy to the point of merging their hearts and souls with others, Earth types seek to establish connections with many different people. You accept everyone into your world, for you do not ask people to be anything but themselves.

Earth is the serene, stable center of gravity around which the rest of the world gratefully gathers. In contrast to Fire types, who fascinate others with their charismatic charm, people are attracted to Earth types because they accept them for who they are and make no attempt to change them to suit their needs or preferences.

Tolerance for differences guides relationships in every aspect of your life. You adore your children because of their quirks (and not in spite of them); your friends include many different types of people from all walks of life; and your relatives automatically turn to you to settle disputes. You are a natural mediator who thrives on peace and harmony and is thrown off-balance by discord and dissension. Quarreling and bickering disturb your peace of mind; even when you hear strangers arguing, you have an overwhelming desire to step in and help resolve the disagreement.

Stable, quiet, compassionate, and well-grounded, you can move out of yourself to experience another person's pain or joy and with equal ease come back home to yourself. Your sense of self is so secure and your boundaries so well defined that you can step into another person's shoes without becoming confused about whose shoes you are wearing. You have a keen awareness of the place where you fit and feel at "home," and you suffer deeply when you are separated from familiar comforts.

Imbalances in Earth Energy

The Chinese believe that imbalances in Earth energy arise from and, in turn, are affected by the organ systems associated with Earth: the Stomach and the Spleen.

Western medicine describes the stomach as a muscular structure responsible for storing and digesting food; contractions in the stomach muscles push the partially digested food particles into the small intestine. In Chinese medicine the Stomach ("the Sea of Nutrients") receives food, sifts and sorts through the various nutrients, and then transports pure nutritive energy to the Spleen, where it is transformed into energy (*chi*) and blood. When the Stomach is not functioning properly, you are unable to assimilate the nutrients necessary to enrich and strengthen your body, mind, and spirit, gradually weakening your energy level. Nausea, gastrointestinal pain, bloating, gas, chronic nausea, and rapid weight gain are signs of weakness or disharmony in this vital organ system.

The Western spleen functions as a reservoir for blood and contains a particularly high concentration of red blood cells; when the body requires greater quantities of blood due to emotional stress, pregnancy, severe bleeding, or overexertion, the spleen releases additional red blood cells into the bloodstream. The spleen also removes wastes and other unwanted substances from the blood.

In Chinese medicine the Spleen's primary function is to transform food and drink into *chi* (vital energy) and blood; after completing this transformation, the Spleen distributes the *chi* and blood throughout the body, mind, and spirit. Called "the Official of Transformation and Transportation," the Spleen also keeps the blood flowing in its proper channels. When its energy is depleted or deficient, it cannot keep the blood contained within its vessels, and "reckless blood" symptoms such as nosebleeds, vomiting blood, blood in the stools, or menstrual problems such as breakthrough bleeding, spotting, or flooding may occur. Deficient Spleen *chi* also results in improper nourishment to the cells and tissues and in digestive disturbances, including bloating, bowel problems, and lethargy.

EXCESS EARTH

When the need to solve other people's problems becomes all-consuming, leaving you little time or energy for taking care of yourself, you lose your center of gravity and begin to teeter on your axis. You are literally off-center, for the boundaries separating yourself from others are no longer clearly definable. As Earth's innate need to nurture others is gradually transformed into a smothering overprotectiveness, you find yourself wondering, "Where do I end and you begin?" Your displaced center of gravity leads to feelings of emptiness. What was previously loving support turns into meddlesome behavior, and a natural concern for the welfare of others degenerates into constant fretting and worry.

The worst fear of the excess Earth type is deprivation, which in its most painful form is the severing of connections with other human beings. When they feel empty, lonely, undernourished, and hungry for love or attention, Earth types often turn to food for gratification, filling themselves with those foods associated with the power of Earth—sweets. Eating chocolate, pastries, cakes, and cookies temporarily soothes your fears, nourishing and rewarding you for being a "good" person, but you feel full only when you are literally gorged with food. Even then, you are unable to fill up your center.

An excess of Earth energy contributes to such intense feelings of emptiness and longing that the craving for more—more food, more love, more attention—cannot be satisfied and continues unabated.

Excess Earth: Physical Symptoms
- Excess saliva
- Swollen, tender, or bleeding gums
- Ache in the head and eyes, or a "heavy" feeling
- Thick mucus in the nose, throat, or mouth
- Arms and legs feel "heavy" and unwieldy; moving around takes an effort
- Weak joints, particularly in the ankles, knees, and hips
- Lack of energy and endurance
- Frequent bruising
- Headaches, usually related to conflict or excessive worrying

- Water retention: edema and swelling in the abdomen, hips, legs, ankles
- Premenstrual syndrome (PMS) with lethargy, bloating, soreness, hunger, and swelling
- Heavy menstrual flow with clots
- Fibroid tumors
- Bowel and intestinal disturbances: gas, distended abdomen, constipation, loose stools, diarrhea
- Excess appetite
- Metabolic problems, including sluggish metabolism, difficulty losing weight, and rapid weight gain
- Recurrent abdominal pain and stomachaches
- Heartburn
- Tendency to develop ulcers
- Hypoglycemia: wide fluctuations of blood sugar leading to anxiety, dizziness, difficulty concentrating, lethargy, and exhaustion
- Obesity
- Thyroid problems, especially hypothyroidism (deficient thyroid)

Excess Earth: Psychological and Behavioral Symptoms

- Self-pity
- Fluctuating self-esteem
- Overall heaviness of spirit
- Temper tantrums
- Obsessive worrying
- Craving for love and affection
- Constant need to be needed or included
- Muddled or confused thought patterns
- Tendency to be wishy-washy and ambivalent
- Behavior perceived by others as meddlesome
- Hypersensitivity to criticism
- Craving for sweets and carbohydrates (bread, pasta, pastries, cakes, cookies)
- Compulsive overeating alternating with strict dieting
- Sluggishness
- Difficulty with changes and transitions

• Overpowering need to stay in touch with others, for example, feeling the need to answer the phone when it rings because someone might be in trouble and need your help

DEFICIENT EARTH

Practitioners of traditional Chinese medicine believe that deficiencies in Earth energy begin in childhood, for more than any other type, Earth needs continuous support and nourishment in order to develop feelings of self-worth. If your emotional attachments were somehow strained or ruptured in childhood, you may harbor deep feelings of inadequacy and find it difficult to take care of yourself.

The first symptoms of deficient Earth energy include dependence on others for emotional and physical needs and an insatiable craving for attention and appreciation. Fear of abandonment drives you to cling possessively to relatives and friends, smothering them with your neediness. To protect yourself, you may try to cover up your deep emotional insecurities with an outward display of detachment and indifference.

The Chinese believe that when Earth is out of balance, food and fluids cannot be broken down or eliminated efficiently, and a watery sludge begins to build up in the system that eventually coagulates into a mucuslike substance called *tan*. A buildup of *tan* creates an overall quality of excessive dampness, which can cause loose stools, arthritis (which is aggravated by dampness in the atmosphere and/or barometric pressure changes), and edema (a buildup of fluid, especially in the abdomen). An excess of *tan* also affects the mind and spirit, contributing to lethargy, heaviness of spirit, a sense of being overwhelmed or weighed down by problems, headaches, foggy thinking, difficulty concentrating, absentmindedness, and forgetfulness. The feeling that energy is leaking out at a steady rate also leads to an inability to maintain proper boundaries, and the sinking sensation of losing control over your life.

Deficient Earth: Physical Symptoms
• Constant hunger but often can't decide what to eat
• Difficulty losing weight

- Lack of saliva
- Swallowing difficulties
- Tooth decay
- Bleeding gums
- Swollen glands
- Bloating due to fluid retention (edema)
- Poor muscle tone
- Aching or "heavy" limbs, joints, and muscles
- Arthritis
- Slow healing of cuts
- Tendency to bruise easily
- Dull headaches that feel like a wet towel wrapped around your head; the pain intensifies in damp weather
- Varicose veins
- Hemorrhoids
- Loose stools
- Prolapse of stomach, intestine, bladder, or uterus
- Craving for sugar and heavily sweetened caffeinated beverages
- Tendency to develop blood sugar disturbances: hypoglycemia or diabetes
- Lack of endurance

Deficient Earth: Psychological and Behavioral Symptoms

- Excessive concern for the feelings of others
- Obsessive worrying
- Insatiable craving for attention
- Clinging relationships
- Feelings of inadequacy
- Emptiness, loneliness, feelings of abandonment
- Nervousness
- Flightiness
- Fears of being disconnected or homeless
- Lack of energy
- Difficulty getting started on work projects, exercise regimes, housekeeping chores, etc.
- Lack of aggressiveness

- Unfocused, scattered thought processes
- Addictive relationship to food
- Feelings of loss of control
- Phobias: fear of the unknown, school phobias, separation anxiety

Restoring Harmony

LIFESTYLE

To restore harmony to body, mind, and spirit, Earth types need to remember this key phrase: "Get unstuck." Whenever a relationship or situation feels sticky—thick, dense, inextricable—you need to determine why you feel stuck and make plans to get unstuck. Detaching yourself from sticky situations is always difficult for the Earth type, however, because your major objective in life is to stay connected to your family, friends, co-workers, and the community at large. You want to be everything to everyone, yet you often fail to take care of yourself.

Time of day: An important part of "getting unstuck" is shutting off that recurring, internal voice that says, "I don't deserve time for myself." In order to avoid the many physical and psychological problems associated with Earth imbalances, you need to remind yourself that you not only deserve, but absolutely *need* to take time to relax and nurture yourself. The Chinese believe that Earth's power is at its peak between 7 A.M. and 11 A.M.; this is the time to clear your mind, focus your attention, and prepare yourself for the demands of the day. Take at least an hour during this time, and set it aside for you and you alone. Close your eyes and listen to music—Ravel's *Bolero,* with its repeated crescendos and climactic buildup, is particularly energizing music for Earth types. Keep a daily journal, read a good book, write a letter to a friend, or go for a walk.

Season: Earth's season is primarily late summer (Indian summer), though in the ancient Chinese texts, Earth's season is also said to be the last ten days of each season, when the forces of nature are in perfect balance. Despite the apparent calm of these transitional seasons, great changes are taking place underneath the surface as the energies of Wood, Fire, Earth, Metal, and Water change their ebb and flow. When Earth energy is balanced, we can maintain our equilibrium during the changing seasons of our lives.

Damp or humid weather can contribute to feelings of stickiness and inertia, so on hot, muggy days Earth types would benefit by turning on the air conditioner or going for a swim. Hot, dry weather can be soothing for Earth, because the warmth of the sun helps to dissipate feelings of dampness and lethargy. On cool, damp days light a fire, turn up the heat, take a hot bath, or eat a hot, nourishing meal.

Learn to say no: The inability to say no can be Earth's downfall, for the more you say yes, the more you will feel trapped by your commitments and deprived of time for yourself. To help you *practice saying no,* try this simple exercise, which we've adapted from one developed by Rusian spiritual master George Ivanovitch Gurdjieff. "Remember yourself, always and everywhere," Gurdjieff used to say. His basic philosophy centered on the belief that most of us have forgotten how to respond with conscious awareness and instead simply react to life. Gurdjieff developed this exercise to teach his students how to bring consciousness and awareness to their responses.

> When someone asks you to do something, respond by saying, "Let me think about it and I'll get back to you in twenty-four hours."
>
> Use those twenty-four hours to determine if you have the time and energy to commit yourself to another project (no matter how simple it may be). If you feel torn between the need to help others and the need to take care of yourself, choose your own needs. Practice saying no clearly and without equivocation. The more you say it, the easier it gets.

Deep breathing exercises: Deep breathing exercises help to open up blood vessels, allow the heart to pump more efficiently, increase blood flow to the head, improving thinking and reasoning, and reduce hot flashes in menopausal women. For Earth types, the Belly Breath is particularly appropriate.

THE BELLY BREATH

- Sit in a chair with your back straight.
- Close your eyes, and imagine that your diaphragm (the muscle separating the lungs and abdomen) is an accordion. When you have completely exhaled all

the air from your lungs, the accordion is tightly compressed; when you take a deep breath, it expands.

• Place one hand just below your belly button and the other just below your breasts. Slowly breathe in, imagining that your lower hand is pulling down on the accordion while the upper hand is pulling up.

• Feel your lungs fill up from top to bottom. When the accordion is fully expanded, slowly exhale, and feel the accordion relax.

• Continue for 2–3 minutes, and repeat twice daily.

DIET

Earth types love to eat, and you will spend a significant amount of time thinking about food, shopping for the freshest produce and highest-quality meats, cutting, chopping, cooking, and then—the best part of all—eating. Mealtimes are without question one of the most important times of the day.

A tendency to overeat and a penchant for sweets are the major dietary weaknesses for Earth. While the Chinese believe that the natural sweetness of grains, fruits, and vegetables is nourishing and stimulating to the Spleen and Stomach, overindulgence in sweet foods is considered damaging to these and other vital organs. "Too much sweet taste can disturb the heart *chi,* causing it to become restless and congested, as well as cause imbalance of kidney energy," cautions Qi Bo. Modern nutritional science uses different words and concepts to describe the disturbances excess sugar can create in the body, but few people doubt that our high-sugar and refined-carbohydrate diets are contributing to the rising incidence of chronic disease and disorder.

To help you control your sweet tooth and eat more nutritious foods, try these simple strategies:

• Drink plenty of water, at least eight to ten 8-ounce glasses every day. Water helps us to eat less because it "bulks" the food we eat, softening and expanding the food particles and making them easier to digest. Because water also makes you feel full, you'll tend to eat less when you drink more. Important: While it won't hurt you to sip a glass of water at mealtimes, drink the bulk of your water in between meals. Many nutritionists believe that water taken with the meal dilutes the digestive enzymes and interferes with the digestive process.

• Avoid iced beverages, because extreme cold inhibits enzyme activity and interferes with digestion. Room temperature water will lessen the burden on your digestive system. If you feel hot, feverish, or experience hot flashes, cold drinks won't hurt you, but always try to avoid iced drinks and frozen foods.

• Never fill your plate to the brim. Take small portions and eat slowly. If you are still hungry, take a small second helping. (Some people find it helps to use a smaller plate, which makes it appear as if you have more food to enjoy.) Smaller, more frequent meals also help to stabilize blood sugar levels and reduce cravings for sweets.

• Increase your intake of whole foods (whole grains, vegetables, and fruits), which are low in calories yet occupy a lot of bulk and give the feeling of fullness. Because whole foods are high in fiber, they pass through the digestive system quickly, and your body actually absorbs fewer calories.

• Whenever possible, substitute fruit for a sweet dessert. A diet high in sugar and refined carbohydrates can injure Earth energies and contribute to blood sugar abnormalities such as hypoglycemia (low blood sugar) and diabetes (high blood sugar). For more information on diabetes, see pages 324 to 338.

• If your Earth energies are deficient, you may have trouble digesting raw foods. Steaming and wok frying (with extra-virgin, cold-pressed olive oil) help to break down a vegetable's cellulose covering, which makes it easier for the digestive system to metabolize the food, thereby increasing the body's absorption of nutrients.

• Legumes (lentils, chick peas, split peas, kidney beans, fava beans, soybeans, and soybean products such as tofu, miso, soy sauce, and tempeh) and root vegetables (carrots, celery, onions, turnips, parsnips, radishes, potatoes, and sweet potatoes) help stabilize blood sugar levels, which in turn reduces sugar cravings.

• Avoid fatty foods (particularly red meat and dairy products, including yogurt, milk, butter, cream, ice cream, cheese). These foods are often difficult to digest and create dampness (mucus) in the system, which can slow down digestion and increase the burden on the stomach and intestines. Substitute fish, chicken, or turkey (with the skin removed) for red meat.

• Warm, dry condiments like ginger, pepper, parsley, cinnamon, garlic, and cardamom help eliminate moisture in the system, easing digestive complaints such as gas, water retention, indigestion, nausea, diarrhea, and abdominal pain. In addition to their warming qualities, these spices support digestion in general and increase metabolism—a nice bonus for Earth types.

• Reduce your consumption of coffee, alcohol, refined breads and pastas, and pastries, cakes, or cookies. These foods interfere with digestion, which can lead to inefficient or incomplete metabolism. When undigested food particles accumulate in the system, they coagulate into *tan,* which contributes to excess dampness, water retention, loose stools, lethargy, headaches, and mental confusion.

• The most important strategy for Earth types is also the simplest to obey: Don't deprive yourself. When Earth types feel deprived, they're unhappy, and when they're unhappy, they tend to overindulge themselves. Restricting sweets, rich cream sauces, and fatty foods is always a good idea, but giving up sweets completely is unrealistic for Earth types. Moderation, as always, is the key. An occasional (once-a-week) sweet or rich dessert won't hurt you.

NUTRITIONAL SUPPLEMENTS

To prevent illness and maintain general good health, take the following vitamins and minerals every day:

General Formula for Maximum Immunity

Vitamin A: 25,000 I.U. (in the form of beta-carotene or mixed carotenes)
Vitamin C: 2,000–3,000 mg.
Vitamin E: 400–800 I.U. (take the higher amount if you are over 50)
Magnesium: 500 mg. (chelated with amino acids)
Multivitamin and mineral supplement: Choose a formula with 100–200 percent of the RDA for various vitamins and minerals

For Extra Protection Add:

Selenium: 200 mcg. (take with vitamin E)
Coenzyme Q-10: 30 mg.
Pycnogenol (pine bark or grape-seed extract): 50 mg.
Zinc: 30 mg. (15 mg. of zinc is included in many multivitamin and mineral supplements)

EXERCISE

Earth types enjoy exercise that is slow, easy, and not too strenuous. A leisurely walk, a long bicycle ride on relatively flat ground, swimming laps, yoga, and light aerobics appeal to Earth's gentle, noncompetitive nature and desire for smooth, fluid movements. If you exercise with friends (always a good idea for Earth), be sure to find partners who share your desire to exercise for the joy of it, rather than to prove how strong or capable they might be.

The biggest problem for Earth in terms of exercise is finding the energy to get going. Given a choice, you would rather sip a cup of tea with a friend or putter around in the garden than walk a mile or two. Once you start exercising, however, you'll quickly recognize its physical and emotional benefits as your thoughts clear, your spirits lift, and your body feels lighter and more flexible. Even if it feels as if you're pushing the limit, set aside ten or fifteen minutes every day to walk the dog, play tennis with a friend, or practice your yoga postures.

The graceful movements and slow tempo of tai chi ("great energy") offer Earth types a gentle form of exercise that develops and strengthens both mind and body. Inner awareness is the central goal of this ancient art, which encourages self-control and self-discipline rather than outward displays of strength. Because the knees are always bent and the arms and legs move gracefully in curved, flowing movements, tai chi helps us feel grounded and centered—Earth's favorite way to be.

Yoga exercise: This simple yoga *asana* (exercise) is specifically recommended for Earth types and will invigorate the Stomach and Spleen *chi* (energy).

Important note: Use this exercise as an adjunct to your regular yoga class. If you have never taken yoga, please find a certified instructor and attend classes to learn the proper techniques. Be sure to warm up with stretching and limbering exercises before trying this or any other yoga *asana*. Never force your body into any position or movement. If you feel pain, your body is telling you to back off. If you are not sure what you are doing, ask your yoga instructor for guidance.

RECLINING HERO

Reclining Hero is simple but often not easy, especially if your legs and back are tight. Go slow, and don't force yourself. If you have knee problems, be very cautious.

Kneel on a soft mat, and sit back on your heels. Place your palms on your legs, and take in a deep breath. Separate your legs so you can sit between your feet with your buttocks on the mat. (If that position is uncomfortable, sit on a cushion.) Open your knees wider, to the point where they are comfortable, then slowly bring them closer together. You will feel stretching in the tops of the legs (and perhaps other areas of your body as well). Bring the knees as close together as they can comfortably go—*do not force them.*

Now place your palms on the soles of your feet. Take five full, slow breaths. You can stop at this point, or you can continue by reclining back onto your elbows and forearms. Keep your chin down, and breathe five breaths. Come up slowly, and rest on your back, with the knees up and feet flat for one minute.

Repeat one more time if you feel up to it.

HERBS

Western

The following herbs can be used alone or in combination.

Ginger *(Zingiber officinalis):* Ginger is a wonderful warming herb traditionally used to relieve nausea and vomiting. (Modern researchers have discovered that powdered ginger root is more effective than Dramamine in preventing the nausea, dizziness, and general discomfort of motion sickness.) Ginger's antispasmodic and antinausea actions help to relieve gas, heartburn, diarrhea, and indigestion. In experiments with laboratory animals, ginger reduces blood serum cholesterol levels; many herbalists claim to have similar results with their patients.

Dandelion *(Taraxacum officinalis):* Dandelion acts as a natural diuretic, increasing the flow of urine and relieving the bloated feelings so common to Earth. Dandelion also stimulates the flow of bile, which supports the Liver and Gallbladder and aids the digestive system.

Ginseng: Ginseng stimulates the immune system, which increases resistance to disease. It also supports digestion and metabolism, improves physical stamina, increases mental alertness, and counteracts the effects of stress and fatigue. We particularly like Siberian ginseng, which is less stimulating and less expensive than the Panax varieties. *Caution:* Ginseng can have a stimulating effect in large amounts. Do not exceed the recommended dosage.

Dosage: If you purchase your herbs in a health food store (either in tincture form or, as dried herbs, in capsule or pill form), follow the dosage instructions on the label. Because herbs in dried form tend to lose their potency rather quickly, be sure to check the label for the expiration date.

For information on preparing your own herbs from the root, bark, leaves, flowers, or seeds of a plant, see Appendix II.

Chinese

Bu Zhong Yi Qi Wan ("Support the Center, Benefit Energy Pills" or "Ginseng and Astragalus Combination"): This Chinese patent remedy is a gentle, balanced formula often prescribed for Earth imbalances, particularly when symptoms include lethargy, bloating, "heavy" limbs and head, hypoglycemia, poor digestion, or prolapses of any kind, from hemmorhoids to hernias. Ginseng and astragalus share Emperor status, working with eight attending herbs (dong quai, licorice, atractylodes, citrus peel, bupleurum, jujube fruit, cimicifuga, and ginger) to balance metabolism, improve digestion, invigorate the immune system, increase energy, and nourish the blood.

Unless otherwise directed, take eight pills three times daily or twelve pills twice daily.

In Appendix I we offer a list of mail-order sources for high-quality herbs and herbal preparations.

ACUPOINTS

CONCEPTION VESSEL 12 ("Sea of Nutritive Energy"): This is a well-known acupoint in traditional Chinese medicine that is frequently used to restore balance in the Stomach and Spleen. When the Stomach energies are out of balance, this point will feel tender and sore to the touch. Firm pressure on this point will support digestion and metabolism, easing many digestive disturbances.

Common Uses

• Nourishes and supports the Spleen, aiding assimilation of food and easing symptoms such as lethargy, fatigue, inability to eat or enjoy food, and loose stools

- Strengthens and balances Stomach energy (*chi*), easing such symptoms as nausea, vomiting, hiccups, and acid taste in the mouth
- Helps move food quickly and efficiently through the digestive system, breaking through obstructions to relieve gas, cramping, bloating, and stomachaches
- Resolves dampness and phlegm in the digestive tract; often used for "Damp" symptoms such as heaviness of body and limb, muddled thinking, lethargy, slurred speech, forgetfulness, dull, throbbing headaches, and sinus stuffiness

Location: Conception Vessel 12 is located on the midline of the body, approximately two inches below the sternum or five or six inches above the belly button.

SPLEEN 3 ("Great Brightness"): This acupoint helps the digestive "fires" work efficiently to extract energy from food and eliminate waste products. Imagine that you have just taken a hot shower, and the bathroom mirrors are fogged up with steam; pressing Spleen 3 acts like a powerful hair dryer to dissipate the dense fog and eliminate humidity.

Common Uses

- Supports and strengthens the Spleen and Stomach, increasing energy, improving appetite, relieving food cravings (especially the craving for sweets), and easing chronic nausea, abdominal discomfort, sluggish digestion, loose bowels, and constipation
- Transforms and resolves dampness, easing such symptoms as sluggishness, "heavy" limbs, water retention, bloating, gurgling sounds in stomach and intestines, muddled thinking, headaches, and muscle cramps
- Supports the pancreas, helping to balance blood sugar levels and easing symptoms associated with hypoglycemia and adult-onset diabetes
- Promotes the Spleen's ability to increase energy, alleviating problems such as hemorrhoids and varicose veins

Location: Spleen 3 is located on the inside of the foot, just below the joint at the base of the big toe. Slide your finger down the big toe and over the joint, then stop at the natural depression. You'll know you've found the point because it is more sensitive to the touch than the surrounding areas.

INVIGORATING THE SENSES

Vision: Earth's color is yellow, which the Chinese identify as the color of the middle. Because yellow is the color of the sun, the Chinese also believe it represents longevity. Although yellow is considered a healing color for Earth types, a pale, sickly yellow or an intense orange hue around the mouth or temples is said to be a clear sign that Earth energies are out of balance.

If you have an excess or deficiency of Earth energy, add more yellow to your life. Buy yellow fruits and vegetables—bananas, grapefruits, lemons, yellow squash, yellow cucumbers—and place them in an attractive bowl on your kitchen counter or dining room table. (Don't forget to eat them, too!) Plant sunflowers, yellow daisies, or yellow roses in your garden. Put a slice or two of lemon in your water glass. Drink lemon balm tea, which will soothe your nervous system and improve digestion. Buy a pair of sunglasses with a yellow tint. Wear a yellow blouse or scarf.

Sound: The Chinese believe that the sound of Earth is singing. When Earth's energy is balanced, the voice has a melodious quality that is pleasant to the ear and calming to the spirit. An exaggerated or artificial singsongy voice might signify excess Earth, while a dull or monotonous vocal tone would suggest deficient Earth energy.

The traditional Sanskrit mantra *om* or *aum,* which is said to be the primordial sound of the earth as it moves through the heavens, is deeply soothing for Earth types. "*Om* is the sound nature makes when it's pleased with itself," mythologist Joseph Campbell explained. "The secret to having a spiritual life as you move in the world is to hear the *aum* in all things all the time. If you do, everything is transformed. You no longer have to go anywhere to find your fulfillment and achievement and the treasure that you seek. It is here. It is everywhere."

What does *aum* sound like? Cover your ears with the palms of your hands, and you can hear the blood moving through the capillaries—the blood says "*aum.*" Put a seashell to your ear, and you can hear the ocean roar—the ocean says "*aum.*"

Try this breathing exercise that incorporates the mantra *om:* Find a comfortable position with your back erect but not stiff. Place your hands on your upper abdomen, about a hand's width above the navel—this is the point the Chinese call *tantien* or "the center." Breathe in deeply, and when you exhale, say, *"Aummm-mmmmmmmmmmm,"* continuing the sound for as long as possible without straining yourself. Repeat this exercise for five minutes every day.

Smell: Rub together two leaves of *lemon balm,* inhale the mintlike fragrance, and feel the anxiety and tension drain away. A particularly mild and gentle herb (which suits Earth's sensitive nature), lemon balm is often used in children's remedies, to treat symptoms of colds and flus. Nursing mothers can safely drink lemon balm tea to soothe the irritability and restlessness of their colicky babies. If you suffer from indigestion or gas, a lemon balm tea or tincture will relax your digestive system and ease your discomfort.

Peppermint has been used for hundreds of years to treat colds, flus, and digestive disturbances including gas, nausea, vomiting, heartburn, and diarrhea; this safe, gentle herb also relieves anxiety and insomnia. To stimulate your digestive system and ease gastric discomfort, drink peppermint tea or gently rub peppermint-scented massage oil onto your stomach and abdomen. Another way to enjoy the soothing comfort of peppermint (and one that will immediately appeal to Earth's sweet tooth) is to suck on a sugar cube flavored with one drop of peppermint oil. Don't try substituting an after-dinner mint—most mints contain only the flavoring of peppermint and not the essential oil.

Taste: The sense organ associated with Earth is the mouth, and the taste associated with Earth is sweet. The natural sweetness of grains and vegetables—oats, wheat, barley, carrots, and root vegetables such as potatoes, yams, and artichokes—nourish and support Earth energies. Sugar-rich sweets such as candy, cookies, cakes, ice cream, and refined carbohydrates can cause imbalances in Earth energies by interfering with digestion; sugary foods also play a role in hyperactivity, hypoglycemia, mood swings, and anxiety.

Sunflower seeds, almonds, pumpkin seeds, grapes, grapefruits, and pineapples have bitter, bland, or salty properties that will curb your sweet cravings. Lemon balm tea will also help relieve the craving for sweets, relax the digestive system, and soothe irritability, restlessness, and nervous tension. (Some herbalists claim that lemon balm makes wrinkles disappear!)

Touch: A full-body massage is a wonderful stress-reducing remedy for Earth types, who love to touch and be touched in gentle, loving ways. If your Earth energies are out of balance, you may feel so overburdened or scattered that you neglect to satisfy this fundamental need. Indulging in a massage once a week or even once a month will help you feel nourished and invigorated. The soothing kneading strokes used by Swedish massage therapists may be more appropriate for Earth types, as compared with a very gentle, light massage (which would appeal to Metal and Water types), a sensual massage with candles, romantic music, and scented oils (which Fire types would love), or a deep connective-tissue massage (enjoyed by most Wood types).

QUESTIONS TO ASK YOURSELF

For Earth, the greatest fear is to be lost or wandering aimlessly, removed from the familiar comforts of home. Relationships, family, and friends balance Earth's energy, while conflict and abrupt changes make Earth feel unsteady and unstable. If you feel off-balance or out of sorts, use these questions to identify the source of your distress. Focus on one or two questions that seem to relate most directly to your current problems or emotional state of mind.

- I often wonder what my *real* role in life should be: How many roles do I have? Which of these roles nourish my own needs?
- I love to be with people, yet I also need time to be by myself: How can I create some time and space to think, reflect, and replenish my energies?
- I often get bogged down in details: What can I do to keep myself focused on the task at hand?
- My boundaries are always shifting: How can I be a good friend without letting other people's problems become my own?
- I can be manipulative and interfering: How can I show my affection and concern for others without meddling in their affairs?
- I am obsessed with safety and stability: What dangers lurk in the dark? What fears prevent me from taking risks?
- I have difficulty with change and transition: How can I learn to yield to the constantly changing demands of life?

- I avoid conflict: Why do disagreements with—as well as between—people throw me off-balance? What can I do to stay centered?
- I often feel homesick: How can I take "home" with me and learn to feel stable and secure wherever I am?
- I fear emptiness: How can I fill myself up with nutritious activities, food, and relationships yet avoid overstuffing myself?

A Story for Earth

The power of Earth calls us "home"—that place inside where we feel centered and balanced, at peace with the world. The following story reminds us that we do not have to leave home to find fulfillment, for "heaven" is contained within:

> God created the world and was happy. On the seventh day, he decided it was time to rest, but Adam called out: "God, I've got a problem!" and then Eve called with problems of her own ("God, Adam is trying to feed me this apple, what should I do?"), and then that quarrelsome pair had hundreds of children who had hundreds of children, and God was thoroughly exhausted with all their problems and demands for his time. Calling a meeting of his ministers, he announced, "I'm afraid I've created a monster, and I must find a place to hide."
>
> "How about the top of the Himalayas?" suggested one of his ministers.
>
> "No," God replied, "I'm afraid you don't understand what I've created . . . in just a few moments measured by my time they will be there."
>
> "What about the moon?" suggested another.
>
> "No," God replied wearily, "in just a few minutes more they will be there, too."
>
> Suddenly a smile spread over God's face. "I know where they will never look! I'll hide inside human beings themselves."
>
> And to this day, that is where God is hiding.

Famous Earth Types

Eleanor Roosevelt

Albert Schweitzer

Julia Child

Dr. Joyce Brothers

John Candy

Oprah Winfrey

Gautama the Buddha

George, from the TV show *Seinfeld*

Winnie the Pooh

Woody Woodpecker

5. METAL: THE ARTIST

The mountain rests on the earth. When it is steep and narrow, lacking a broad base, it must topple over. Its position is strong only when it rises out of the earth broad and great, not proud and steep. So likewise those who rule rest on the broad foundation of the people. They too should be generous and benevolent, like the earth that carries all. Then they will make their position as secure as a mountain in its tranquillity.

—The I Ching

When Ken told his dermatologist that he was concerned about the long-term effects of the steroid creams he used for his eczema, the doctor admitted that he had no other treatment options. "Eczema is a baffling condition, with no known cure," the doctor explained. "Most people simply try to find a way to live with it."

Thirty-eight-year-old Ken, a loan officer at a local bank, walked into my office promptly on time. He was dressed very neatly in a gray pinstripe suit, a light blue shirt, and a silk tie with gray and blue stripes. His hair was perfectly in place, with a tinge of gray around the temples exaggerating the whitish hue emanating from his skin. Tall and slim with long hands and fingers, he appeared to be a fairly pure Metal type: the precision and clarity of his speech, the sad, tearful quality to his voice, his meticulous appearance, and the fact that he suffered from skin and lung disorders confirmed a strong affinity to Metal.

"I'm extremely frustrated with this skin condition," Ken began. He sat very straight in the chair, his legs crossed, hands folded in his lap. "I've had allergies all my life, so I'm somewhat accustomed to chronic illness, but the constant itching is beginning to drive me insane. I've dabbled in alternative medicine, taking nutritional supplements every day and an herb now and then, but I must admit that I'm a bit uneasy with the conflicting opinions about herbs and the medical world's disdain for unorthodox techniques. Nevertheless, Western medicine seems to have reached a dead end with my disease, and I'm not willing to admit that there's nothing more I can do."

Ken developed allergies and sinus problems when he was four years old. Allergic reactions to pollen and mold during the spring and fall caused a persistent postnasal drip, which often developed into a raging sinus infection. While multiple courses of antibiotics temporarily relieved his symptoms, they didn't cure the problem; Ken estimated that he averaged three or four sinus infections every year.

Ken's naturally dry, flaky skin had always been sensitive to various allergens. In his youth he'd been a swimmer, and all year round his skin was covered with a fine rash caused by an allergic reaction to chlorine. In his junior year at college he began to develop patches of dry, itchy skin on his arms and legs that became larger and more inflamed as time went on.

Stress had an obvious and immediate effect on Ken's eczema. With his two teenage daughters rebelling against every rule he tried to enforce, Ken felt as if his neatly ordered, carefully organized world was in danger of imminent collapse. When I mentioned the wealth of scientific research verifying the connection between stress and chronic illness, Ken showed immediate interest. After our first meeting, he went to the library and checked out several books and articles on stress and stress-related diseases.

In our second session, we talked about the connection between allergies and skin disorders. I explained how the Chinese call the Skin "the Third Lung," and that like the Lungs, the Skin is involved in the process of respiration. It breathes in nutrients, oxygen, and sunlight to be used by every cell in the body, and it breathes out numerous toxins through the pores via perspiration. In emotional and spiritual terms, the Skin and Lungs work together to help us let go of unnecessary or useless thoughts, behavior, and routines and take in new ideas and perspectives. Like the Skin, I said, we have to learn how to be flexible and adaptable to changing situations.

Ken and I talked for a long time about the Five Element System and his strong affinity to Metal. The metaphors of traditional Chinese medicine fascinated Ken, particularly the image the ancient texts often associate with Metal energy: the tranquil and serene mountain. A backpacker and mountain biker, Ken had always enjoyed the serenity of the mountains and loved to think of himself as intimately connected with their solid yet graceful power.

Of all the strategies we pursued in treatment, including herbs, dietary changes, nutritional supplements, and stress-reduction techniques, Ken responded immediately and most powerfully to acupuncture. The darkened room, the silence, and the opportunity to close his eyes and meditate on the underlying meaning of his illness always seemed to refresh and invigorate his body, mind, and spirit.

If you are guided by the power of Metal, you feel drawn to the core issues, essential structures, and guiding principles of life. You are attracted to beauty, pleased by symmetry, and inspired by purity. Art, philosophy, and religion intrigue you, and you thrive on intellectual discussions with like-minded friends and acquaintances. Small talk bores you to tears. You'd rather be stranded in the wilds with only the vast stretches of the heavens to keep you company than crammed in a room crowded with strangers discussing superficialities. Quality, not quantity, is what matters most.

Disciplined and precise, strong-willed yet flexible, you also search for the higher truths of art and philosophy. Your keen aesthetic sense and high moral standards guide you in understanding that the true meaning of life lies in the inner substance and not the outer form. With great powers of concentration, you seek to develop your character by devoted attention to ethics, morality, and the acquisition of knowledge.

Of all the emotions, you are most powerfully affected by grief. You have a special appreciation for the temporary nature of life, yet your grief is alleviated by the knowledge that within every ending is contained the promise of a new beginning. By focusing on the enduring structures and underlying meaning of life, you are able to mourn what is gone while patiently awaiting what is yet to arrive. Letting go of the past, you eagerly anticipate what the future has to offer.

A majestic, snow-capped mountain is the image that best captures the power of Metal. Broad-based, firmly grounded in the earth, reaching with power and authority toward the heavens, the mountain stands as a symbol of inner strength, endurance, and tranquillity. Like the mountain, Metal types are grounded by earth and inspired by heaven. When all the superficialities are stripped away, the core structures remain as enduring symbols of life's beauty and grace.

> *The most perfect grace consists not in external ornamentation but in allowing the original material to stand forth, beautified by being given form.*
>
> —*The I Ching*

Imbalances in Metal Energy

The Chinese believe that the organs associated with Metal—the Lung and Large Intestine—"know" when to let substances in and when to let them go, a wisdom that is considered essential for health and happiness.

Western medicine describes the lungs as the organs of respiration, responsible for supplying the blood with oxygen inhaled from the outside air and disposing of waste carbon dioxide in the exhaled air. In Chinese medicine the Lung ("the Official of Rhythmic Order") rules the ongoing interaction between the interior and exterior world. Expanding to inhale and contracting to exhale, the Lung joins the energy of Heaven (air) with the energy of Earth (essential nutrients), instilling the body, mind, and spirit with a sense of rhythm and order based on the understanding that for every ending, there is a new beginning.

In emotional and spiritual terms, the Lung balances the ability to yield and demand, give and take, hold on and let go. When the Lung (Metal) energy is out of balance, order and discipline are rigidly maintained, the emotions are kept under tight control, rules and routines become inflexible, and the body begins to stiffen up.

In Western terms the large intestine is a digestive organ approximately five and a half feet long, consisting of the cecum, colon, and rectum. Indigestible parts of food pass from the small intestine into the large intestine; there, the body gradually reabsorbs the liquid from the wastes through the intestinal walls, and the solid waste products are eliminated through the rectum.

In the Chinese classification system the Large Intestine ("the Dust Bin Collector") is responsible for making distinctions between harmless and harmful elements. The ability to discriminate between substances the body can and cannot use is extremely important in creating an uncluttered environment in which the organs can work efficiently. A breakdown in this power inevitably leads to overcrowding and congestion, with such physical symptoms as abdominal pain, cramping, diarrhea, and/or constipation, all of which deplete our vital energy (*chi*). Emotional and spiritual symptoms of a breakdown in this organ system include the inability to discriminate between what is right and wrong, a lack of originality or creativity, and a growing sensation of rigidity and inflexibility.

EXCESS METAL

If the power of Metal becomes dominant or exaggerated, your ability to give and take—from the inhalation and exhalation of breath, to the ingestion of nutrients and the release of wastes, to the ability to maintain loving relationships while relinquishing harmful associations—gradually erodes, and you become increasingly inflexible and dogmatic. The less balanced your energies, the more you will feel the need to create some semblance of control in your life by imposing order and discipline on yourself and others. Any deviation from your normal routine will create intense anxiety, which will inevitably affect your physical health and emotional well-being.

Excess Metal creates a hardening effect, in which your molten nature cools down, becoming solid and unyielding. You find it difficult to compromise or yield to opposing viewpoints, and inevitably, your belief system ossifies. Over time, the absence of fresh ideas corrodes your energy, like an abandoned car left out in the rain to rust.

When your Metal energy is too strong, a basic lack of self-esteem governs your thoughts and actions. Because you don't feel innately valuable or worthy of respect, you try to increase your self-worth by collecting material possessions. As your self-respect continues to deteriorate, you become greedy and possessive, hoarding your belongings while jealously guarding your personal relationships. When you encounter someone who possesses more than you do, whether it is beauty, wealth, power, or love, you experience intense envy. You also hold on to grief, refusing to let go of those people and possessions that you have already lost and cannot recover, clinging possessively to all that you "own," including people, material possessions, and rigid adherence to a fixed set of beliefs.

You have forgotten the basic wisdom intrinsic to Metal: Quality emanates from within and cannot be imposed from without.

Excess Metal: Physical Symptoms
- Stiff, tight muscles
- Unnaturally stiff posture and awkward movements
- Inflexible spine and neck
- Spine and joint problems: chronic joint pain and stiffness, "frozen" shoulder, arthritis, calcification of spinal column
- Tendency to develop allergies, especially hay fever and allergies to mold, chemical fumes, and animal dander; excess symptoms tend to manifest in acute flare-ups
- Sinus problems: acute sinus infections and sinus headaches
- Nasal polyps
- Poor circulation
- Lack of perspiration
- Respiratory symptoms, which tend to be acute (*yang*) in nature: shortness of breath, chronic dry cough, tight chest, and tendency to develop asthma
- Intestinal problems that flare up suddenly: bloating, constipation, diarrhea, colitis, irritable bowel syndrome
- Extremely dry skin, hair, nails, lips, nasal passages, and other mucous membranes
- Acne
- Eczema and/or psoriasis, with acute flare-ups
- Sensitivity to odors
- Sensitivity to climate changes (particularly to humid or excessively dry climates)

Excess Metal: Psychological and Behavioral Symptoms
- Domineering personality
- Tendency to maintain emotional distance from others
- Difficulty with conflict and disorder
- Flat, mechanical emotional responses

- Self-righteousness
- Fear of losing control
- Overly critical and judgmental attitude
- Formal, stuffy, overbearing presence
- Natural tendency to be prejudiced, judging others by their appearance or beliefs
- Intolerant of opposing viewpoints or those who deviate from your strict ethical standards
- Strict disciplinarian
- Inability to adapt to changing circumstances
- Emphasis on order
- Obsession with cleanliness
- Ritualized routines
- Unable to form new or lasting relationships
- Lack of originality and creativity
- Tendency to collect various items (coins, knickknacks, rare gems) and form strong attachments to them
- Tendency to be possessive of both people and material goods

DEFICIENT METAL

Because the power of Metal rules rhythm and order, a deficiency results in a general state of confusion and disarray. In a metaphorical sense, your energy is liquefying and spilling out of your pores. As a result, the need for outside support dominates your thoughts and actions; only when others are openly and consistently approving of your behavior do you feel good about yourself. Criticisms, no matter how gently offered, wound you deeply, and even casual comments are taken personally, resulting in persistent hurt feelings and damage to self-esteem.

Like the excess Metal type, you have lost the ability to "let go," and you cling tenaciously to your opinions, relationships, self-image, and various possessions. Plagued by self-doubt, you are no longer certain of what is right and what is wrong. Your lack of inner resolve forces you to rely on social conventions for personal guidance. Good manners, proper etiquette, and superficial beauty begin to mean more to you than inner qualities and substance. The underlying structure that girds your character starts to deteriorate, and eventually, your system of energy collapses.

The deficient Metal type would do well to heed this commonsense advice, thousands of years old, from *The I Ching:*

> We cannot lose what really belongs to us, even if we throw it away.
> Therefore we need have no anxiety. All that need concern us is that
> we should remain true to our own natures and not listen to others.

Deficient Metal: Physical Symptoms

- Congested nose, throat, and sinuses
- Food and environmental allergies that tend to be *yin* (chronic, dull, and persistent) in nature: hay fever, and allergic reactions to cats, dust, chemicals, and dairy products and other foods
- Contact dermatitis or hives; tendency to be severely allergic to poison ivy, oak, or sumac
- Respiratory problems that tend to be *yin* in nature: chronic feelings of pressure in chest, difficulty breathing, tight chest, bronchial spasm
- Chronic asthma, especially allergy-induced asthma
- Chronically dry skin, hair, lips, and nasal passages
- Moles and warts
- Cracked, dry, or soft nails
- Sneezing or coughing bouts caused by changes in temperature or humidity
- Difficulty adapting to climate changes; tendency to feel excessively hot or cold
- Eczema or psoriasis, with chronic itching and/or low-grade inflammation
- Headaches, typically experienced in reaction to loss or disappointment
- Chronic, recurring bowel disturbances: constipation, loose stools, irritable bowel syndrome (alternating diarrhea and constipation)
- Depleted immune function, characterized by persistent colds and flus, a tendency to sinus congestion and postnasal drip, and immunodeficient disorders such as chronic fatigue syndrome and lupus

Deficient Metal: Psychological and Behavioral Symptoms

- Tendency to be petty, judgmental, and critical of others
- Emotional numbness and lack of feeling

- Chronic anxiety
- Difficulty letting go of the familiar
- Low self-confidence and self-esteem
- Hypersensitivity to criticism
- Tendency to wallow in past grief
- Obsessive relationships (in which friends and family are considered possessions)
- Lack of inspiration and creativity
- Tendency to accumulate junk and clutter, in the belief that such items will be useful (or valuable) someday
- Fear of failure, which results in anxiety or phobias about engaging in new pursuits, meeting new people, or becoming involved in new situations
- Phobias, particularly school phobias or agoraphobia

Restoring Harmony

LIFESTYLE

Time of day: The Chinese designate the hours between 3:00 A.M. and 7:00 A.M. as the time when the power of Metal is most keenly felt. Many religions use these early morning hours for prayers or meditation, believing that this is the time when we are most receptive to spiritual energies. In China, men, women, and children of all ages gather together between 5:00 and 6:00 A.M. for tai chi exercises, because this is the time when Metal's spiritual energies are thought to be most abundant and powerful.

Season: The season of Metal is autumn, when we compress our energies and eliminate all that is unnecessary and extraneous. Autumn reminds us that flexibility and adaptability are crucial for staying healthy and balanced during the difficult months ahead. During these months you will want to prepare for the challenges of winter by completing unfinished projects, clearing away clutter and debris, setting extra food and fuel aside, and making sure that you are physically and emotionally prepared for the cold, dark months ahead. For Metal types, autumn is often the best time to do "spring cleaning" and get rid of all extraneous and unnecessary items in your life (see the "Get organized" section).

The Yellow Emperor has this to say about the season of autumn:

> In the three months of autumn all things in nature reach their full maturity. The grains ripen and harvesting occurs. The heavenly energy cools, as does the weather. . . . One should retire with the sunset and rise with the dawn. Just as the weather in autumn turns harsh, so does the emotional climate. It is therefore important to remain calm and peaceful, refraining from depression so that one can make the transition to winter smoothly. This is the time to gather one's spirit and energy, be more focused, and not allow desires to run wild. One must keep the lung energy full, clean, and quiet. This means practicing breathing exercises to enhance lung qi [*chi*]. Also, one should refrain from both smoking and grief, the emotion of the lung. This will prevent kidney or digestive problems in the winter.

Let yourself feel the special poignancy of the season, epitomized by the leaves drying up and falling off the trees, but always try to balance the sense of loss with this bit of wisdom from the *The I Ching:*

> Like the day or the year in nature, so every life, indeed every cycle of experience, is a continuity by which old and new are linked together.

Get organized: Nothing will drive a Metal type crazier than a closet filled with dirty, crumpled clothing, a desk piled high with unpaid bills, a garage stuffed with junk, or a kitchen strewn with breakfast crumbs, open cereal boxes, and dirty dishes. Rubbish and clutter are obstacles that prevent Metal from getting down to the core issues that give meaning and purpose to life.

When the junk piles up, it's time to get organized. Organization is one of Metal's natural talents, and you can regain control of your life by rearranging your desk, closets, drawers, and filing cabinets. Making order out of chaos is inherently creative because in a short period of time you are forced to make dozens of decisions about where to file, how to label and categorize, what to keep, and what to toss. Even more important, learning how to let go of useless items is an important skill for Metal types to learn because of their tendency to hoard their possessions.

As you work to organize your life, try to focus on what you have accomplished rather than fretting about all the work that remains to be done. Give yourself a task that you can finish in less than an hour, and then chip away at the mess and clutter one step at a time.

Make lists: When you make daily to-do lists (such lists are common among Metal types), don't expect to cross off every item by the end of the day. Congratulate yourself for finishing three or four items on the list. In her book *Everyday Sacred,* Sue Bender (definitely a Metal type) writes: "I do not want to spend my life making a mess and then cleaning it up. These incomplete tasks weigh on me—my mind often focuses on what I'm *not* getting done rather than on what I am doing." To impose order on her life, Bender set aside one hour every day to sort through the mess and create order. "Having a limited time frame, and without rushing, I was able to approach each job with focused attention. . . . That one hour, no matter what else I had chosen to do that day, was as sweet and satisfying as anything I could have imagined doing."

Don't go overboard. In their attempt to impose order on chaos, Metal types have a tendency to go overboard, tightly scheduling the day so that each hour overflows with duties and responsibilities. Such inflexible boundaries inevitably diminish creativity and spontaneity. When rigidity enters Metal's life, passion is lost; as the Chinese would say, Metal "humiliates" Fire. As the Control Cycle of the Five Element System shows (see page 6), Fire restrains Metal by heating and melting it; however, if Metal becomes excessive, it "insults" Fire by taking over control and upsetting the natural order of things.

To warm up the Metal energy and return some flexibility to your life, you will need to "apologize" to Fire and invite its passion back. Keep your mind open and receptive to new ideas. Put yourself in situations that demand quick, even impetuous responses. Let go of strict discipline, and learn how to enjoy the rhythms of give and take.

Practice breathing exercises. Breathing exercises, which strengthen the Lungs, increase energy, still the mind, and lift the spirits, are particularly appropriate for Metal types. In all breathing exercises, make sure you focus on exhalation; when you exhale completely, the inhalation phase of breathing will occur naturally and spontaneously. The following breathing technique was created by F. M. Alexander, the originator of a unique form of bodywork called the Alexander technique. He believed that we can reestablish a natural breathing rhythm when we focus our attention on exhalation. (For additional breathing techniques, see pages 59, 80, and 126).

THE WHISPERED AH

Focus on the exhalation phase, saying *"Ahhhhhhhhh"* until your outgoing breath feels complete. Do not consciously focus on the ingoing breath, but simply wait and "watch" as the breath comes in, a natural response to full exhalation.

Meditation: Anything that inspires you and appeals to a higher truth or moral order—transcendental meditation, philosophy, music, church services, spiritual retreats, climbing a mountain, watching a sunset—will help you loosen and lighten up. Meditation is especially appropriate for Metal types, who naturally gravitate to solitary activities that involve the search for unifying principles and spiritual truths.

Of all the different meditative techniques, Zen meditation is the most suited to Metal because it involves a willingness to let go of everything and reduce your experiences to the "wonder of being." Zen techniques instruct you to sit and breathe in and out, counting from one to ten on the exhalations; if your mind strays or you lose count, you simply go back to one and start over again. The point is not to get to ten (or indeed to get anywhere), but only to immerse yourself fully in the moment.

Zen meditative techniques are extremely challenging because they're completely unadorned and don't promise anything—no supernatural experiences or visits from angels are sought or experienced in Zen. If you keep on sitting, however, you'll experience a deep sense of connection with the world around you. As Zen teacher and author Perle Besserman puts it: "Zen leads you away from isolation and seclusion and brings about the experience of interdependence, the knowledge that you are no different from the other, whether that other be the air in the room, a sneezing neighbor, or the dog barking next door."

Metal types have a natural tendency to be self-righteous, judging people by their lifestyle, ethics, or beliefs, and they should always be on the lookout for perfectionist tendencies.

DIET

Metal types tend to have strong, even hypermetabolism, and as a result they seem able to eat as much and as often as they want without gaining weight. Paradoxically, food simply isn't very important to them, and they often skip meals without even thinking about it. "What did you have for breakfast?" an Earth type might ask (for Earth types love to think about food), to which Metal would respond, "I don't remember—in fact, I'm not sure if I ate at all!"

Ironically, Metal types tend to be most vulnerable to food allergies and sensitivities. Food allergies, which create an immediate and obvious effect (hives or welts, red, itchy eyes, and a wide range of respiratory problems), are relatively easy to diagnose. Much more difficult to detect, however, are food sensitivities, which develop slowly and feature diverse and seemingly unconnected symptoms that can occur hours, or even days, after consuming the offending food.

Symptoms of Food Sensitivities
- *Digestive symptoms:* bloating, cramps, diarrhea, constipation, nausea, gas, loss of appetite, vomiting
- *Respiratory problems:* coughing, wheezing, sinus or nasal congestion, bronchial congestion, frequent colds or earaches
- *Skin disorders:* hives, rashes, eczema, psoriasis
- *Emotional and behavioral symptoms:* tension, fatigue, headaches, insomnia, depression, mood swings

If Metal is an important or dominant part of your nature and you regularly experience any of these symptoms, you might consider consulting with a naturopathic physician, an acupuncturist trained in nutrition, or a physician who practices complementary medicine (integrating ancient healing techniques with modern medical science). One way to test for food sensitivities is the Elimination Provocation Diet, in which suspected food allergens are avoided for three to four weeks and then reintroduced, with careful attention paid to any recurrence of physical, emotional, or behavioral problems.

Common Food Allergens

- Dairy products: milk, butter, cheese, yogurt, cottage cheese, ice cream, etc.
- Wheat or gluten products: bread, cereal, gravies, crackers, cookies
- Eggs
- Chocolate
- Citrus (particularly oranges and orange juice)
- Soy products
- Peanuts and other nuts
- Shellfish (lobster, crab, shrimp)
- Sugar
- Yeast

To avoid potential problems with food sensitivities and keep your digestive system in good working order, follow these general guidelines:

- Eliminate or drastically cut back on dairy products, the primary food allergen. Dairy products also produce excess mucus in the system, which can aggravate Metal's tendency to respiratory problems. Some people are allergic to the proteins in milk (lactalbumin or casein), while others are allergic to the fat (beta-lactoglobulin). If you're allergic to fat, always use nonfat milk products; if you're allergic to the proteins in milk, avoid milk products completely.
- Avoid spicy and greasy foods, which are difficult to digest.
- Vary your diet by using different foods from all the basic food groups. Although this advice may seem obvious, most of us tend to stick to our favorite foods, eating variations of the same five or six meals over and over again. If you are allergic or sensitive to a particular type of food and eat it several times a week, your problems will intensify.
- Beware of persistent cravings for particular foods; food cravings are often symptoms of an underlying food sensitivity.
- Avoid sweet, sticky, or cold foods because they tend to overburden Earth energies, leading to incomplete digestion. This, in turn, creates excess mucus, which is stored in the Lungs (the source of Metal energy), and it can contribute to asthma and other respiratory problems. A malfunctioning digestive system is also unable to completely break down proteins in the foods we eat; "renegade"

(undigested) proteins leak into our body fluids, where they are attacked by the immune system, causing allergic reactions.

◆ Increase the fiber in your diet with whole grains, fruits, and vegetables. Even if you don't experience intestinal problems, we recommend that you use a daily fiber supplement. Yerba Prima's Daily Fiber Formula is an excellent, completely natural product that contains no artificial colorings, flavorings, sugar, or sugar substitutes.

◆ To eliminate toxins that may have accumulated in your body, fast periodically, eating just fruits, vegetables, and juices. Some Metal types like to fast for a week every autumn (a fall cleaning), while others fast one day every week, or even one meal every day. While most people find it difficult if not impossible to fast, Metal types are not overly concerned with food and find it easier to stick with a strict regime.

◆ Drink eight to ten 8-ounce glasses of fresh, filtered water every day. Water helps to "bulk up" the intestinal contents and flush everything through the system quickly and efficiently.

NUTRITIONAL SUPPLEMENTS

To prevent illness and maintain general good health, take the following vitamins and minerals every day:

General Formula for Maximum Immunity

Vitamin A: 25,000 I.U. (in the form of beta-carotene or mixed carotenes)
Vitamin C: 2,000–3,000 mg.
Vitamin E: 400–800 I.U. (take the higher amount if you are over 50)
Magnesium: 500 mg. (chelated with amino acids)
Multivitamin and mineral supplement: Choose a formula with 100–200 percent of the RDA for various vitamins and minerals

For Extra Protection Add:

Selenium: 200 mcg. (take with vitamin E)
Coenzyme Q-10: 30 mg.
Pycnogenol (pine bark or grape-seed extract): 50 mg.

Zinc: 30 mg. (15 mg. of zinc is included in many multivitamin and mineral supplements)

EXERCISE

Metal types tend to be introverted and prefer exercises that can be done alone. Walking is a wonderful way to gently exercise your muscles, practice your breathing techniques, and enjoy the silence and serenity of nature. Metal types often enjoy jogging, but running on hard surfaces can damage the joints (a vulnerable area for Metal). If you jog, we recommend running around a track or on a soft, dirt surface. Since mountains symbolize the power of Metal, obvious exercise choices for Metal types also include backpacking in the mountains, mountain climbing, and rock climbing.

The deep breathing, gentle stretching, and meditation involved in yoga exercises are perfectly suited to Metal. Deep abdominal (belly) breathing pulls energy into the body, nourishing the muscles and organs with oxygen and helping you relax. The physical poses work to stretch and strengthen muscles, improving posture and increasing blood flow to the vital organs.

Yoga exercise: These simple yoga *asanas* (exercises) are specifically recommended for Metal types and will benefit your Lungs and Large Intestine; the Standing Squat is particularly beneficial for the Large Intestine.

Important note: Use these exercises as adjuncts to your regular yoga class. If you have never taken yoga, please find a certified instructor and attend classes to learn the proper techniques. Be sure to warm up with stretching and limbering exercises before trying this or any other yoga *asana*. Never force your body into any position or movement. If you feel pain, your body is telling you to back off. If you are not sure what you are doing, ask your yoga instructor for guidance.

YOGA MUDRA

Stand on your mat, and take a few deep breaths. Stand with your feet two inches apart, and look straight ahead. Put your hands behind your back, and hook your thumbs together. Stretch the arms back and up, taking a full breath in. Feel your chest expand. As you exhale, elongate up and out of the waist and fold forward slowly. Look at your big toes as you descend. Bend your knees if your lower back is tight. Try bringing your abdomen in, and extend your arms up and forward. Bring your chin in, and keep your eyes open. Take five breaths, feeling the energy flow through your body.

To come up, place your palms on the lower back and rise up *slowly*. As you stand erect, close your eyes and breathe ten soft breaths.

Repeat two times if you feel up to it.

STANDING SQUAT

Stand on your mat with your feet straight, hip width apart. Look ahead, and bend your knees slightly. Corkscrew your feet into the floor, and feel your leg muscles contract. Raise your arms up in front of you to shoulder height with palms down. Take a full breath in, and squat an inch lower if you can. Take another breath, and as you exhale, squat down another inch. Stay right there for two more breaths if you can, then come up *slowly,* feeling the strength in your legs. Bring your arms down to your sides, close your eyes, breathe, and feel the energy in your body.

Repeat two more times if you feel up to it.

HERBS

Western

Elecampane (*Inula helenium*): The Greeks and Romans relied on elecampane for its digestive healing powers, while Chinese and Ayurvedic practitioners have used this herb for hundreds of years to treat bronchitis and asthma. Because its neutral nature can be either relaxing or stimulating, depending on your particular needs, elecampane can be used for any condition involving lung weakness or inflammation, from wet, cold, congestive coughs to hot, dry, irritating coughs.

Red Clover (*Trifolium pratense*): This herb's expectorant qualities make it extremely useful for upper respiratory problems, including bronchitis, colds, and persistent coughs. Red clover's antitumor activities make it a valuable supplement in the prevention and treatment of cancer, and it is frequently prescribed for skin ailments such as rashes, eczema, and psoriasis. Red clover is gentle enough for children to use.

Elecampane and red clover are often mixed together to make a gentle but powerful Lung tonic.

Dosage: If you purchase your herbs in a health food store (either in tincture form or, as dried herbs, in capsule or pill form), follow the dosage instructions on the label. Because herbs in dried form tend to lose their potency rather quickly, be sure to check the label for the expiration date.

For information on preparing your own herbs from the root, bark, leaves, flowers, or seeds of a plant, see Appendix II.

Chinese

Ba Xian Chang Shou Wan ("Eight Immortals Long Life Pills"): This is a wonderful Chinese patent remedy for Metal imbalances. If your Lung energies are weak or deficient and you suffer from a persistent dry, hacking cough, stuffy nose, congested sinuses, tightness in the chest, or breathing difficulties of any kind, this formula will work wonders to restore your health and vigor. The formula consists of eight herbs, with rehmannia root and ophiopogon sharing Emperor status; rehmannia root is a kidney *yin* (fluid) supporting herb, and ophiopogon directs the *yin* energy to the Lungs, where it mists and cools the entire system. Attending herbs include cornus, dioscorea, moutan, alisma, poria fungus, and schisandra.

Unless otherwise directed, take eight pills (actually tiny pellets) three times daily or twelve pills twice daily.

In Appendix I we offer a list of mail-order sources for high-quality Chinese and Western herbs and herbal formulas.

ACUPOINTS

LUNG 9 ("Great Abyss"): This point is thought to offer a direct line to the Lungs, where it activates and energizes the Lung energy. The energy circulating throughout the Lungs can be imagined as a waterfall that plunges from high atop a mountain into the "great abyss" of the body's interior. There it surges and swells in the deep, hidden caves, the site of an abundant, powerful source of healing.

Common Uses

- Supports the *wei chi* (immune energy), which originates in the Lungs
- Supports and strengthens Lung energies, helping to resolve Lung diseases and disorders, including colds, bronchitis, asthma, and sinus infections
- Supports and moves the blood to stop heavy ("reckless") bleeding and regulates the steady flow of blood
- Eases anxiety, irritability, and heart palpitations

Location: Lung 9 is located on the crease on the palm side of the wrist in the depression at the base of the thumb (about half an inch in from the side of the wrist).

LUNG 1 ("Central Palace"): The Chinese believe that the energy of Earth (considered "the Mother of Metal") provides a stable and secure home for precious minerals and ores. At Lung 1 Earth and Metal energy join forces to nourish the Lungs and invigorate the *wei chi.*

Common Uses

- Supports the Lung function by producing additional energy and blood and moving the energy throughout the body
- Promotes the manufacture and distribution of the *wei chi,* the defensive energy of the body, which supports immune function and prevents disease
- Clears heat from the chest and Lungs, resolving such conditions as dry cough, fever with bronchial symptoms, tuberculosis, pneumonia, bronchitis, chronic respiratory colds and flus, chronic sinusitis, asthma, pneumonia, and tuberculosis

Location: Slide your finger along your collarbone to the outer end, just above the armpit. Central Palace is in the natural depression just under the collarbone and just above the armpit.

INVIGORATING THE SENSES

Sight: The color associated with Metal is white, which in traditional Chinese texts connotes simplicity. At Chinese funerals, for example, mourners wear unbleached muslin robes to signify humble grief. (Black, which is seen as the mark of wealth and career, would be considered highly inappropriate at a Chinese funeral.)

White is also the color of snow, clouds, the full moon, and the sun reflected on water—reminders of the purity and dignity of Metal. Surround yourself with the heavenly color of white. Use cream or ivory fabrics, paints, and furnishings to decorate your home and office. White or beige clothing will remind you of the need to clear away the fluff and frills and stick to the basics.

When you feel stressed and drained of energy, try this exercise: Go outside and sit for five minutes with your eyes closed, face turned to the sun (or the moon). Imagine that the heavenly light is filtering into your body, mind, and spirit, warming and inspiring you. Breathe deep, feeling your muscles relax and your tension dissipate. As you exhale, remind yourself of your strong affinity to the heavens and your solid roots on earth.

Sound: The sound associated with Metal is weeping; if your voice always sounds weepy or whiny, as if you are constantly on the verge of tears, you may be expressing a disharmony in Metal.

The sound "Sssssssssss," like a tire slowly leaking air, is soothing for Metal types, because you can actually hear the air escaping and imagine "letting go" of all that is extraneous and unnecessary in your life. Metal types often enjoy the following "sound meditation": Find a comfortable sitting position, with your back straight but not stiff. Place a hand on your chest, and breathe in several times, gently filling your lungs with oxygen. When you exhale, say, "*Sssssssssss,*" and imagine that you are letting go of all your pent-up grief and pain. Then inhale, and imagine that you are breathing in a pure white light that spreads from your lungs to every cell of your body.

Listening to music is another way to balance your Metal energy. Numerous studies show that music can reduce stress, improve memory, and relieve pain. For Metal types the most soothing sound of all is the music of nature: the wind rustling through pine trees, river water splashing over rocks, dried autumn leaves crunching underfoot, pine cones dropping in the forest. Whenever you feel grief-stricken or off-balance, take a walk in the wilds, breathe deeply, and listen to nature sing.

Smell: The nose, which connects through the sinuses to the Lungs, is the sense organ associated with Metal. Metal types tend to be extremely sensitive to odors, and imbalances in Metal energy often affect the sense of smell.

Eucalyptus, a refreshing scent used by aromatherapists to treat asthma, bronchitis, colds, and chronic coughs, works well for Metal types. Most cough drops contain the chemical eucalyptol, which is found in the eucalyptus leaves; eucalyptol is also an active ingredient in such over-the-counter products as Sine-off, Vicks VapoRub, and Dristan decongestant. To soothe upper respiratory ailments (colds, flus, bronchitis), put two or three drops of this sweet-smelling oil in a pot of hot water and breathe deeply.

You don't have to be sick to use eucalyptus. When you're feeling healthy and balanced, the scent of fresh eucalyptus can serve as a reminder to breathe deeply and rhythmically. You can find fresh eucalyptus leaves, which release a crisp, clean fragrance for months, in florist shops and many large department stores. Place several sprigs of eucalyptus in a strategic spot in your house, and take a deep, invigorating breath whenever you enter the room. (You can also comfort yourself with this thought: According to a report in *Science News,* the chemical eucalyptol may help rid your house of cockroaches!)

Caution: Never take eucalyptus internally; just one teaspoon can be fatal.

Taste: Spicy or tangy foods such as curry, peppery cheese, pepper sauce, lemon, vinegar, and vinaigrette salad dressing often appeal to Metal types. In moderation, these foods are considered good for you and balancing for your Metal energies, but in excess, these foods can disturb Metal, injuring the Lungs and Large Intestine. As Qi Bo told the Yellow Emperor: "Overly excessive consumption of sour foods can make the skin rough, thick, and wrinkled, and cause the lips to become shriveled."

A craving for sour or spicy foods may be a sign of an imbalance in Metal. If this is the case, be sure to balance these foods with mild or bland foods such as whole grains, steamed yellow or green vegetables, fresh fruit, and fish.

Another benefit of spicy foods is that they provide heat and digestive fire, supporting the digestion and increasing the production of stomach acid. The latter is essential, as people with low levels of stomach acid are more likely to develop food allergies. Once again, however, moderation is recommended because spicy foods can dry out the Lungs and create imbalances in Metal energy.

Touch: Traditional Chinese medicine views the Skin as the Third Lung and the Skin's condition as a reflection of the health of the Lungs. Like the Lungs, the Skin breathes, exhaling toxins via perspiration and inhaling sunlight and nutrients from the air. If the Lungs are vigorously healthy, the Skin has less work to do; if the Lungs are weak and Metal energy is deficient, the skin must work harder to eliminate excess toxins.

Just as your skin benefits from strong, sturdy Lungs, so do your Lungs thrive when your skin is healthy. Whenever you take a bath or shower, use a special skin (loofa) brush to remove dead skin cells and allow the toxins to exit easily through the pores. Sauna and steam baths are wonderful, purifying therapies for Metal, assisting the skin in its efforts to release toxins with the sweat.

A full-body massage will stimulate blood circulation and improve the condition of your skin, but avoid exotic massage oils featuring "mystery" ingredients because these products often cause allergic reactions in Metal types. To ease the symptoms associated with upper respiratory infections, try this gentle massage: Lightly oil your hands (use plain vegetable oil, almond oil, sesame oil, or a non-allergic massage oil), and massage your chest and abdomen, using long, gliding strokes and gentle pressure. Continue for several minutes.

If you have an active or painful skin disorder such as eczema or psoriasis, regular massage may help. If massage aggravates your skin condition, try a soothing baking soda bath instead: Add a cup of baking soda to a tub of lukewarm water, and soak for as long as an hour.

QUESTIONS TO ASK YOURSELF

If you feel off-balance or out of sorts with the world, these questions will help you discover the source of your distress and guide you to potential solutions. Focus on one or two questions that seem to relate most directly to your current problems or emotional state of mind.

- I hold myself and others to impossibly high standards: How can I lower my expectations and still devote my energies to excellence?

◆ I tend to enmesh myself in organizational details to the point that I lose sight of the core issues: How can I maintain order in my life without getting bogged down in technicalities?

◆ Etiquette and formality appeal to my sense of decorum, and yet I am sometimes overly concerned with propriety and protocol: How can I loosen up and stop being such a prig?

◆ I find myself upset and disturbed by spontaneous, impulsive behavior: How can I learn to be comfortable with the unexpected?

◆ I like to be in control, but I have a tendency to be domineering: How can I maintain order in my life without bossing other people around?

◆ I am often judgmental and critical of others: How can I continue to ask the most of myself without expecting everyone else to deliver a hundred percent? What can I do to become more tolerant and compassionate?

◆ I am addicted to being right: How can I do what I feel is right without requiring everyone else to agree with me?

◆ My greatest fear is being corrupted or falling apart: What can I do to maintain my basic integrity?

◆ I crave distance and solitude, yet I need close, meaningful relationships: How can I balance my need to be alone with time devoted to my friends and family?

A Story for Metal

The quest for meaning preoccupies Metal. In a very real sense your life is devoted to the search for the Holy Grail, which in mythologist Joseph Campbell's words "represents the fulfillment of the highest spiritual potentialities of the human consciousness." Earth grounds you, but Heaven inspires you, and you long to escape the boundaries of the human world to discover the deeper meanings of life.

Certain wise men and women have been blessed with that transcendent experience of awareness that emerges when time stops, movement stills, and the wholeness and holiness of the world are suddenly revealed. Through their experiences we can learn about our own spiritual quests. When Black Elk of the Oglala

Sioux was a young boy, he had a prophetic vision of standing on a mountaintop and seeing the sacred hoop at the center of the world. His description of that event speaks to the sacred interdependence of life that is the high point of the Metal experience:

> Then I was standing on the highest mountain of them all, and around about beneath me was the whole hoop of the world. And while I stood there I saw more than I can tell and I understood more than I saw; for I was seeing in a sacred manner the shapes of all things in the spirit, and the shape of all shapes as they must live together like one being. And I saw the sacred hoop of my people was one of the many hoops that made one circle, wide as daylight and as starlight, and in the center grew one mighty flowering tree to shelter all the children of one mother and one father. And I saw that it was holy. . . .
>
> But anywhere is the center of the world.

Famous Metal Types

Abraham Lincoln

Prince Charles

Mother Teresa

Mahatma Gandhi

Owl, from *The House at Pooh Corner*

The Tin Man, from *The Wizard of Oz*

Bing Crosby

Barbra Streisand

6. WATER: THE PHILOSOPHER

Water . . . flows on and on, and merely fills up all the places through which it flows; it does not shrink from any dangerous spot nor from any plunge, and nothing can make it lose its own essential nature. It remains true to itself under all conditions.

—The I Ching

Pale and thin, with prematurely gray hair, puffy skin, and dark circles under her eyes, Ann looked much older than her thirty-five years. After years of feeling tired and run down, she had been recently diagnosed with Chronic Fatigue Syndrome. The fatigue was so overpowering that she had taken a leave of absence from her job as a Latin teacher at the community college.

"I feel like my life is over," Ann said, her voice low and lifeless. "All I do is lie in bed, aching all over and thinking about the past, when I had more energy than I could handle. It wouldn't be so bad if I could read all the wonderful classics I've been dying to read, but I can't concentrate, and I can't remember anything I just read. If my mind no longer works, what's the point of living?"

The moaning sound of Ann's voice, the translucent quality of her skin, her dark complexion, sculptured features, and deep-set eyes, the plainness of her clothes (she was always dressed in black), and her passion for knowledge and insight into her condition all signified a strong affinity to Water. She lived alone and had never married, choices that suited her basic nature ("I need my solitude"), yet her illness forced her to be dependent upon her family and friends, which intensified her feelings of weakness and inadequacy.

During our first acupuncture session, Ann listened to a violin concerto tape; after a few moments she began to cry. Although she tried to stop the tears and initially seemed embarrassed and even ashamed for opening up in front of a relative stranger, eventually she acknowledged the need to express her sadness and fear. Once the dam had opened, the river flowed freely; she cried for over an hour that day.

For the next seven months Ann came to my office for twice-weekly acupuncture sessions. When I inserted the needles, she claimed she could feel the energy flowing through her, and as time went on, the benefits seemed to last longer and longer. Chinese and Western herbs, nutritional supplements, weekly psychotherapy sessions, daily yoga exercises, and breathing techniques progressively strengthened her body, mind, and spirit. Just a month after we started working together, she was able to read for half-hour stretches, and within three months she felt strong enough to go back to work part time. Recently she moved into an apartment complex near the Hudson River; she takes great joy in watching the water flow by, a symbol of her own power and potential.

Like Metal, Water represents a spiritual type of energy, and both Metal and Water types tend to be interested in art, ethics, religion, and philosophy. Unlike Metal, however, Water types are particularly fascinated by the underlying meaning and mechanics of the world they inhabit, and in their perpetual pursuit of knowledge, they tend to be more introspective than Metal types. If Water defines your nature, you like to retreat into a quiet, still place where nothing distracts you from thinking about the meaning and mystery of life. Insatiably curious and blessed with a vivid imagination, you are an intellectual and a visionary. The world of logic and analysis appeals to your naturally reflective nature, and you spend a significant amount of time trying to figure out how things work, from solving complicated mathematical problems to analyzing the strengths and weaknesses of various political systems to unraveling the structure of the universe itself.

Like a stream flowing down a mountain, Water types hold firm to their course in life, refusing to fret over setbacks or worry about past defeats. Water energy is fearless and directed—it knows where it's going, and it has the intelligence and inner drive to get there, similar to the way a river flows around a boulder rather than try to remove it. Every action Water takes, even the nonaction of pooling up and reserving strength, is filled with potential and readiness to continue onward toward the goal.

Yet Water knows its limitations. When obstructions block the way, Water yields by retreating, refusing to waste energy in vain pursuits. When danger threatens, Water does not shrink in fear or give up the struggle in hopeless resignation; it remains true to its basic nature, knowing when to pool up and reserve its strength and when to continue on with force and determination. When the time is right, Water does not hesitate but follows its course with strength and purpose.

Imbalances in Water Energy

The power of Water nourishes the body, mind, and spirit with real and potential energy, which is stored in the Kidneys. In Western medicine these bean-shaped glandular organs, located on either side of the spinal column in the lower back area, are responsible for regulating the content of water and other substances in the blood and for removing wastes from the blood through the urine. Several thousand quarts of blood pass through the kidneys every day, from which approximately 160 quarts are extracted for further filtration. Most of this liquid is reabsorbed into the body by the kidneys, leaving only one to two quarts to be eliminated through the urine.

In Chinese medicine the Kidneys ("the Storehouse of the Vital Essence") are mainly responsible for creating and dispersing warmth and energy throughout the body. The Chinese like to think of the Kidneys as the body's pilot light; steady and slow-burning, they provide warmth and fuel for every cell in the body. Kidney Fire ("the Fire of Ming Men") provides energy to the vital organs, allowing them to function at peak level. On a metaphorical level, the Fire of Ming Men supplies the driving energy and resolute willpower needed to press forward, overcome obstacles, and reach our goals in life.

Balancing the warming energy of Kidney Fire is the cooling energy of Kidney Water, which is responsible for storing *jing,* the inherited essence that creates the bone marrow, which in turn contributes to the development of the brain, spinal cord, bones, teeth, blood, and hair. Thus the Kidneys are said to rule our bones and skeletal structure as well as our ability to reason, remember, and imagine. The spirit of the Kidneys, the *zhi,* determines the strength of our ambition, willpower, and survival instincts.

The second organ associated with Water is the Urinary Bladder, which Western medicine describes as a hollow container with muscular walls, joined to the kidneys by the ureters and to the body's exterior by the urethra. Every few seconds urine is passed from the kidneys to the bladder, where it is stored until eliminated through urination. In Chinese medicine the Urinary Bladder ("the Official in Charge of Eliminating Fluid Waste") is compared to a reservoir where the waters of the body collect. "The bladder is where the water converges and where, after being catalyzed by the *chi,* it is eliminated," Qi Bo explains in *The Yellow Emperor's Classic.* When the Bladder is "leaky" or somehow not functioning properly, the entire system is in danger of bogging down and filling up with toxic wastes. Depression, coping difficulties, inability to adapt to new or unusual circumstances, fatigue, and a general sense of foreboding are considered symptoms of an energy imbalance in this vital organ.

EXCESS WATER

When Water energy builds up, it tends to congeal and harden, contributing to physical and mental inflexibility. Practitioners of traditional Chinese medicine look for solidified Water energy in a person's posture (stiff or frozen), musculature (rigid and bunched up, particularly in the shoulders and neck), and body movements (awkward and inflexible).

This hardening process also causes physical problems—Kidney and bladder stones, lumps, tumors, stiff joints, arthritic conditions, hardening of the arteries, and high blood pressure are common in excess Water types. When Water solidifies, it can no longer moisten the tissues and organs, which leads to a general drying-out process and such symptoms as dry nose and sinuses, lack of sexual secretion (vaginal dryness in women, painful intercourse for men), lack of sexual interest, lack of perspiration, and urinary problems.

On the emotional plane, excess Water types tend to be opinionated and intolerant of viewpoints that diverge from their own. You cling to fixed goals, and you refuse to stray from your course. If others challenge your opinions, you are likely to maintain a deep and lasting resentment toward them. In general, you tend to blame others for your problems, and you find it hard to for-give an insult.

When under stress, you can be aggressive and even belligerent, but your be-havior is a thin cover-up for feelings of inadequacy and a mounting sensation of fear. Forceful and defiant on the outside, you are filled with trepidation on the inside. If steps are not taken to break up and divert the excess energy, you may become suspicious of others, imagining that they are talking about you or con-spiring behind your back. Paranoid tendencies and a fear of persecution become pronounced if the imbalance continues undetected and untreated.

Excess Water: Physical Symptoms

- Dry nose and throat
- Deterioration of gums and teeth
- Shallow breathing
- Sleep problems: difficulty falling asleep, insomnia
- Severe lower back pain
- Stiff joints, particularly in the knees and hips
- Acute flare-ups of arthritis (both osteoarthritis and rheumatoid arthritis)
- Lack of perspiration
- Bladder problems: difficulty urinating, low flow, urinary infections that ap-pear suddenly and cause extreme pain or discomfort
- Kidney and bladder stones
- Prostate problems: prostate infections, burning urination, urinary infections
- Sexual problems: overexcitement, premature ejaculation, promiscuity
- Headaches, often severe behind the eyes or in the occiput, where the skull and neck meet
- Hypersensitivity to light and loud noises
- Tendency to neurological disturbances or disorders: attention deficit disor-der, inability to concentrate, intense anxiety, multiple phobias
- Vertigo, dizziness, loss of equilibrium
- High blood pressure, with a tendency toward heart attacks and strokes

Excess Water: Psychological and Behavioral Symptoms

- Emotional inaccessibility and withdrawal
- Antisocial tendencies

- Irritability
- Insecurity
- Apathy
- Cynicism
- Pessimism
- Depression
- Suspicious of other people's motives
- Paranoid tendencies
- Obsessive thoughts about sex and a tendency to become overstimulated
- Hypochondriac tendencies
- Tendency to be unforgiving
- Lack of interest in food
- Preoccupation with inner thoughts and feelings, paying little attention to others
- Tendency to withdraw and isolate yourself when stressed or overwhelmed
- Tendency to equate love with loyalty
- Fanaticism
- Inflexibility

DEFICIENT WATER

The old gray donkey Eeyore, Winnie the Pooh's friend, offers a vivid portrait of the deficient Water type. Standing with his head bowed low, nose just barely above ground, tail dropping straight down without a bend, tilt, or wag to signal even an iota of excitement, Eeyore is the embodiment of melancholy. Sudden outbursts of spontaneous joy are not going to emerge from this donkey. Plodding ahead, he puts one foot in front of the other, having no idea where he is headed or even why he happens to be going in that direction.

Whereas an excess in the power of Water leads to an engorged sense of self (like a river at flood stage overflowing its boundaries), a deficiency creates a gradual contraction of the self. Like Eeyore, you begin to feel as if everything you do is a chore, and nothing that you do matters to anyone else. As time passes and your Water energy continues to dissipate, you lose the ability to interact naturally and spontaneously with others. Relationships are difficult to maintain, for you lack the deep reserves of concern and compassion that are essential for true friendship and love, and your feelings of disconnectedness and isolation intensify. Much of the time you feel arid and empty, and you fear that you might be drying up inside and that all your motivation and creative juices will slowly evaporate.

As your insecurity, fear, and indecision grow, you neglect the essential wisdom of Water: to stay focused, refuse to shrink from danger, keep your goals in sight, and stand firm against all temptations to stray from your true nature.

Deficient Water: Physical Symptoms

- Lack of energy or stamina
- Loss of appetite
- Excessive dryness and thirst
- Brittle, dry, split hair; thinning or balding hair; prematurely gray hair
- Prematurely wrinkled skin
- Weak abdominal muscles
- Chronic lower back pain
- Achy, weak knees
- Cold extremities: hands and feet
- Tendency to ear infections or tinnitus (ringing in the ears)
- Hearing and visual deterioration
- Dark (blue-black) hue around the eyes, indicating a weakness in Kidney and adrenal function
- Urinary problems, including frequent urination and chronic, low-grade urinary infections
- Vaginal infections
- Yeast infections
- Amenorrhea (unusual menstrual bleeding, in which menstruation has never occurred, or a sudden cessation in menstruation after years of regular bleeding)
- Sexual problems: impotence, infertility, lack of interest in sex, diminished sex drive
- Weak, stiff spine with degeneration of disks and cartilage
- Brittle joints and bones
- Osteoporosis
- Chronic fatigue immune deficiency syndrome

Deficient Water: Psychological and Behavioral Problems

- Absentmindedness
- Procrastination
- Laziness
- Excessive criticism of other people's behavior, thoughts, or feelings
- Deep feelings of impotence and frustration
- Lack of confidence and loss of faith in self
- Lack of trust in others
- Tendency for goals and sense of direction to be unfocused or poorly defined
- Gloomy, cheerless demeanor
- Self-centeredness
- Hypochondria
- Paranoia
- Phobias regarding intimacy, exposure, emotional involvement, water, new situations, sexuality, closed spaces, heights, the unknown, death
- Depression, often accompanied by hopelessness
- Lack of motivation and willpower
- Loss of will to live
- An aversion to cold and intense dislike of winter

Restoring Harmony

LIFESTYLE

Time of day: The Chinese designate the hours between 3:00 P.M. and 7:00 P.M. as the time when Water energy is most powerful. In countries all over the world these are the "siesta" hours, when shops close and people regenerate their energies by napping, relaxing, or enjoying a cup of tea. If you consistently feel tired or drained of energy during these hours, your Kidney battery pack may be running low and need recharging. Use the hours between 3:00 P.M. and 7:00 P.M.to focus or redirect your energies, concentrating on the healing remedies described in the remainder of this chapter.

Season: Water's season is winter, the time of year when the natural world contracts and condenses, conserving its energy for the season of renewal and regeneration that lies ahead. Just as the waters of the earth freeze over, Water energy may also harden and solidify during this season, becoming passive and inward-directed. Anyone who dreads the winter months or suffers from restless, pent-up energy during this season may be experiencing an imbalance in Water energy.

The Yellow Emperor has this to say about the season of winter:

> During the winter months all things in nature wither, hide, return home, and enter a resting period, just as lakes and rivers freeze and snow falls. . . . Retire early and get up with the sunrise, which is later in winter. Desires and mental activity should be kept quiet and subdued. Sexual desires especially should be contained, as if keeping a happy secret. Stay warm, avoid the cold, and keep the pores closed. Avoid sweating. The philosophy of the winter season is one of conservation and storage. Without such a practice the result will be injury to the kidney energy.

Find a cause to believe in: Water types need a cause to believe in and a direction to follow, something outside themselves that they can flow in and through. Earth types experience a similar need, but while Earth craves relationships with human beings or the community as a whole, Water yearns for connections that are more spiritual or cerebral. If not actively pursuing knowledge and wisdom, Water types are the community activists who donate their time and energy to worthy causes, the philanthropists who give generously to those in need, or the idealistic visionaries who seek to create a better world.

Whenever the connection to something greater than the self is severed or weakened, Water types suffer deeply. To restore harmony, you will need to rediscover your goal and purpose in life and establish pathways that will allow you to fulfill your ambitions. Choose a cause that you can believe in passionately and completely. Volunteer in a homeless shelter, nursing home, or public school. Write a book. Work for a political campaign.

If you can keep in mind that your health depends on your happiness, you will have the necessary motivation to make changes in your life. Follow Water's example, and be thorough and consistent in all that you do, completing one task before moving on to another and always keeping your goals in sight. Just as it takes a long period of time and a continuous flow of energy to create a new river channel, so does it require patience and persistent effort to make significant changes in your lifestyle.

Listen to music: Water types often enjoy listening to classical compositions by the great masters—Mozart, Bach, Beethoven, Wagner, Vivaldi, Chopin. The passion and pathos of tragic operas also appeal to Water types, who share the operatic philosophy that life is inherently dramatic. Attending concerts, ballet performances, or choral recitals will remove you from your self-imposed isolation and offer you an occasion to interact with others who share your interests.

Take up a musical instrument: Playing a musical instrument is another way to keep your energy flowing smoothly. If you always wanted to play the piano, violin, or cello, now is the time to take lessons and set time aside for practice.

Breathing exercises: Breathing exercises help to reestablish a sense of rhythm and flow. For extra energy and vitality, try this breathing exercise, which we've adapted from Andrew Weil's wonderful book *Spontaneous Healing*:

Invigorating Breath

- Keeping your mouth closed, breathe in and out rapidly through the nose, concentrating on fast, mechanical breathing similar to a bellows pumping air; the breath should be audible on both inhalation and exhalation.
- Rapid breathing is the goal, with as many as three inhalation/exhalation cycles per second.
- Begin with twenty to thirty seconds of rapid breathing, eventually working up to a full minute; repeat three or four times daily.
- End with a deep cleansing breath: Inhale fully through your nose, then exhale slowly through your mouth.

When you are anxious, tense, or need to relax, try the Calming Breath (see page 59). During the phase when you hold your breath, place your hands on your abdomen, and imagine that you can feel the energy concentrating there, waiting for you to exhale so that it can be dispersed to all the vital organs. The main acupoint used to support the Kidney *yin* (fluid) energy is Conception Vessel 3, located directly in the center of your body between the belly button and pubic bone. (See page 134 for a detailed discussion of the many benefits associated with stimulating this acupoint.) Breathing techniques used by many different cultures and spiritual traditions emphasize breathing into this central point rather than into the chest.

Meditation: Meditation appeals to Water's yearning for silence, solitude, and spiritual growth. Meditation is simply the art of letting your thoughts come in and go out, feeling your emotions but not being attached to them. Think of meditation as a mental form of bullfighting. Thoughts and emotions come rushing at you, your attention is completely focused, and at the last moment you step aside, letting them pass by without harming you. In meditation you are an observer, and Water types are exceptionally keen observers of life.

Like Metal, Water types have the internal discipline and desire for spiritual enlightenment that allows them to pursue successfully more demanding meditative techniques. Water types often respond well to Zen meditation (see page 104) and Vipassana-style meditations. Vipassana is an Eastern meditation technique that involves both sitting and walking in silence; for example, you might sit for forty-five minutes, then walk for forty-five minutes. Students are often advised to place their hands over the lower belly and concentrate on breathing into the center (the *tantien*) as they walk in silence.

Psychotherapy: Group or individual psychotherapy sessions can be extremely beneficial for Water types, who often need help breaking up rigid behavior patterns or emerging from their protective shell and risking emotional involvement. It's essential, however, that you choose a psychotherapist or counselor who focuses on the present rather than the past. When your energy is out of balance, you will have a tendency to look back to the past and brood on what once was or could have been, or you may be drawn forward into the future, experiencing fears of the unknown or imagining disasters that might take place. Ask your therapist to help you live in the present moment, stay true to yourself (which, for Water, is often an eccentric, unorthodox way of being), and gain the confidence and courage to face whatever challenges and adventures might await you.

Stay warm: Because of your affinity to Water, which in its natural, flowing state is cold, you will have a tendency to get chilled during every season, especially in winter. Cold, wet weather often aggravates arthritic conditions, and depression, lethargy, and mood swings are common during the winter. If you tend to get depressed during the winter months (a common affliction for Water types), you may be suffering from seasonal affective disorder (SAD), which is caused by the lack of natural light and is common in the dark months of winter. SAD can be eased or even reversed by using full-spectrum light, which stimulates a chemical reaction in the pineal gland and contributes to a sense of joy and well-being. Read under the light for an hour every day, or simply close your eyes and bathe in it.

Ultimately, it is important for Water types to take care to conserve energy and stay warm in every season. Turn up the thermostat, light a fire, and drink warm (but not steaming-hot) drinks such as tea, cocoa, or apple cider. For a real treat on a cold day, try a hot ginger foot bath, which works wonders for circulatory problems, aches and pains in the legs or lower back, insomnia, and tense, bunched-up muscles. The most invigorating of all the acupoints on the Kidney meridian, Kidney 1, is located on the soles of your feet; when you soak your feet, the ginger stimulates Kidney 1, dispersing warmth throughout the entire body.

HOT GINGER FOOT BATH

Fill a rubber tub with comfortably hot water, throw in some crushed or shaved ginger (it doesn't matter how much you use), and soak your feet until the water begins to cool.

DIET

When Water energy is excessive or deficient, it's common for Water types to crave salty foods such as potato chips, pretzels, McDonald's french fries, hot dogs, salami, or sausage. (It's also not uncommon for someone with a Water imbalance to have an excessive dislike for the taste of salty foods.) While sodium (salt) is essential for proper body functioning and in moderate amounts strengthens Water energies, excess salt in the diet can contribute to menstrual irregularities, constipation, water retention (edema), high blood pressure, congestive heart failure, and osteoporosis.

Because the staples of the average American diet—canned, processed, refined, and fast foods—are already loaded with salt, it's a good idea to avoid adding extra table salt to your food. Common table salt is heavily refined and treated with numerous chemicals to brighten its appearance and prevent clumping. If you feel that you need additional salt, use natural sources such as seafoods, seaweeds, kelp, and sea salt (available in most health food stores and many supermarkets).

Strictly limit or avoid coffee, soft drinks, and sweet foods because their stimulant qualities, in Chinese terminology, "deplete the *yin* by causing false Fire." In other words, the quick spark of energy provided by caffeine and sugar starts a little brushfire, which draws the water from the Kidneys and gradually depletes the fluid reserves. Chocolate is perhaps the worst offender, because it contains both sugar and caffeine.

If your Water energy is out of balance, try to avoid cold, raw foods such as raw vegetables, lettuces, and other roughage, which can have a chilling, dampening effect on the body. Gently steam or wok-fry your vegetables to make them easier to digest.

Perhaps the most important dietary suggestion for Water is to drink eight to ten 8-ounce glasses of fresh, filtered water every day. Water helps flush out the system, easing the burden on your Kidneys and Bladder and assisting these organs in their ongoing efforts to detoxify the blood and eliminate toxic wastes. Drinking plenty of water every day will help prevent and treat urinary infections, kidney stones, and bladder stones.

NUTRITIONAL SUPPLEMENTS

To prevent illness and maintain general good health, take the following vitamins and minerals every day:

General Formula for Maximum Immunity

Vitamin A: 25,000 I.U. (in the form of beta-carotene or mixed carotenes)
Vitamin C: 2,000–3,000 mg.

Vitamin E: 400–800 I.U. (take the higher amount if you are over 50)

Magnesium: 500 mg. (chelated with amino acids)

Multivitamin and mineral supplement: Choose a formula with 100–200 percent of the RDA for various vitamins and minerals

For Extra Protection Add:

Selenium: 200 mcg. (take with vitamin E)

Coenzyme Q-10: 30 mg.

Pycnogenol (pine bark or grape-seed extract): 50 mg.

Zinc: 30 mg. (15 mg. of zinc is included in many multivitamin and mineral supplements)

EXERCISE

As we age, our skin, flesh, blood vessels, and mucous membranes thin out and lose water, forcing the Kidneys to work harder and eventually contributing to Kidney deficiencies. Tendons and muscles gradually lose shape and elasticity, and even our bones, which Water energy feeds and nourishes, may become porous and brittle, increasing our susceptibility to broken bones, hip fractures, and spinal fractures. The Chinese believe that osteoporosis, a progressive disease characterized by a decrease in bone mass and an increase in bone brittleness, is caused by inactivity and lack of appropriate exercise as well as diminished Kidney *yin* (fluid) energy.

To keep your bones healthy and strong, incorporate into your daily routine exercises such as jogging, bicycling, aerobics, stair-stepping, cross-country ski machines, and *weight-bearing exercises,* including brisk walking while carrying light weights. Even if you're not a fitness fanatic, you can keep your bones strong by parking your car a distance away from your destination, carrying your groceries to the car rather than using a cart, or walking up and down the stairs rather than taking the elevator.

Toning and stretching the muscles, tendons, and ligaments is essential for Water types, who have a tendency to become inactive when their energy is out of balance. With inactivity comes inflexibility; as the muscles, tendons, and bones stiffen up, aches and pains increase.

Exercises that emphasize flow and fluidity are particularly well suited to Water: Swimming, snorkeling, scuba diving, fly fishing, canoeing, kayaking, sailing, and river rafting are all invigorating activities for Water types who enjoy both solitude and direct connection with their primary element.

Any exercise that involves silence and solitude will appeal to Water: Jogging, brisk walking, and cross-country skiing help to build endurance, tone muscles, and contribute to feelings of inner strength and flexibility.

Yoga and tai chi are wonderful exercises for Water types, not only because they can be practiced alone (Water's favorite way to be), but also because they focus the body's energy and the mind's attention in ways that encourage spiritual awareness (an important goal for Water). Both tai chi and yoga can be considered "exercise acupuncture," because the body movements are designed to focus and disperse the energy in the meridians, opening up blocked channels and redirecting the energy to the places where it is needed.

Yoga exercise: This simple yoga *asana* (exercise) is specifically recommended for Water types and will directly benefit both the Urinary Bladder and the Kidneys. If you have high or low blood pressure, check with your doctor first.

Important note: Use this exercise as an adjunct to your regular yoga class. If you have never taken yoga, please find a certified instructor and attend classes to learn the proper techniques. Be sure to warm up with stretching and limbering exercises before trying this or any other yoga *asana*. Never force your body into any position or movement. If you feel pain, your body is telling you to back off. If you are not sure what you are doing, ask your yoga instructor for guidance.

STANDING FORWARD BEND

Stand on your mat with your feet together, or as close as you can get them. Take a full breath. Stand tall, and extend your arms out to shoulder height, palms down. Bend your knees slightly, and elongate forward, placing your chest on your thighs and your hands on the ground at the sides of your feet. Bring your forehead into your knees, and keep your butt up. (You are not down in a squat.) Breathe long and slow. You will feel your back stretching.

If the back stretch feels okay, try straightening your legs. This is the full forward bend, and it opens the bladder meridian from the little toe up the legs and back to the crown of the head. Hold for five breaths, and then come up *slowly* by placing your palms on the lower back and rising up one vertebra at a time. When you are standing erect, close your eyes and breathe relaxed.

You can repeat this exercise two times.

Other recommended yoga *asanas* for Water types include the Butterfly (see page 38) and Yoga Mudra (see page 108).

We recommend a minimum of twenty minutes of exercise daily. The goal for Water types is to feel that you've accomplished something, pushing yourself a little harder than you did the day before while gradually developing your muscles and increasing your strength. Never push yourself to exhaustion (as Wood types tend to do), or you'll quickly drain your energy reserves.

HERBS

Western

Ginseng (*Panax ginseng, Panax quinquefolium, Eleutherococcus senticosus*): Ginseng is an ancient herbal remedy that stimulates the immune system, increases energy, relieves general weakness and exhaustion, eases physical and emotional stress, improves physical stamina, and stimulates the appetite. A strong brew of ginseng root in the morning might be just what you need to relieve stress, dispel tension, and gradually build up your strength and endurance.

Vervain (*Verbena officinalis*): Herbalists frequently use the soothing herb vervain to relieve mild pain, reduce inflammation, ease everyday tension and stress, and promote sleep. Vervain has a tranquilizing effect and is often used to alleviate everyday stress.

Dosage: If you purchase your herbs in a health food store (either in tincture form or, as dried herbs, in capsule or pill form), follow the dosage instructions on the label. Because herbs in dried form tend to lose their potency rather quickly, be sure to check the label for the expiration date.

For information on preparing your own herbs from the root, bark, leaves, flowers, or seeds of a plant, see Appendix II.

Chinese

Two Chinese patent remedies, one for deficient Kidney *yin* (Water) and the other for deficient Kidney *yang* (Fire), will help diminish your aches and pains and renew your energy:

GejieTa Bu Wan ("Gecko GreatTonifying Pills"): This superlative tonic is used to support the *yin, chi,* and blood and therefore is extremely valuable for general signs of deficiency—lethargy, fatigue, lower back pain, aching knees and joints, diminished sex drive, frequent urination, and benign prostate enlargement with diminished force of urinary flow. The Emperor ingredient in this formula is actually not an herb at all but dried, crushed, and powdered gecko lizard. The Chinese believe (and long experience with this herbal remedy confirms) that the gecko lizard cannot be rivaled in its ability to replenish Kidney energy; if the geckos are caught and killed while copulating, the *yang* (Fire) energy is considered even more potent (and the price goes up).

Attending herbs include rehmannia, polygonatum, dioscorea, ligustrum, poria fungus, dipsacus, cibotium, chaenomeles, morinda, atractylodes, ginseng, eucommia, astragalus, lyceum, drynaria, dong quai, and licorice.

Take four capsules three times daily or five to six capsules twice daily, unless otherwise directed by a qualified herbalist

Liu Wei Di HuangWan ("Six Flavor Rehmannia Pills"): When the *yin* (Water) reserves are depleted, the Chinese say "The *yin* is unable to embrace the *yang*," which results in false or deficient heat symptoms. If you suffer from signs of "deficient heat"—irritability, hot hands and feet, low-grade fevers, hot flashes, night sweats, or dark, strong-smelling urine—this Chinese patent remedy will gently cool your system and disperse the damp humidity that causes these symptoms. The Emperor herb is rehmannia root, a powerful Kidney *yin* tonic, which is supported by five additional Kidney-supporting herbs: cornus, dioscorea, moutan, poria fungus, and alisma.

Take eight pills (actually tiny pellets) three times daily or twelve pills twice daily, unless otherwise directed by a qualified herbalist.

Shou Wu Chih ("Polygonum Multiflorum Juice"): The herbal beverage Shou Wu Chih is unparalleled in fortifying the blood, nourishing the Kidneys, supporting the tendons and muscles, and helping you "age gracefully." Polygonum (*shou wu*), the Emperor herb in the formula, is supported by six attending herbs—dong quai, polygonatum, rehmannia root, ligusticum, amomum, and citrus seed. Shou Wu Chih is commonly used in China for problems associated with aging, and many elderly men and women take several tablespoons of this tasty concoction before dinner—an unusual but extremely effective herbal cocktail.

In Appendix I we offer a list of mail-order sources for high-quality Eastern and Western herbs and herbal preparations.

ACUPOINTS

CONCEPTION VESSEL 3 ("Central Pole"): Conception Vessel 3 is considered a powerful supporter of the *yin* (Water) energy and is traditionally used to restore sexual desire, enhance libido, "cool" hot flashes, and ease anxiety and general irritability. Also known as the *mu* (supportive) point for the Urinary Bladder, Conception Vessel 3 is commonly used for many bladder dysfunctions.

Common Uses

- Supports Kidney function, particularly the *yin* energy
- Promotes urination and helps to prevent and cure cystitis and incontinence
- Supports and nourishes the uterus, relieving menstrual disturbances including premenstrual syndrome (PMS), pelvic inflammatory disease, fibroids, and irregular menses

Location: Conception Vessel 3 is located on the midline of the lower belly, approximately one inch below the midpoint between the umbilicus and the top of the pubic bone.

KIDNEY 3 ("Great Mountain Stream"): This point is considered the generator and root of both Kidney *yin* (Water) and *yang* (Fire) energies. Stimulating this point generally supports and nourishes the Kidneys, relieving Kidney conditions characterized by depletion of energy.

Common Uses

- Relieves low back pain, knee pain, urinary incontinence or retention, and lack of sexual vigor and/or interest

- Restores energy, willpower, and motivation
- Indirectly supports the Liver *yin* and is used for depleted conditions where "heat" symptoms are prevalent, such as agitation, hot flashes, night sweats, insomnia, restless sleep, or "hot" (itchy or irritated) eyes

Location: Kidney 3 is located in the depression between the inside ankle bone and the Achilles tendon; use your fingers to poke around in the valley until you feel the tender spot.

In addition to these points, we'd like to mention an acupuncture technique that relies on an herb rather than needles or acupressure. When a patient complains of being cold or feeling chilled, the acupuncturist may use moxa, the dried flowers of the mugwort plant. The Chinese believe moxa is capable of penetrating deep into the system to disperse warmth and vital energy to all the vital organs. Moxa rolls, which look like cigars, are lighted with a match and held an inch or so above the areas that require warming. This ancient technique works wonders for dispelling dampness and cold and relieving the patient's discomfort.

INVIGORATING THE SENSES

Vision: Black or a deep bluish-black is the color associated with Water, and a strong attraction or repulsion to this color may indicate an imbalance in Water energy. In the West we associate the color black with grief and mourning, but in China black is considered an auspicious color signifying money, wealth, knowledge, career, and family. Wearing a black jacket or coat when applying for a job, strategically placing a black vase in your office, or arranging a series of black and white ink drawings in the central room in your house may bring you good fortune.

Imagery techniques can be helpful for backaches and lower back pain, common afflictions for Water. San Diego psychiatrist Dennis Gersten suggests the following exercise for back pain: Close your eyes, and imagine that you are carrying a hundred-pound bag on your back. Let the bag drop off your shoulders and fall to the ground. Spend a moment thinking about how light and carefree you feel without all that weight on your shoulders. Now sit down next to the bag and start rummaging through it, removing everything that is unnecessary, including painful memories, anger, resentment, grief, anxiety, and fear.

Sound: The ears are the sense organs governed by Water, and many hearing problems are the result of an imbalance in Water energy. Hypersensitive hearing as well as difficulty in hearing, a constant ringing in the ears (tinnitus), and vertigo (often caused by pressure in the inner ear) are common problems experienced by Water types. If you have hearing difficulties, your problem may signal an imbalance in Water energy rather than an actual physical defect. Before you invest in expensive diagnostic tests or hearing aids, you might want to make an appointment with an acupuncturist or herbalist to determine if your problems result from a Water imbalance.

The herb gingko, which increases the blood flow to the brain, can relieve tinnitus, although it may take two to three months before you notice any improvement. Magnesium deficiencies can also lead to tinnitus, so eat foods rich in this essential mineral—nuts, wheat germ, pumpkin seeds, seafood, potatoes, spinach, broccoli, and bananas—and take a daily magnesium supplement (500 mg., chelated with amino acids).

Water's sound is groaning or moaning. When the power of Water is out of balance, this vocal quality turns into an unconscious, persistent tone of whining that becomes pervasive and exaggerated.

The sound *"Whooooooooo"*—the mysterious, haunting sound associated with the wise owl's nightly call—can be soothing for water. Find a comfortable position with your spine erect, yet relaxed. Place your hands on your lower belly, just above Conception Vessel 4 (located halfway between the belly button and the pubic bone), and inhale deeply, imagining that you are breathing in a soft blue light and filling your cells with healing energy. Upon exhaling, say *"Whooooooooooo,"* imagining that you are releasing your fears into the infinite stretches of space. Continue this breathing exercise for five minutes.

Smell: A putrid, stagnant smell similar to the scent of flowers left to rot in a vase of stale water is associated with an imbalance in Water energy. To counteract Water imbalances, surround yourself with fresh flowers, making sure to replace the water every day.

Clean, fresh-smelling drinking water is also important for balancing Water energies. If your home is on a city water line, your drinking water is probably treated with chlorine and other disinfecting chemicals. We strongly recommend that you drink fresh spring water, distilled water, or properly filtered water. See Appendix I for information on purchasing water-filtering devices.

Frankincense and *myrrh,* both plant resins, are said to induce a spiritual state of consciousness, an appealing goal for Water types. If these incense fragrances do not appeal to you, experiment with different scents until you find one that seems to inspire you or soothe your spirit. Aromatherapists use lavender for many Water-related problems, including anxiety, depression, backaches, foot pain, hair loss, and muscle and joint pain.

Taste: If you suffer from a Water imbalance, you will probably love (or hate) the taste of salt. Salt cravings can also be a symptom of adrenal exhaustion, diabetes, and high blood pressure, so be sure to check with your doctor if you experience an unrelieved craving for salt.

Avoid indulging in salty foods, which can stress your Kidneys. Excess salt intake causes the Kidneys to excrete calcium, eventually draining the body's calcium stores and contributing to the development of osteoporosis. Swollen ankles, legs, and fingers and a bloated abdomen are signs of water retention, which is often the result of Kidney dysfunction.

If you crave salty foods, add seaweeds to your diet or use sea salt to season your food. Avoid using regular table salt. Vitamin C, potassium, and magnesium supplements can also help restore balance and reduce salt cravings.

Touch: Water energy provides the essential spark needed to maintain sexual desire and perform sexually. Infertility, frigidity, impotence, insufficient lubrication, and loss of libido are all associated with Water imbalances. Public displays of affection—kissing, holding hands, even sitting close to someone—can create intense anxiety and discomfort for Water types, as can a simple gesture of friendship such as an arm around the shoulder, a handshake, or a quick hug.

Water types need to have their boundaries respected, but an intense fear of touching signals an imbalance of energy that should be corrected. Learning how to risk contact with others, form attachments, and openly express affection are critical skills for Water types, particularly given your natural inclination to retreat into solitude.

Massage offers a means of safe and impersonal touching. Reiki massage, magnetic healing, and polarity therapy all appeal to Water types, but self-massage may be Water's preferred method. A simple foot massage is a wonderful way to invigorate Water energy—nine of the twenty-seven acupoints on the Kidney meridian are located below the calf, with six on the foot itself. (See the illustrations in Appendix III to locate these points.) When you massage your feet and ankles, use gentle pressure and circular motions, concentrating on the areas on or around the Kidney points. If certain points are more sensitive than others, spend a few extra minutes massaging them.

To reduce lower back pain, a common Water symptom, give yourself a backrub using tennis balls tied up in a sock. Lie down, and place the sock underneath the small of your back, with a tennis ball on either side of your spine. Move around gently to massage the lower back, gradually shifting your weight around to move the balls up your back, and then shifting again to move them back down.

You might also try massaging Kidney 10 ("Yin Valley"), the master point on the Kidney channel, located on the inner part of the knee crease between the two tendons. It is often used to replenish depleted Water supplies. We also recommend massaging Urinary Bladder 40 ("Bend at the Middle"), the master point on the Urinary Bladder meridian, which cools down fires raging anywhere in the body and relieves lower back pain. Urinary Bladder 40 is located behind the knee in the center of the crease. Be sure to use gentle pressure and rhythmic, circular motions with your fingers, as these points are located in soft, easily penetratable areas.

QUESTIONS TO ASK YOURSELF

If you feel off-balance or out of sorts with the world at large, these questions will help you discover the source of your distress and guide you to potential solutions. Focus on one or two questions that seem to relate most directly to your current problems or emotional state of mind.

- I spend a great deal of energy searching for "the truth": Why is truth so important to me? Is there just one truth, or can there be many truths? Is truth an absolute, or can there be such a thing as an ambiguous, imperfect truth?

- My greatest virtue is honesty, but I can be tactless and insensitive: How can I balance my innate need to be honest with sensitivity to the needs of others?
- I am often critical of other people, particularly those I consider uninformed or superficial: What can I do to become more tolerant of other people's flaws and imperfections?
- I detest having my space invaded by others: How can I firmly establish my boundaries without pushing people away?
- I yearn for connection to others, and yet I become extremely uncomfortable when someone touches me or is openly affectionate with me: How can I let people know I care about them while maintaining a physical distance?
- I need to be alone, and yet I fear being abandoned: How can I find a way to balance my need for solitude with time devoted to the people I love and respect?
- I can't have faith in something that can't be proven, yet I long for spiritual enlightenment: How can I convince myself that life has meaning and purpose, even though I may never discover what the meaning is?
- My greatest talent is my vivid imagination, but I often get carried away by my desire to penetrate the mysteries of the future or the secrets of the past: What can I do to keep myself centered in the present moment? How can I use my imagination creatively and constructively?
- My greatest fear is death: How can I accept my mortality without living in fear of it?

A Story for Water

If you have an affinity to Water, you are blessed with a deep sense of the power of silence, patience, and introspection. You have the strength of mind to know that "the right way" is your way, even if your way is not the "usual" or "normal" way. ("They will say that you are on the wrong road," Antonio Porchia warned, "if it is your own.") The balance for Water lies in keeping an open mind and studiously avoiding the tendency to proclaim that your path is "the one and only way" to truth, wisdom, or enlightenment.

If you keep yourself open to new interpretations and approaches, you will be able to avoid the traps of rigidity and inflexibility. As long as you respect your limitations and remain true to your basic nature, you will meet with good fortune. A wonderful Hasidic story shows us one way to maintain balance:

Two disciples of an old rabbi were arguing about the true path to God. One said that the path was built on effort and energy. "You must give yourself totally and fully with all your effort to follow the way of the Law. To pray, to pay attention, to live rightly." The second disciple disagreed. "It is not effort at all. That is only based on ego. It is pure surrender. To follow the way to God, to awaken, is to let go of all things and live the teaching: 'Not my will but thine.'"

As they could not agree on who was right they went to see the Master. He listened as the first disciple praised the path of wholehearted effort and when asked by this disciple, "Is this the true path?" the Master said, "You're right." The second disciple was quite upset and eloquently described the path of surrender and letting go. When he had finished, he said, "Is this not the true path?" and the Master replied, "You're right."

A third student who was sitting nearby said, "But Master, they can't both be right!"

The Master smiled and said, "You're right, too!"

Famous Water Types

Richard M. Nixon

Anne Frank

Woody Allen

Susan Sarandon

Bette Davis

Joan of Arc

Napoleon Bonaparte

Jimmy Carter

7. A DELICATE BALANCE

The Five Elemental Phases are always in a delicate balance.

—*The Yellow Emperor's Classic*

Every human being on this planet has a natural affinity to one of the Five Elements, an abiding connection that determines thoughts, feelings, needs, and desires. Gathering around this central organizing force, like planets circling the sun, are the four other elements, each exerting its own unique gravitational force on the planetary orbits. Just as the earth wobbles on its axis, at times tilting away from the sun and at other times leaning closer, so do the elements shift their positions through the seasonal cycles. In this dynamic, ever-changing system, the Five Elements are in constant movement, interchanging their energies in predictable patterns and rhythms, each element influencing the others and in turn influenced by them.

As the stars and planets in our solar system are guided by the universal laws of gravity, relativity, and thermodynamics, so is the orbiting dance of the Five Elements dependent on laws determined by the Control and Generation Cycles. The Generation Cycle regulates the nurturing, supportive relationships between the Five Elements, in which one element gives birth to and nurtures another. In this Mother/Child Cycle, Fire gives birth to Earth, Earth to Metal, Metal to Water, Water to Wood, and Wood to Fire in a never-ending cycle of regeneration and renewal. Refer to the generation cycle illustration on page 5.

When all Five Elements are in balance, each feeding into and being nourished by the others, health and harmony reign. If one element becomes dominant, however, the energy is gradually drained from the other elements, disrupting the delicate balance. The Control Cycle (page 6) keeps the elements in equilibrium, creating a system of checks and balances so that no one element dominates the others. In this cycle, Wood controls Earth by rooting the soil in its place and preventing erosion, while Earth contains Water by providing secure boundaries to prevent flooding. Water controls Fire, preventing it from blazing out of control, Fire controls Metal by keeping it flexible and allowing it to be molded into different forms, and Metal controls Wood by chopping down overgrowth to provide sufficient space for all forms of life to grow and thrive.

When the Generation and Control Cycles are combined, every element is connected to the others. Water, for example, generates Wood and is generated by Metal, while it controls Fire and is controlled by Earth. If Water is excessive, Wood becomes waterlogged, making it difficult to ignite the Fire. If the floodwaters keep rising, Earth's boundaries are gradually eroded away, and Water begins to spread and disperse its energies. As Earth becomes soggy, Metal drains away and can no longer invigorate Water with essential minerals and nutrients, eventually leading to a depletion of Water energy that, in turn, drains energy from the other elements.

Although the Generation and Control Cycles may seem ethereal and impractical, the delicate balance among the Five Elements directly influences your personality, emotional balance, physical vulnerabilities, and spiritual cravings. To illustrate the real-life implications of the Five Element System, let's look at the role Wood, Fire, Earth, Metal, and Water play in the lives of the authors of this book.

Jason's strong affinity to Earth was evident early in his childhood. Blessed with a cast-iron stomach and a sunny disposition, his greatest childhood pleasures centered on frequent family gatherings featuring dozens of laughing, chattering relatives and tables loaded with delicious food. Like many Earth types, food has always played a central role in his life. His mother loves to tell the story of flying with seven-year-old Jason to Miami Beach to visit relatives. In mid-flight Jason announced he was going to take a walk around the cabin; unbeknownst to his parents, he took the expensive box of chocolates intended for the Florida rel-

THE CONTROL CYCLE AND
GENERATION CYCLE COMBINED

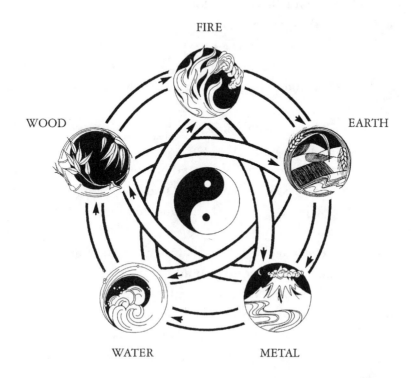

FIRE

WOOD

EARTH

WATER

METAL

atives and offered them to the passengers. "What a sweet boy you have!" several passengers complimented Jason's mother as they exited the plane.

Feeding others with food, compassion, and emotional support is a central theme in Jason's life. One of his favorite activities is cooking for his family and friends, and mealtimes are definitely the highlight of the day. Because he periodically experiences metabolic problems and tends to gain weight easily, he keeps a careful eye on his food intake and concentrates on eating healthy, nutritious foods. Other solid Earth traits include a profound need for peace and harmony, a natural talent for mediation, difficulty with changes or transitions, and a tendency to lethargy and sluggishness, particularly in humid weather conditions.

Water also has a significant effect on Jason's body, mind, and spirit. Knee injuries, joint pains, and back problems represent Water's influence on his physical makeup, while a lifelong fascination with spiritual issues, a profound need for silence and solitude, and an aversion to the cold, bleak landscapes of winter speak to Water's influence on his emotional and spiritual nature. Jason's Fire is also strong and steady, evident in his passion for his work and his desire to communicate his knowledge and experience to others.

Kathy is powerfully influenced by Fire, which tends to blaze out of control because of her strong secondary affinity to Wood. Her excess Fire drains her Water energy, which causes Wood to become brittle and dry, leading to periodic emotional flare-ups.

When Kathy was four years old, she also had a chocolate experience, but hers was very different from Jason's. At a family gathering at her grandmother's house, she took a large box of chocolates and hid under the dining room table. Her uncle loved to tell the story of finding her underneath the table, surrounded by empty candy wrappers, a guilty but contented smile on her chocolate-smeared face.

That tendency to consume life in large gulps rather than small nibbles is characteristic of everything Kathy does. Unafraid to take risks and confident in her abilities, she barges ahead with contagious enthusiasm, often neglecting to plan ahead. Affectionate, creative, empathic, and intuitive, she seeks out the vibrant colors and experiences of life. When agitated or stressed, she tends to overheat, which leads to emotional outbursts and physical problems like heart palpitations, anxiety attacks, and insomnia.

Her fiercely competitive nature, forceful personality, outspoken manner, and frustration when she doesn't get her way are all characteristic of strong Wood energy. Water also plays an important tertiary role, evident in her need to work alone, her idealism, her fascination with ancient religions and spiritual traditions, and her tendency to go her own way regardless of what others think. A craving for order and discipline (and an inability to maintain it due to the frenetic, scattered energy of excess Fire) suggest a deficiency in Metal, while a deficiency in Earth can be seen in her tendency to worry obsessively as well as her inability to let others take care of her.

Kathy and Jason have worked together for four years and have never had a major disagreement; their working relationship is characterized by deep respect, frequent laughter, and great affection. In large part they credit their harmonious working relationship to the fact that their affinities complement rather than compete with each other. Jason's strong Earth grounds Kathy's excess Fire, absorbing the heat of her energy without smothering the flames, while Kathy's blazing Fire brings joy and enthusiasm to Jason's Earth, sparking his underlying desire to communicate with others. Jason's natural attraction to Water also keeps Kathy's Fire under control, while Kathy's affinity to Water allows them to share their interests in spiritual matters and their profound respect for the natural world.

While the Five Elements combine and interact in hundreds of different configurations, they tend to join together in fairly predictable patterns determined by the Generation and Control Cycles. Earth/Water (Jason's type) is a common combination because Earth controls Water in the Control Cycle. Wood/Fire (Kathy's type) is another common type because Wood generates Fire in the Generation Cycle.

COMBINATIONS BASED ON THE GENERATION AND CONTROL CYCLES

Generation Cycle:
Wood/Fire
Fire/Earth
Earth/Metal
Metal/Water
Water/Wood

Control Cycle:
Fire/Metal
Earth/Water
Metal/Wood
Water/Fire
Wood/Earth

Of these ten combinations, six types—Wood/Earth, Wood/Fire, Earth/Water, Metal/Wood, Water/Fire, and Metal/Water—are the most common, representing approximately ninety percent of the patients Jason sees in his practice. In the remainder of this chapter, we'll take a closer look at these six combinations, illustrating each with a real-life case. After discussing the individual's primary and secondary affinities, we will briefly outline the different strategies used to restore harmony to body, mind, and spirit.

The purpose of this chapter is not to be exhaustive—the possible combinations are simply too numerous and diverse to cover adequately—but to give you a better sense of the inherent flexibility of the Five Element System. Once you understand how Wood, Fire, Earth, Metal and Water can combine and interact, changing shape and form through the seasons of your life, you will have a much better appreciation for the sensitivity of this system to individual differences. Every one of us is influenced by all of the Five Elements, yet the rhythm and flow of the energy is distinctly individual.

The Five Element System was never intended to "type" or categorize people, establishing rigid boundaries that narrowly define their personality and temperament; its sole purpose is to make you aware of your deep and abiding connections to the cycles and phases of the natural world and the need to live, in Qi Bo's words, "in accordance with the rhythmic patterns of the seasons: heaven and earth, moon, sun, and stars."

Wood/Earth

Wood is an aggressive, forceful energy that likes to strike out on its own, taking risks and engaging in wild, unpredictable adventures, while Earth tends to be docile and agreeable, most comfortable at home in a peaceful setting surrounded by friends, family, and plenty of good food. In the Control Cycle, Wood is said to restrain Earth, literally rooting the earth in its place to prevent the soil from eroding away. If Wood becomes excessive, however, it can take over Earth and gradually deplete its energies. Imagine a forest in which the trees continue to grow and spread until every inch of ground space is covered. Sunlight can't penetrate the dense canopy of leaves, and the soil can't support the entangled root systems. Saplings wither and die from lack of sun and insufficient nutrients in the soil, while the older, more established trees must continually compete for space.

This is the basic underlying scenario for thirty-nine-year-old Daniel. Relatively young and healthy, Daniel's problems did not extend beyond his two primary elements, Wood and Earth. If he had ignored his physical and emotional symptoms, however, the other elements eventually would have been compromised. When Wood becomes excessive, it can back up on the Control Cycle (somewhat like a clock that malfunctions and starts running backward) and control its controller—Metal. As Metal weakens, it is no longer able to nourish and regenerate Water, which is already near depletion because of its constantly demanding child (Wood). Deficient Water can't properly control Fire, which begins to blaze out of control, drying out and eventually exhausting Wood. Without proper checks and balances, an excess in any element eventually leads to imbalances of energy in all the elements.

I'm almost forty years old, and I'm fed up," Daniel said, his hands chopping at the air as he spoke. "I've got a nervous stomach and periodic bouts of diarrhea, which create all sorts of problems, but the migraine headaches are the worst. I take prescription drugs to deal with the pain, but they irritate my stomach, which leads to more digestive problems, and the cycle just goes on and on."

Daniel's chief complaints—migraine headaches and "nervous stomach" (irritable bowel syndrome)—are often associated with excess Wood energy; his no-nonsense, let's-get-down-to-business approach to life, general irritability, and tendency to erupt in anger, particularly when frustrated, are obvious signs of the aggressive, forceful energy of Wood. Stocky and muscular, with shoulders hunched up to his neck and knots of muscles in his chest and back, he demanded to be fixed up quickly so he could get on with his life—the classic Wood approach to most problems.

But as Daniel relaxed and opened up, another side of his nature began to emerge. An extremely sociable man, Daniel was driven by a strong need to be in the thick of things (Earth qualities). A school psychologist, he never stopped worrying about the students he counseled and constantly battled his own tendency to step in and solve their problems for them. A "wicked sweet tooth," a tendency to gain weight easily, and an intense aversion to being alone confirmed a strong undercurrent of Earth energy.

RESTORING HARMONY

Lifestyle: Daniel agreed to take five minutes between student appointments to practice breathing and relaxation techniques. Although he was familiar with these exercises and often suggested them to the teenagers he counseled, he claimed he had always been too busy to take his own advice. He particularly enjoyed the progressive relaxation exercise, Tense and Release (see page 32), in which he tensed and released each major muscle group beginning with the facial muscles and working down to the toes. The entire process, which took about five minutes, left him feeling relaxed and refreshed.

Diet: Daniel cut back on spicy, greasy, and fried foods, as well as alcohol and caffeine, all of which can trigger migraine headaches and irritate the intestinal tract. To help control his craving for sweets, I suggested he take a healthy snack (fruit, whole-wheat bread or crackers, juice) to work. For meals he concentrated on "Earth-friendly" foods such as rice, potatoes, whole-grain breads and pastas, and steamed vegetables. Although Daniel initially balked at the mention of organic (nonchemically treated) food, after reading John Robbins's eye-opening book *Diet for a New America,* he gave up meat altogether and became something of an expert on organic gardening.

Exercise: Daniel was an admitted "couch potato" (definitely an Earth quality). He did enjoy a competitive game of racquetball, however, and began to play twice a week after work at the local YMCA.

Chinese herbal formulas: Hsiao Yao Wan ("Relaxed Wanderer Pills") helped support Daniel's Liver (the organ associated with Wood) by breaking through obstructions and restoring the free flow of energy and blood. Bu Zhong Yi Qi Wan ("Support the Center, Benefit Energy Pills") strengthened his Stomach, Spleen, and Pancreas (the organs associated with Earth) by improving his digestion and stimulating his metabolism.

Western herbs: Daniel's herbal tonic consisted of dandelion root (a digestive aid and liver tonic), milk thistle (a liver tonic), feverfew (a digestive aid and extremely effective migraine remedy), St. John's wort (a nervous system tonic with antidepressant and anti-anxiety actions), and lemon balm (a gentle, relaxing herb often used to treat digestive disorders).

Acupoints: Spleen 6 ("Three Yin Meeting") and Stomach 36 ("Walks Three Miles") are often used together to restore balance, increase energy, and revitalize digestive functions. Daniel also liked to press Liver 3 ("Great Rushing"), which is viewed as a physical, emotional, and spiritual Roto-Rooter, breaking up internal blockages that can lead to such symptoms as migraines and irritable bowel syndrome.

Invigorating the senses: Of all the senses, Daniel responded most immediately to touch, so it didn't take much prodding to convince him to schedule a weekly massage. After a few weeks he insisted that this was the healing remedy he couldn't live without.

Wood/Fire

In the Generation Cycle the aggressive, forceful energy of Wood keeps the passionate energy of Fire burning. If Wood becomes excessive, however, Fire tends to flare up and create excess heat throughout the body, mind, and spirit. While everyone periodically experiences Fire flare-ups when excited or agitated, the fires usually cool down fairly quickly. Wood/Fire types, on the other hand, tend to have difficulty controlling the thermostat, and their fires often flare up and blaze out of control.

Water is almost always a tertiary influence for Wood/Fire types, because Water is responsible for restraining Fire in the Control Cycle and nourishing Wood in the Generation Cycle. When Wood becomes excessive and stokes up Fire, the alarm goes off and the sprinkler system goes on. If this condition continues, the diminished Water reservoirs are unable to nourish Wood (Water's "child" in the Generation Cycle), leading to symptoms like migraine headaches, tense muscles, frustration, and explosive anger. As Wood weakens, Fire sputters and sparks, with brief explosions of energy followed by signs of deficiency like anxiety, nervousness, exhaustion, and depression.

In twenty-eight-year-old Natalie's case, excess Wood and Fire had drained her Water energy, leading to a "deficient *yin,* False Fire" condition. Her blazing Fire signs were actually symptoms of insufficient Water reserves rather than signs of excess Fire, for the Fire had burned too hot for too long, creating a condition of deficient water. The recent birth of a child had further drained Natalie's Water energy, which was unable to feed and nourish Wood, leading to problems in many areas.

Am I dying?" Natalie asked, her voice trembling. "Everything I eat goes right through me. I feel sick to my stomach all the time, and I'm scared to death."

Extremely thin with a pleasantly rosy complexion that deepened to bright crimson when she was agitated, Natalie's main complaint was a long history of food intolerances, which she had handled for years by avoiding all wheat and dairy products. After the birth of her first child ten months earlier, however, the tell-tale symptoms of overwhelming fatigue, mood swings, depression, muscle weakness and pain, insomnia, diarrhea, nausea, vomiting, and hives returned, and nothing she ate or stopped eating seemed to make a difference. "I'm just completely stressed out," she said, tears streaming down her cheeks.

I offered Natalie the Chinese explanation for her symptoms: The stress in Natalie's life was causing her Liver to work too hard, drying out her Wood energy, which, in turn, caused her Fire energy to burn too quickly and, at times, flare out of control. With brushfires blazing everywhere, her Water reserves were nearing depletion.

"That makes a lot of sense," Natalie said, wiping away her tears. "Now tell me—where can I find a fire extinguisher?"

RESTORING HARMONY

Lifestyle: An artist with a successful silver jewelry business, Natalie mourned the loss of the time she used to spend in her studio creating new designs for her collection. Although initially reluctant to hire a baby-sitter (as a child she had often been left alone with a housekeeper and vowed she would never do the same to her child), she eventually found a loving elderly woman to watch her baby for two hours every weekday morning. With just those few hours to herself, she felt completely rejuvenated.

Natalie loved music, so we created a meditation exercise in which she spent half an hour every day simply holding her baby and listening to her favorite CDs. Practicing the Belly Breath (see page 80) also helped her cope with the stresses of motherhood and chronic illness.

Diet: Because of her "hot" (Fire) nature and her tendency to flare up physically and emotionally, Natalie agreed to eliminate caffeine and spicy foods. When she learned that bitter foods are supportive of the Liver (Wood) and the Heart (Fire), she started adding bitter greens (endive, kale, Swiss chard, and dandelion greens) to her daily salad; in the spring and summer she sprinkled her salads with pansies and nasturtiums, both of which are edible. Rice, tofu, and deep sea fish (salmon, mackerel, halibut, tuna) were all safe and enjoyable foods for her. She continued to avoid dairy and wheat products.

For three months Natalie concentrated on this fairly restrictive diet, and during that period she discovered that she enjoyed finding creative ways to cook these nourishing foods. After three months she slowly added different foods back into her diet and found that she could tolerate wheat products in small amounts. Even an occasional ice cream cone didn't cause any problems for her.

Exercise: Both Wood and Fire types thrive on constant movement to maintain physical health and emotional well-being, but due to the constraints of motherhood Natalie found it difficult to find time to exercise. One day she came into my office and in her usual exuberant style announced that she had found a solution: "I put on some great boogie music, pick up my baby, and dance like a mad fool around the living room. The baby laughs out loud the whole time!"

Chinese herbs: Hsiao Yao Wan ("Relaxed Wanderer Pills") is the standard remedy for "constrained Liver *chi*" (obstructed Wood energy), especially when digestive symptoms are present. To support her Kidneys and replenish her diminished Water reserves, Natalie also took Tian Wang Bu Xin Wan ("Heavenly Emperor, Tonify the Heart Pills"), a Chinese patent remedy often used to harmonize the spirit, resolve restlessness and anxiety, and ease insomnia.

Western herbs: Natalie's herbal formula consisted of dandelion root (a liver and digestive tonic), hawthorn berries (a heart balancer and digestive aid), gentian (a cooling herb with supportive digestive qualities), lemon balm (a gentle, relaxing digestive herb), and licorice (an anti-inflammatory, liver-supportive herb that helps balance the actions of different herbs in a formula).

Acupoints: Liver 3 ("Great Rushing") and Pericardium 6 ("Inner Gate") are often used together to resolve "constrained Liver *chi*." When Wood (Liver) energy builds up, it can invade the Stomach and Spleen, causing problems like nausea, excess gas or bloating, irritable bowels, and colitis; pressing and massaging these two points provided Natalie with significant relief from these problems. (These points are also recommended for patients who are agitated or anxious or seem to have lost hope.)

Invigorating the senses: Touch—specifically *being* touched—was the one sensual area that was consistently neglected in Natalie's life. One day when I commented on how much she seemed to enjoy holding her baby, she burst into tears. "My husband and I never touch each other anymore," she said. "Since the baby was born, we're so exhausted at the end of the day that we just roll over and go to sleep."

Once again Natalie's creative energies helped her find a solution to her problem. She bought some lavender-scented massage oil, and two or three nights a week just before bedtime, she and her husband give each other a light massage. "I light the candles, turn off the light, and lo and behold—we aren't tired anymore!"

Earth/Water

In the Control Cycle the solid, stable qualities of Earth provide a natural boundary for Water's forceful, directed energy. When Earth is strong, it can contain raging rivers and withstand the relentless ebb and flow of the sea. If Earth weakens, however, Water begins to erode the riverbanks and coastal areas, gradually undermining Earth's control. Eventually, Water overflows its boundaries, spreading and dispersing its natural energy.

When its natural boundaries collapse, Water loses its direction; spread out over the landscape, its energy is dissipated. As Water weakens, it can no longer adequately nourish Wood, which begins to shrivel and wilt from neglect. Imagine a swampy area where the water ponds up in stagnant pools, the trees are covered with fungus and mold, and the air smells of decay. This is a vivid image for the problems that confronted forty-two-year-old James, whose depleted Earth energies were unable to restrain Water, leading to digestive problems, difficulties setting boundaries in his relationships, and escalating fear and worry.

Tears filled James's eyes when he talked about having to give up his job as an advertising design specialist. A year earlier, he'd been involved in a serious moped accident while on vacation in Bermuda and had injured his back. At times the pain was so severe that he couldn't sit up for an hour at a time, let alone work for eight hours a day. Eventually, James was forced to move in with his mother, whom he adored but who smothered him with love, food, and unwelcome advice.

A strong affinity to Earth was evident in James's stocky build, soft muscle tone, problems with weight control, and history of digestive problems. Even his close but stifling relationship with his mother suggested an Earth imbalance, for Earth types often have difficulty setting firm boundaries in their relationships. Yet the persistent moaning quality to his voice, a lifelong proclivity to lower back and knee pain, sexual problems that had inhibited his relationships with women, and an intense fear bordering on a phobia of intimacy confirmed that Water was equally influential in his makeup.

James enjoyed discussions about Chinese medicine and immediately grasped the metaphors associated with both Earth and Water. When I explained that his Earth energy was depleted and could no longer contain or control his Water energy, he thought for a moment and then said: "Kind of like the creek by our house that periodically floods the property," he said. After another moment, he added, "I can see that—I definitely feel like my feet are stuck in the mud."

RESTORING HARMONY

Lifestyle: Without a steady job and daily work responsibilities to direct his energies, James spent his days brooding about the future. We talked about the activities he used to enjoy, and he mentioned a lifelong love of classical music. "I always used to get great ideas when I listened to Wagner or Beethoven—my two favorite composers—but now I'm so depressed that I can't even find the energy to turn on the radio." Agreeing that music might help him emerge from his funk, he set up a stereo system in his room and often retreated there when he was feeling overwhelmed by his mother's constant attention and concern. James also decided to keep a daily journal, carefully recording all the activities he wanted to pursue when he recovered.

Diet: James loved to eat, and it was the one part of his life that had not been affected by the accident. Although at first I was concerned about his intense love affair with food, it turned out to be his salvation. Searching for healthy gourmet recipes, James bought dozens of cookbooks and created elaborate meal plans and seven-course dinners for his family and friends. A year after he began treatment, he opened a small gourmet delicatessen and soon developed a successful catering business.

Exercise: Although James intensely disliked physical exercise ("Walking up and down the stairs is more than enough for me"), he agreed to try tai chi, a perfect exercise for Earth/Water types—Earth types appreciate the gentle, nonjarring movements, the lack of competition, and the camaraderie of the classes, while Water types respond to the spiritual emphasis on grounding and centering. After just a few classes he realized the positive effects of exercise on his digestive system and his emotional stability, and he made a commitment to exercise on a regular basis.

Chinese herbs: Earth/Water types often benefit from combining two Chinese formulas: Bu Zhong Yi Qi Wan ("Support the Center, Benefit Energy Pills") and Gejie Ta Bu Wan ("Gecko Great Tonifying Pills"). James absolutely refused to have anything to do with dried gecko lizards, however, so I suggested Shih Chuan Ta Bu Wan ("Ten Ingredient Great Tonifying Pills") as a substitute.

The patent formula Yunnan Pai Yao ("Yunnan White Powder") helped speed up the healing process and relieve his pain. I often use Yunnan Pai Yao for acute pain immediately after an accident or injury and for chronic pain from an old injury; the results can be quite dramatic.

Western herbs: James's formula consisted of eleutherococcus ginseng (to support both his Earth and Water energy), ginger (a warming digestive herb), crampbark (a nervine tonic herb, with muscle-relaxing qualities), meadowsweet (a natural anti-inflammatory herb often used for digestive problems), and licorice (an anti-inflammatory herb).

Acupoints: Kidney 3 ("Great Mountain Stream") helped replenish the depleted Water reserves, while Spleen 3 ("Great Brightness") invigorated his Earth energy. I also suggested that James massage the areas around the inside and outside ankle bones. The Kidney and Urinary Bladder meridians run through this area and extend to the lower back, and massaging these points can help relieve many kidney and bladder disorders.

Invigorating the senses: When James learned that yellow—Earth's color—represents longevity in Chinese medicine, he resolved to add more yellow to his life. Yellow fruits and vegetables were prominently displayed in the windows of his delicatessen, and yellow daisies graced the tables during every season of the year. Lemon balm tea soothed his digestive system, and his water glass always contained a slice of fresh lemon.

Metal/Wood

In the Control Cycle the sharp, cutting edge of Metal restrains the aggressive, expansive energy of Wood. If Metal is too strong, it inhibits Wood, leading to a lack of growth, spontaneity, and sense of adventure, various physical and emotional obstructions, and a general inflexibility of body, mind, and spirit. If Metal energy is deficient, Wood becomes aggressive and overfeeds Fire. Fire, in its turn, overheats Metal, liquefying its hard-edged power and further weakening its control over Wood.

In Chinese terminology an excess in any element can create a Humiliation Cycle in which the dominant element turns around and controls its controller. In the case of Wood and Metal, excess Wood backs up and "humiliates" Metal, which then loses control over its domain (the Lungs, Large Intestine, nose, body hair, and Skin), leaving these areas vulnerable to insult and injury. Excess Wood energy also demands too much from its energy source, Water, which can create depression, insomnia, fatigue, and irritability. This is what happened to forty-eight-year-old Suzanne, whose natural affinities to Metal and Wood were gradually weakened by overwork, inadequate exercise, and general neglect of her emotional and spiritual needs.

A psychology professor specializing in women's studies, Suzanne appeared as if she were on the verge of collapse. Although nearly six feet tall and sturdily built, with well-developed muscle tone, her shoulders sagged as she walked slowly to the chair and sat down with a heavy sigh. Suzanne's physical problems—chronic fatigue, intestinal problems (abdominal pain, bloating, diarrhea), recurrent sinusitis, and general immune depletion—were complicated by premenopausal symptoms, including periodic bouts with depression, mood swings, and insomnia.

An affinity to Metal was immediately obvious from her fastidious appearance, the soft, sad quality of her voice, the high standards she set for her work and personal life, her formal, somewhat distant manner, and her physical symptoms. A strong connection to Wood was also evident in her sturdy body type, in the way her voice began to rise, escalating to a near-shout whenever she talked about equality for women and other issues close to her heart, and in her ability to continue teaching, writing, and organizing conferences despite her overwhelming fatigue.

RESTORING HARMONY

Lifestyle: Suzanne enjoyed working under pressure, and deadlines tended to excite her rather than stress her out (Wood qualities), yet as her reputation spread and she became more involved in the university's political battles, she began to feel stifled. "I'm sick of all these committee meetings and bureaucratic red tape," she said. "I need room to breathe." Lifestyle changes included resigning from several committees and board positions, establishing stricter office hours, and making a firm commitment to concentrate her attention only on those issues that meant the most to her. Ridding her life of clutter, both physical and emotional, helped her feel more in control.

As Suzanne intuitively realized, she needed room to breathe, both literally and figuratively. Breathing exercises helped ground her, and she particularly enjoyed the Calming Breath (see page 59), which involves inhaling, holding your breath, and then exhaling, all to a specific count. When she exhaled, she liked to say, "Ssssssssssss," the sound of the snake, which, she carefully explained, was worshipped by ancient goddess societies as a symbol of physical and spiritual renewal.

Diet: A vegetarian and gourmet cook, Suzanne was well versed in nutrition and healthy eating. I was concerned, however, about her dependence on milk, cream, cheese, cottage cheese, and yogurt for her protein and calcium needs. She agreed to eliminate dairy products from her diet for a four-week trial period. When her clogged sinuses and intestinal complaints improved dramatically, she enthusiastically eliminated milk products from her diet altogether and claimed that her general outlook on life was also much improved.

Exercise: When Suzanne got caught up in her various projects, she forgot to exercise, often for weeks at a time. Because she loved to walk and claimed that it cleared her head and helped her organize her day, she decided to change her schedule to wake up half an hour earlier every morning and take a brisk two-mile walk. She recently purchased a treadmill for those days when the weather prohibits her from exercising outside.

Chinese herbs: Hsiao Yao Wan ("Relaxed Wanderer Pills") strengthened Suzanne's overstressed Liver (the Wood organ), and Bi Yan Pian ("Benefit the Nose Tablets") quickly cleared up her sinuses.

Western herbs: Suzanne's formula included dandelion root (a gentle but powerful liver tonic), elecampane (a soothing Lung tonic and gentle expectorant), echinacea (an antimicrobial and immune-supportive herb), osha root (an antimicrobial herb with specific anti-allergy actions), licorice root (a gentle expectorant and support for the mucous linings of the respiratory tract), and a small amount of ephedra, also called *ma huang* (a powerful herb often used for treating asthma, allergies, and upper respiratory infections).

Acupoints: The Liver meridian is said to carry Wood energy, while the Large Intestine is a Metal channel. Pressing Liver 3 ("Great Rushing") helped move

Suzanne's "stuck" energy, while massaging Large Intestine 4 ("Great Eliminator") and Large Intestine 20 ("Receiving Fragrance") helped open and clear out her sinuses.

Invigorating the senses: Suzanne grew up in the suburbs of San Francisco in a house surrounded by eucalyptus shrubs, and the pleasant aroma of eucalyptus immediately brought back happy childhood memories. During her morning shower, she put a few drops of the essential oil of eucalyptus (the chemical eucalyptol) on a wet washcloth and hung the washcloth in the shower. As the steam built up, the vapors filled the shower stall, and she took deep, long breaths of the sweet, healing fragrance. Suzanne also purchased a forty-dollar aromatic diffuser, which she uses regularly in her office to the delight of her students and colleagues.

Water/Fire

In the Control Cycle the cooling, liquid energy of Water controls the hot, passionate energy of Fire. When the body's Water reserves are sufficient, the fires are easily contained, but if Water weakens and is not replenished, even a small brushfire can quickly become a major conflagration. The problem is compounded by the fact that Water generates and nourishes Wood. Without sufficient Water, Wood becomes brittle and dry. The excess Fire feeds on the dwindling wood, and it doesn't take long before the fires die out, having exhausted their available supply of Wood energy.

This is the general background for fifty-five-year-old Mary, whose long history of kidney problems and urinary tract infections weakened her Water energy to the point that it could no longer nourish Wood or control Fire. For years her Fire had blazed out of control, further draining her Water reserves and depleting the available supply of Wood energy. By the time she came to see me, both her Water and Fire energies were nearing depletion.

Ten years ago Mary was diagnosed with lupus, an autoimmune disease that was attacking her joints and, to a lesser extent, her kidneys. Her history of urinary tract infections complicated her life to the point that she decided to try acupuncture and, possibly, herbal therapy. "I'm afraid that all the antibiotics I take for the urinary infections are weakening my immune system," she said, "but I'm also afraid to take herbs because the doctor said they might harm my kidneys. I don't know where to turn."

Mary was thin, almost emaciated looking, with a pale complexion, dark circles under her eyes, and a distinct moaning quality to her voice (all Water qualities). Her physical symptoms were also Water-related; in addition to lupus and chronic urinary tract infections, she had a history of lower back pain and stiffness, especially in the mornings and after exertion, and extreme fatigue in the late afternoon (Water's hours).

I also noted an affinity to Fire in her history of panic attacks and heart palpitations, her tendency to become agitated and anxious when she was stressed, and her exceptionally serious demeanor (indicating a deficiency in Fire). When I tried to get her to laugh by telling a joke, she became very cross with me. "This is serious," she said, tears in her eyes. "Please—can't you help me?"

RESTORING HARMONY

Lifestyle: A deeply spiritual person—before she became a social worker, she had considered joining a religious order—Mary often had trouble separating her own problems from other people's miseries. "The Chinese would say that the gates to your heart are stuck open," I said, "and you are being consumed by emotions. You need to bring more Fire into your Water, which is simply another means of saying that you need more joy and light in your life."

Bringing more light into her life was important both literally and figuratively. As Mary talked about her problems, she expressed a long-standing hatred for winter, explaining that her lupus symptoms often intensified during the winter months, when she suffered from mood swings and periodic bouts of depression as well. We talked about seasonal affective disorder (SAD), a depressive illness caused by a lack of exposure to natural light, and Mary decided to purchase a full-spectrum light; her health insurance company eventually reimbursed her. Within two weeks she noticed a distinct improvement in her moods and general outlook on life.

After she began to feel better physically and emotionally, Mary talked about her relationship with her husband of thirty years. Although she loved him dearly, their relationship had settled into a "rather boring" routine of coming home from work, eating dinner (without much conversation), watching the news, and going to bed by 9:00 P.M. When I asked her what they used to do for fun, she laughed and said, "Tango—we always loved to tango!" The next day she signed up for ballroom dance classes at the local community college.

Diet: Mary was basically a vegetarian, although she occasionally ate fish, cheese, and eggs. Her one weakness was salty foods, especially pretzels and tortilla chips. When she splurged, she could eat an entire bag of chips at one sitting.

I explained that while some salt in her diet was fine, too much could create problems, increasing the risk of high blood pressure and congestive heart failure. ("Overindulgence in salty foods will coagulate the blood circulation and will change the color of the blood," Qi Bo warned nearly five thousand years ago.) When she craved salt, I suggested she eat seafood, use sea salt, drink lots of fresh, filtered water (at least eight 8-ounce glasses daily) to replenish her Water reserves, and concentrate on eating water-rich foods, especially fruits and vegetables.

To help prevent the chronic urinary infections, I recommended cranberry extract mixed with water and a teaspoon or two of maple syrup to sweeten it. I strongly advised her to avoid store-bought cranberry juice, which is loaded with sugar.

Exercise: Ballroom dancing proved to be wonderful exercise for Mary and her husband, although they quickly realized the importance of stretching and limbering exercises before dance class. Fifteen minutes of yoga every day combined with deep breathing exercises increased her flexibility, and a three-mile walk with her husband every morning firmed and toned her muscles.

Chinese herbs: I suggested Mary take the patent formula Tian Wang Bu Xin Wan ("Heavenly Emperor, Tonify the Heart Pills"), which nourishes and supports both the Kidney (Water) and Heart (Fire) energies.

Western herbs: Mary's formula consisted of hawthorn berries (a heart balancer and digestive aid), motherwort (a heart tonic with relaxing qualities), vervain (a

Kidney tonic with anti-inflammatory and tranquilizing actions), uva ursi (a natural diuretic with soothing effects on the urinary tract), barberry (a natural antibiotic with immune-boosting and liver-supporting actions), and couchgrass (a soothing, lubricating herb for the mucous linings of the urinary tract).

Acupoints: Pressing or massaging Conception Vessel 3 ("Central Pole") supported Mary's Kidney *yin* (Water) energy, while Kidney 3 ("Great Mountain Stream") restored her energy and willpower, and Heart 7 ("Spirit Gate") soothed her spirit, reduced her anxiety, and helped her sleep.

Invigorating the senses: To reignite Mary's Fire—her love of life and her will to live—I suggested that she try to laugh more often. I loaned her my copy of Norman Cousins's book *Anatomy of an Illness,* and the next time I saw her, she announced that the book had inspired her to try a "laugh cure." Every Friday night she and her husband rented movies featuring comedians such as the Marx Brothers, Charlie Chaplin, the Three Stooges, Robin Williams, and Steve Martin.

"Once I started to laugh again," Mary recently told me, "I realized how much I missed it. My husband and I promised each other we wouldn't let a day go by without telling a few jokes or watching a funny movie."

Metal/Water

In the Generation Cycle the disciplined yet malleable energy of Metal gives birth to the yielding yet strong-willed power of Water. If Metal energy becomes unbalanced for any reason, Water is immediately and powerfully affected. When Metal is excessive, it will overnourish Water, which like a spoiled child continues to demand everything it can get from its doting parent. Eventually the mother (Metal) weakens, and the deprived child (Water) becomes even more demanding. As Metal continues to weaken, Water begins to languish from neglect, leading to anxiety, phobias, and feelings of being overwhelmed or inundated. As Water begins to flow sluggishly and erratically, Wood (Water's child in the Generation Cycle) becomes irritable and inflamed, contributing to high blood pressure, migraine headaches, irritability, and explosive outbursts.

Thirty-five-year-old Lenny had a natural constitutional affinity to both Water and Metal. His high-stress job and fast-moving lifestyle eventually depleted his natural energies, leading to increasingly serious physical and emotional problems.

My wife has been after me for years to come see you because she hates all the drugs I have to take for my asthma," Lenny told me in our first session. "But I kept putting it off until I started having prostate problems and my blood pressure began to rise. 'Okay,' I thought, 'now it's time.'"

An architect by profession, Lenny was a handsome man who reminded me at different times of Clint Eastwood and Woody Allen. With his deep chiseled features, piercing eyes, and rare but winning smile (all Metal qualities), he looked like Eastwood in his younger days; but when he talked, I could hear Woody Allen's voice, a kind of moaning, whining quality indicating a deficiency in Water. Lenny's interest in art and philosophy, his perfectionist tendencies, and the intense grief he experienced as he approached middle age spoke to a strong Metal constitution, but Water clearly played an important secondary role. Lower back pain, tinnitus (ringing in the ears), soft, puffy skin, and prematurely gray hair indicated a Water imbalance, and Lenny was definitely overwhelmed by Water's primary emotion (fear), talking at length about his precarious financial situation and fears of being trapped forever in his architectural firm, which he claimed was run by "immoral and unscrupulous" people.

RESTORING HARMONY

Lifestyle: Lenny took a three-pronged approach to changing his lifestyle— short-term counseling to help him deal with his irrational fears and phobias; meditation to help him relax and cope with the stress of his chronic illnesses; and long-term financial planning to ease his mind and allay his fears about the future.

Of the three strategies, he credited the financial planning with bringing him the greatest peace of mind. After receiving advice from several experts, Lenny diversified his stock holdings, increased the amount he put into retirement savings, and updated his will, which was nearly fifteen years old. "Now I feel prepared for anything," he said.

Diet: When Lenny was in his twenties, his sister, a nutritionist, suggested that he eliminate dairy products; the immediate improvement in his health convinced him to strictly avoid those foods. He had a fondness for meat and a weakness for foods high in nitrates like sausage, pepperoni, salami, and ham. When I explained that smoked and nitrate-treated foods can convert to carcinogenic substances in the body, Lenny held up his hands and said, "Say no more." Lenny needed no convincing when it came to cancer: Both sets of grandparents had died of it, his mother had just been diagnosed with breast cancer, and he was deathly afraid that his recurring prostate problems might lead to prostate cancer.

A diet rich in complex carbohydrates, featuring lots of fresh vegetables, fruits, fruit juices, legumes (beans, lentils, peas), and deep sea fish (salmon, trout, tuna), kept Lenny healthy and happy. Every day without fail he drank ten 8-ounce glasses of water to replenish his Water reserves and help his kidneys flush the accumulated toxins from his system.

Exercise: Always looking for the most efficient way to do things, Lenny decided to incorporate exercise into his daily routine by parking his car half a mile from work and walking up and down the stairs to his fourth-floor office. The only sport he really enjoyed was golf, and on weekends he promised to set time aside to play eighteen holes with his wife.

Acupoints: Lenny liked to press Lung 9 ("Great Abyss"), which is often used to support the *wei chi* (immune energy) and strengthen the *chi* to prevent upper respiratory infections and asthma. Located on the crease on the palm side of the wrist, this point also helped him "let off steam" when he was cooped up in a meeting or stuck in a traffic jam.

Kidney 3 ("Great Mountain Stream") helped support his Water energy, easing his prostate problems, stabilizing his blood pressure, and increasing his energy and motivation.

Invigorating the senses: Lenny's high-pressure job and active social life left him little time to enjoy the silence and solitude that most Metal/Water types need to rejuvenate their energies. Although he wasn't immediately aware of the loss, he admitted that he rarely took the time to sit down and be still, soaking in his surroundings. "I don't know when I last saw the sun set or the moon rise," he said.

The sense organs associated with Metal and Water are the nose and the ears. To invigorate his sense of hearing, Lenny bought several meditation tapes featuring the sounds of a river, a waterfall, and the sea. Listening to the tapes in his car on the way to work, he found that he enjoyed them so much that he set up a tape recorder in his room and used the tapes to help him fall asleep at night. Lenny's sense of smell had always been acute, and he enthusiastically experimented with aromatherapy oils. His favorite was white flower oil; every morning he put a drop of the oil on his nostrils, claiming that it helped cool the air and open up his nasal passages.

Daniel, Natalie, James, Suzanne, Mary, and Lenny are real people whose cases help us understand how different elements combine and interact to create specific constellations of symptoms. Practitioners of Chinese medicine approach every patient as an individual and view each symptom in the context of that patient's personality, relationships, lifestyle, emotional makeup, spiritual needs, and physical strengths or weaknesses. While you may have an affinity to Earth/Water like James or Wood/Fire like Natalie, your symptoms will be unique, and your strategies for healing will be wholly individual.

Now that you have a basic understanding of how the Five Elements combine and interact, you can see that even though you may have a natural affinity to one or two elements, that connection is either strengthened or weakened by the flow of energy from the other elements. This might be a good time to refer back to the questionnaire in Chapter 1, noting the strengths and weaknesses of your affinities with each of the Five Elements. You might also want to review Chapters 2 through 6, taking special note of physical, emotional, or behavioral symptoms that may indicate an excess or deficiency in a particular element.

As you read through the chapters and consider the various healing remedies, don't be afraid to try out different combinations of herbs, exercises, acupoints, dietary strategies, and breathing techniques. All the healing strategies offered in this book are safe and gentle and can be used without fear of harm. Use what works for you, remembering that each of the Five Elements holds a special place in the vast landscape of your life.

At certain times in our lives we have all been blessed with images of a world in which the Five Elements are perfectly balanced. In a scene from a movie or a still photograph, or perhaps just by looking out your window, you see the sun (Fire) gently shining on fields of grain (Earth) edged by sturdy pines and graceful birches (Wood). A clean, sparkling river (Water) courses through the landscape, and in the distance snow-capped mountains (Metal) reach upward, beckoning silently to the sun, moon, and stars.

In the splendor of the moment, your breath catches, for the picture before you contains all the elements essential for life. When Wood, Fire, Earth, Metal, and Water nourish and sustain each other to create harmony within your body, mind, and spirit, the delicate balance is equally beautiful to behold.

Part Two

THE HEALING ZONES

Seeing into darkness is clarity.
Knowing how to yield is strength.
Use your own light
and return to the source of light.
This is called practicing eternity.

—*Tao Te Ching*

Introduction to Part Two

More than six hundred years ago, Chinese philosophers and physicians developed a system of classifying diseases based on the degree to which an invading pathogen is able to penetrate the body's defenses ("the Pattern of Four Stages"). In this system, which we have adapted to fit the chronic diseases and disorders of the modern world, the body is imagined as a well-defended kingdom protected by four powerful healing zones. The first level of defense (the *wei chi*) guards the perimeter of the kingdom; the second level consists of an invisible energy force that flows through an underground series of channels or "meridians" traversing the entire kingdom; the third level is ruled by the blood, which courses through another series of underground vessels; and the fourth level is defended by the organs, elite royal guards that stand ready to defend the very heart and soul of the kingdom.

The metaphor of the body as a peaceful but well-defended kingdom shifts the focus from the destructive course of the disease to the miraculous regenerative powers of the body, mind, and spirit. To prevent illness, the vital energy within must be balanced, free-flowing, and continually replenished. Once you learn how to identify the early symptoms of imbalance, you can actively and consciously work to invigorate your energy when it is weak or sluggish, or calm it down when it is rebellious. This system views disease as a temporary breakdown in your internal defenses that can be rectified with proper care and attention.

This subtle, yet radical, shift in metaphoric perspective will help you learn to think of illness as a precautionary warning sign that your body's defenses are vulnerable and need to be strengthened. You will understand that pain is part of the body's early warning system, a symptom of an underlying obstruction or blockage of energy. Rather than living in fear of invasion from numerous malignant agents, you will discover that the most effective way to combat disease is to keep your body, mind, and spirit in harmonious balance. Feelings of passive resignation will give way to active involvement in caring for your body as well as feelings of power and pride as you become fully conscious of the miraculous self-healing capabilities that exist within.

The life-force flows in streams, pools, and oceans deep within the body's kingdom. The challenge is to tap into these inner reservoirs of vital energy to strengthen your defenses against disease.

8. LEVEL ONE: THE *WEI CHI*

Be aware when things are out of balance.

—*Tao Te Ching*

The *wei chi,* an invisible but extremely powerful form of vital energy, rules the body's first level of protection against disease and disorder. Think of the *wei chi* as a combination of sentries stationed in the outposts and scouts roaming the fields and forests that keep watch over the empire. The *wei chi* guards the perimeters of the body's kingdom from external invasion by maintaining strong, impregnable defenses. Fiercely protective, the *wei chi* stands ready to evict any foreigner that dares enter the castle walls and threatens to disturb the peace.

To keep the body's kingdom safe from harm, the *wei chi* depends on a steady stream of supplies and reinforcements. The Chinese point to four basic sources of energy that feed and invigorate the *wei chi*:

- *Jing chi* is an inherited form of energy passed from mother to child in utero and stored in the Kidneys; *jing chi* is usually depleted by the time you reach middle age.
- *Gu chi* derives from food and drink and is distributed throughout the body by the digestive organs (the Stomach, Spleen, and Pancreas).
- *Shen chi* is obtained from our relationships with family, friends, and the natural world and is distributed throughout the body by the Heart.

• *Da chi* is acquired from the air we breathe and is circulated throughout the body by the Lungs. When *jing chi, gu chi, shen chi,* and *da chi* converge in the Lungs, they are synthesized into *wei chi.*

Only *jing chi* is inherited and fixed from birth; all other vital energies depend on external influences (food, air, water, relationships) and internal conditions (the health and vitality of our vital organs). As long as you eat properly, breathe deeply of fresh, clean air, avoid excessive physical and emotional stress, and live in harmony with the world around you, you will maintain a stable internal environment in which the *wei chi* can live and thrive.

When the *wei chi* is strong, the body's kingdom is virtually impregnable. "Pathogenic energy cannot invade if the castle doors are closed," explained the Yellow Emperor. The castle doors creak open, however, when you neglect your diet, breathe polluted air, become involved in unhealthy relationships, or otherwise upset the balance within. After months or years of neglect, the *wei chi* will weaken, and when turmoil erupts either from within or outside the castle walls, the *wei chi* will be ill-equipped to suppress the insurrection.

Of all the pathogenic forces that can overcome the *wei chi* and threaten the inner kingdom, the Chinese are most concerned about the Five Devils and the Five Destructive Emotions.

The Five Devils

If the body is attacked by evil energy, its own energy will become stuck,
just as when the clouds cover the sky, obscuring the sun and moon and
causing darkness.

—*The Yellow Emperor's Classic*

While most Western doctors would agree with Chinese doctors that various lifestyle choices affect the immune system's ability to maintain physical health and well-being, they would no doubt scratch their heads in confusion at the theory of the Five Devils (also called "the Evil Energies," "Exogenous Pernicious Factors," or "External Pathogenic Influences"). The Five Devils refer to external climate conditions—Wind, Heat, Damp, Dryness, and Cold—that the Chinese believe directly affect the strength and vitality of the *wei chi*. These climates do little or no harm in moderation, especially if the *wei chi* is strong and vigorous. When the *wei chi* is progressively weakened by an unhealthy lifestyle or long-term neglect, however, the Five Devils are able to gain entry into the body's kingdom, and disease and disorder become more difficult to combat.

The danger that the Devils present to the *wei chi* varies according to the individual's affinity with a particular element. Wind is the climate associated with Wood, and Wood types often experience various aches and pains when exposed for any length of time to extreme wind. Excessive heat can be injurious to Fire types, excess dampness or humidity creates problems for Earth types, extremely dry weather can adversely affect Metal types, and extreme cold damages Water energy.

The Five Devils can also be generated from within. When the Liver is over-burdened for a long period of time, it cannot perform its duties of maintaining a smooth flow of blood and energy. *Chi* and blood back up and stagnate, leading to "internal Wind" conditions and typical migrating "Wind" symptoms like muscle tics, muscle spasms, tremors, seizures, or strokes. (The Chinese view any symptom that moves unpredictably from one place to another or that creates a flutter or tic, like leaves stirring in the breeze, as a sign of internal Wind.) Excessive stimulation or excitement can eventually stress the Heart, leading to internal Heat conditions and such symptoms as manic behavior, heart palpitations, flushing, and acne rosacea. Excessive worrying unleashes the Damp Devil, which causes dull, throbbing headaches, digestive bloating, lethargy, and a "heavy" spirit. When Metal energies are out of balance for long periods of time, the Lungs are vulnerable to invasion by the Dry Devil, which leads to dry throat, dry skin, and lack of sexual secretions. And when the Kidneys are overburdened with excessive fear, the Cold Devil causes problems such as cold hands and feet, muscle spasms, lower back pain, and difficulties with urinary retention.

THE WIND DEVIL

The Chinese (and many other cultures) are particularly wary of the Wind. Called "the Chariot for One Hundred and One Evils," the Wind enters the body through specific "Wind Points," just as the wind finds its way into a house through cracks in windows and doors. Located on the neck and shoulders, the Wind points are considered both entry points for Wind and areas you can stimulate to expel the Wind and prevent further penetration of the body's kingdom.

Acupoints commonly used to expel the Wind Devil include:

Triple Burner 17 (also known as Triple Heater 17) ("Shielding Wind"): This point is located on the neck in the depression just below the lower tip of the ear. An extremely sensitive point, it often becomes spontaneously sore to the touch when you catch a cold or flu.

Gallbladder 20 ("Wind Pool"): Run your hand from behind your ear onto the base of the skull, then follow the ridge of bone toward the center of the skull, stopping in a natural depression or pit. When you stimulate this point, you help to expel the Wind from the body.

Governing Vessel 16 ("Wind's Palace"): This point is located on the center of the back of the head, just below the base of the skull, about one inch above the hairline. Like the other Wind points, you can use this one to treat Wind diseases such as colds, flus, stiff neck, headaches, aversion to cold or wind, dizziness, seizures, and delirium.

For help locating these points, see Appendix III.

Pathogenic wind is the root of all evil," said the Yellow Emperor. When the Wind Devil invades the body's kingdom, the symptoms migrate from place to place, just as the wind blows erratically and unpredictably in the natural world. When Wind first enters the body, you will know the *wei chi* is under siege by the nature of your symptoms: sore muscles, muscle spasms and twitches, itchy or sensitive skin, skin eruptions (boils, acne, rashes), joint pains, tingling, numbness, and headaches.

As Wind penetrates deeper into the underground channels and tunnels, you may feel dizzy, uncoordinated, and emotionally unstable. Excess or spontaneous sweating, fever, vertigo, tremors, seizures, and strokes as well as emotional problems such as mood swings, explosive anger, and sudden or unexplained grief can result from internal Wind conditions. If the Wind Devil reaches the Lungs, it will cause coughing and shortness of breath; in the Heart, Wind causes speech disturbances and dry, cracked lips and tongue; in the Liver, the symptoms include dry throat and sudden explosive outbursts of anger; in the Spleen, heavy limbs, lack of appetite, and fatigue; and in the Kidneys, back pain and urinary tract problems.

To protect yourself from invasions by the Wind, cover up the Wind Points by wearing a scarf or shawl around your neck and shoulders on windy days. When the wind is extremely cold, hot, damp, or dry, stay inside until it settles down or wear a hat and extra clothing. Because a child's immune system is undeveloped and extremely sensitive to environmental influences, always protect infants and young children from the wind.

You can also protect yourself from the Wind Devil by keeping your emotions balanced and in control. "If one is centered and the emotions are clear and calm," noted the Yellow Emperor, "energy is abundant and resistance is strong; even when confronted with the force of the most powerful, vicious wind, one will not be invaded."

Depending on the nature of the Wind and where it settles in the body, specific herbs and acupuncture techniques can help dispel Wind and invigorate the *wei chi*. To clear Wind from the body, Chinese herbalists often use schizonepeta and ledebouriella (also called siler tuber), while Western herbalists rely on elder flower, linden flower, and boneset.

THE HEAT DEVIL

Heat is associated with Fire and summer (Fire's season); excess Heat is the pathogenic climatic factor associated with Fire and is thought to be injurious to the Heart, the organ system associated with Fire. Because the Heart stores the *shen* (spirit), excess Heat always disturbs the spirit, causing irritability, muddled thinking, delirium, and disturbed sleep.

Heat enters the body externally through the Wind Points on the neck and shoulders, producing symptoms like "hot" colds (sore throat, swollen glands, low-grade fever, dry mouth, dark urine) and skin eruptions (acne, boils, heat rash, patches of eczema). When Heat penetrates deeper into the body's kingdom, you may experience hot, painful joints (often associated with arthritic conditions), rapid pulse, red or swollen tongue, mouth ulcerations, sinusitis, constipation, hemorrhoids, difficulty urinating, burning during urination, "burning" diarrhea, extreme thirst, and a strong craving for cold beverages or a cold climate.

The Chinese believe that excess Heat can also disturb the blood, causing it to warm up and move too fast, overflowing its natural boundaries and contributing to nosebleeds, bleeding gums, excessive bruising, hemorrhages, and blood in the urine or stool. The *wei chi* tries to expel excess Heat through the skin, which can further exacerbate such symptoms as skin eruptions, rashes, welts, sores, or acne. Internal Heat rises upward to the head, causing a red-faced appearance, headaches, and burning or itching eyes.

Sugar, coffee, spicy foods, alcohol, and amphetamines further intensify "rising heat" symptoms; if you suffer from "Heat" symptoms, avoid these foods and drugs whenever possible.

Fire and excess Wood types are most vulnerable to the damaging effects of the Heat Devil and must be exceptionally careful in hot climates or conditions. Make sure you drink plenty of water throughout the day and eat cooling foods like fresh vegetables and fruits, salads, and tofu. Avoid spicy foods, fried foods, and fatty meats (red meat, poultry with the skin, hot dogs, sausage, pepperoni, salami, bacon). Dress lightly, stay in the shade, and avoid strenuous exercise that disrupts the blood flow and puts stress on the Heart. When the temperature rises to uncomfortable levels, stay inside, preferably in an air-conditioned environment.

Depending on the nature of your symptoms, specific herbs and acupuncture techniques are effective in banishing the Heat Devil and invigorating the *wei chi*. To cool down an overheated system, herbalists rely on dandelion, yellow dock, skullcap, honeysuckle, gardenia fruit, gentian, and prunella.

THE DAMP DEVIL

Dampness is associated with Earth and tends to be most prevalent in late summer, when the humidity rises and the air feels heavy and moist, though damp conditions can also develop during any seasonal transition. Feelings of fullness and heaviness, oily skin, sticky perspiration, water retention, and swollen joints often result from dampness.

The Damp Devil rarely appears alone and is usually accompanied by Cold, Heat, or Wind. Damp/Cold causes restricted circulation, stiff joints, tight muscles, and fatigue. Damp/Heat contributes to the development of blisters, herpes, shingles, and inflammatory conditions such as cystitis, jaundice, bronchitis, and ulcers. Damp/Wind produces hives, swollen lymph nodes, gas pains in the stomach and intestines, arthritic aches and pains, and heavy headaches. Mental and emotional disruptions linked to the Damp Devil include foggy thinking, vertigo, memory problems, apathy, lethargy, and passivity.

Dairy products, starchy foods, greasy or fried foods, thyroid medications, and birth control pills can generate Damp conditions internally, especially in Earth types, who are particularly susceptible to dampness. If you suffer from any of the symptoms associated with the Damp Devil, avoid these foods and drugs whenever possible. Certain spices (ginger and cayenne) and spicy foods can help dispel the Damp Devil.

Excessive dampness or humidity can make you feel bogged down, so concentrate on gentle, nonstrenuous forms of exercise like walking, swimming, tai chi, and yoga, which will increase your energy without draining it.

Since damp conditions create an optimal environment for yeasts, molds, and fungi, you might consider purchasing a dehumidifier for your home or office if you live in a perpetually damp (wet, drizzly, or humid) climate.

Keep an eye on your emotional climate as well. The Chinese believe that excessive worrying can generate dampness internally by slowing down metabolism, which leads to the buildup of undigested fluids (*tan*). If you feel bogged down with anxiety, try to find ways to take your mind off your troubles or, better yet, discover solutions to long-standing problems. The healing strategies discussed in the Earth chapter will help restore balance and harmony. Depending on the nature of your symptoms (heavy limbs, aching joints, throbbing headaches, sinus pressure, digestive bloating, loose bowels, yeast infections) various herbs and acupuncture techniques can be used to oust the Damp Devil and invigorate the *wei chi*. To dispel dampness, herbalists frequently rely on poria fungus, barley, cornsilk, agrimony, ginger, and cayenne.

THE DRY DEVIL

Dryness is associated with Metal energy and autumn (the season of Metal). Hot weather and dry winds can create external dryness, which can cause dry, brittle hair and/or nails, dry mouth, dry nasal passages and sinuses, dry skin with a tendency to wrinkle easily, and dry, irritated eyes. As dryness penetrates deeper into the body's kingdom, it can affect the Lungs, leading to thick sputum, a dry, irritating cough, asthma, tightness of chest, constipation, and painful defecation. Low flow of urine and lack of vaginal lubrication are also symptoms of internal dryness.

If you experience any of these symptoms or if you are adversely affected by dry conditions, try to avoid excess heat and drying winds. (Excessively dry climates tend to be especially difficult for Metal types, who are naturally prone to dryness.) If you live in a dry climate, be sure to use creams and moisturizing lotions. Avoid abrasive or excessively drying soaps and detergents. Drink plenty of water throughout the day; if you perspire excessively, be sure to replenish the fluid loss with additional water. Use a humidifier to put moisture back into the air. Forced-air heating and/or cooling systems tend to dry out the air more than other methods, so add a humistat to the system, or place a humidifier in the main room of your home.

Limit your intake of hot and/or spicy foods (Thai, Szechuan, and Mexican dishes as well as heavily peppered or salted foods) and alcohol, coffee, and other caffeinated drinks, as they can exacerbate internal dryness. Avoid certain prescription and over-the-counter drugs (nicotine, diuretics, antihistamines, and stimulants) that also create drying effects in the body.

Depending on the nature of your symptoms, various herbs and acupuncture techniques can help to expel the Dry Devil and invigorate the *wei chi*. Chinese herbs that can be used to support the *yin* (fluid) reserves include rehmannia, dong quai, and fo ti (*shou wu*); Western herbs used to lubricate the system and provide moisture include slippery elm, marshmallow, and comfrey.

THE COLD DEVIL

Cold is associated with Water energy and winter (the season of Water), and excess cold is considered damaging to the Urinary Bladder and Kidneys, the organs associated with Water. When the Cold Devil encounters the *wei chi*, you will initially feel cold or chilled. Tiny goosebumps will cover the skin, and you'll experience a strong desire to wrap yourself in warm blankets or put on extra layers of heavy clothing to keep the Cold Devil at bay. Because Cold generally enters the body through the Wind points on the neck and shoulders, you may also experience pain and stiffness in those areas, headaches centered in the back of the skull that are accompanied by sudden throbbing pains, and toothaches.

The nature of Cold is to contract and congeal, slowing down the flow of energy. If Cold penetrates deep into the system, the blood vessels begin to constrict, which impedes circulation. "Congealed blood" conditions such as clots, lumps, or masses with localized tenderness and pain may result. Kidney stones and gallstones, severe lower back pain, sexual problems (frigidity, loss of libido), prostate problems, and general weakness and lack of stamina offer further proof that Cold is penetrating deeper into the blood and organs.

If you are vulnerable to Cold conditions (Water types are most susceptible), make sure you bundle up when the weather turns chilly, as repeated exposure to cold climates can deplete the *yang* (Fire) energy, contributing to internal cold. If you can't avoid being outside in the cold, make sure you keep moving; continuous movement keeps the *chi* and blood circulating, which in turn supports the *wei chi*.

Prolonged, inadequate nutrition and cold foods like raw vegetables, tofu, and cold or iced beverages can also deplete the body's supply of *yang* energy and further aggravate Cold conditions. Whenever possible, consume warming foods like beans and legumes, complex carbohydrates (whole-grain breads and pastas), and organic meats and poultry.

All medications that counter inflammation and/or fever—antibiotics, aspirin, antacids—have a cold nature; whenever possible, avoid these drugs if you are experiencing Cold symptoms.

Depending on the nature of your symptoms, you can use various acupuncture techniques and herbs to support the body's efforts to eliminate the Cold Devil. Herbalists often use *ma huang* (ephedra), cinnamon, ginger, osha root, and cayenne to provide healing warmth.

The Five Destructive Emotions

Overindulgence in the five emotions—happiness, anger, sadness, worry or fear, and fright—can create imbalances. Failing to regulate one's emotions can be likened to summer and winter failing to regulate each other, threatening life itself.

—*The Yellow Emperor's Classic*

Many Western doctors now agree that our state of mind and emotional balance can influence our susceptibility to disease. Most physicians would have some difficulty, however, with the idea that particular emotional problems affect specific organs; that, for example, unexpressed anger injures the liver, excess joy harms the heart, or prolonged grief damages the lungs. Yet in Chinese medicine unrestrained emotions are considered as dangerous to physical well-being as eating unhealthy foods, smoking cigarettes, drinking too much alcohol, not getting enough exercise, or sleeping only a few hours a night.

Like the Five Devils, the Five Destructive Emotions correspond to the Five Elements. Anger is the emotion associated with Wood, joy with Fire, worry with Earth, grief with Metal, and fear with Water. When one emotion dominates the others, or when you find yourself unable to express your feelings properly, the pressure begins to build, your vital energy weakens, the immune system begins to falter, and you become increasingly vulnerable to disease and disorder.

ANGER

Anger is the emotion associated with the Wood element. In its balanced state, anger is considered a healthy emotional response to stress, frustration, or injustice. When expressed gently and with careful control, anger clears the air, dispels tension, and restores balance.

Problems develop when we repress expressions of anger and allow it to accumulate, which can eventually cause distinct emotional imbalances such as chronic tension, irritability, and frustration, as well as physical problems such as migraine headaches, insomnia, hot flashes, ulcers, and hemorrhoids.

Expressing your anger clearly and forcefully before it builds up to dangerous levels will help you avoid many of these physical and emotional problems. To maintain control over your anger, refer to the healing strategies discussed in Chapter 2.

JOY

Joy is the emotion associated with the power of Fire. The Chinese believe that when the Heart is secure within itself, joy is constant and unwavering, like a steady pilot light that spreads warmth and contentment throughout the body, mind, and spirit. When the Heart is agitated or overstimulated, however, the pilot light flares up and overheats the system. As Fire energy is rapidly consumed, joy turns into mania, leading to symptoms such as constant giggling, chattering, and nervous exhaustion. If this excess joy continues unchecked over an extended period of time, more severe disorders can appear, including hypoglycemia, anorexia, cystitis, eczema, psoriasis, speech disturbances, insomnia, low blood pressure, dizziness, irregular or rapid heartbeat, heart palpitations, and heart attacks.

When you find yourself in a manic or overexcited state, take a few moments to ground the excess Fire. Breathe deep into your lower belly, and imagine that you are pulling up *yin* (fluid) energy from the inner reservoirs and using it to cool down your body, mind, and spirit. For specific healing strategies for Fire types, see Chapter 3.

WORRY

Worry is the emotion associated with Earth energy. A concern for others (a balanced Earth emotion) degenerates into obsessive anxiety, and you become tormented by distressing thoughts and ideas. When Earth becomes "sick with worry," the energies in the Stomach begin to stagnate, creating feelings of heaviness, laziness, and inertia, as well as edema (water retention), inefficient digestion, and ulcers.

Worry is an emotion that focuses only on the past or the future. If you find yourself overcome by anxiety and distress, first try to assess whether you have any control over the outcome of the situation. Accepting the fact that you don't always have control will help you regain your balance and focus your energies in the present. The healing strategies discussed in Chapter 4 will help you correct imbalances within the Earth functions and restore harmony to body, mind, and spirit.

GRIEF

Grief is the emotion associated with Metal. When balanced and openly expressed, grief allows you to experience natural feelings of loss and mourning.

When grief becomes excessive, however, your energy contracts and slows down, and a hardening process sets in that is comparable to the congealing of sap in trees as winter approaches. As grief penetrates deeper into the system, your body stiffens, leading to spine and joint problems, constipation, irritable bowel syndrome, and respiratory diseases such as chronic bronchitis, asthma, and pulmonary fibrosis.

The mind and spirit also become rigid when feelings of grief continue unabated. Imprisoned by grief, you cut yourself off from the rest of the world to avoid the risk of further loss, becoming possessive and greedy. Inflexible and intolerant, you reach out to others only to pull them back into your world, where you maintain ultimate control. You are afraid to let go for fear of losing your most valuable possession: your self.

Grief, like all emotions, should be experienced fully and then passed through. If you find yourself consumed with grief over past losses, give yourself time to grieve and express your feelings of loss. Then make a conscious effort to "let go," gently closing the door to the past and moving back into the present. Breathing exercises are particularly effective in helping to calm your emotions and settle your spirit; refer to the healing strategies discussed in Chapter 5.

FEAR

Fear is the emotion that moves and directs Water types. In its healthy, balanced state, fear allows us to remain alert and attentive, filled with readiness and courage to face whatever situation might present itself. When fear becomes excessive, however, our energy begins to sink and settle, like a stone that is dropped to the bottom of a pond and remains there, submerged in the mud and muck. Fear freezes your ability to think and react; you think only of escape, yet you are unable to remove yourself from your predicament.

To protect yourself, you avoid contact with others, becoming ever more reclusive and solitary. As fear penetrates deeper, anxiety, phobias, and paranoia consume your thoughts. This process can generate physical diseases and disorders, including arthritis, urinary infections, kidney stones, gallstones, various sexual problems, neurological disturbances, high blood pressure, heart attacks, and strokes.

When you feel overwhelmed by fear, ask yourself: What exactly do I fear? Does my fear have any effect on the situation that is causing it? Can I successfully negotiate my way through difficult situations if I am filled with fear? *The I Ching* suggests that you try to avoid two mistakes when confronting danger: haste and hesitation. By avoiding these mistakes and focusing instead on patience and restraint, you will be able to control your fears and rise above them. The healing strategies discussed in Chapter 6 will help you restore balance and harmony.

The Five Devils and the Five Destructive Emotions cannot penetrate the body's internal defenses if the *wei chi* energy is abundant and vigorous. If, however, the *wei chi* is weakened by lack of food, insufficient oxygen, or any number of "miscellaneous factors," including lack of exercise, insufficient rest or relaxation, excessive stress, and unhappy relationships, the Five Devils and the Five Emotions can wreak havoc throughout the body, mind, and spirit.

The first signs of trouble at the *wei chi* level include a persistent cough, a rapid pulse, a reddish tongue, headaches, and fever. When you feel the first sniffles of a cold, the flush of a fever, or the chills and aching joints of the flu, you are receiving a clear and unmistakable message that the *wei chi* is under siege. When the symptoms refuse to go away, you will know that the *wei chi* is unable to expel the intruder. Chronic colds or coughs, persistent infections, minor wounds that take weeks to heal, chronic low-grade fevers, and increasingly severe allergic reactions tell us that the *wei chi* is constantly on alert and therefore in danger of being depleted. Just as untended weeds in a garden eventually choke the life out of healthy plants, chronic illness gradually strangles the life-generating power of the immune system, eventually leading to more serious diseases capable of penetrating deeper into the body's inner kingdom.

In the remainder of this chapter, we'll look at the chronic illnesses associated with a breakdown in *wei chi* energy and show you what you can do to restore balance and harmony. Whenever the *wei chi* is under attack, think of the symptoms as a warning, and remember the words of the ancient Chinese philosopher Lao-tzu:

Think of the small as large
and the few as many.
Confront the difficult
while it is still easy;
accomplish the great task
by a series of small acts.

Recurrent Colds and Flus

"I need to rebuild my immune system," Joseph told me in our first session. "In the last six months I've had three bad colds, and I just got over a miserable bout with the flu. To be truthful, my wife insisted I try Chinese medicine. She claims that I've been so tired lately that I don't give her enough attention, intellectually, emotionally, or sexually."

With his ruddy complexion, magnetic personality, and willingness to discuss the most personal details of his life, Joseph was clearly influenced by Fire energy. Every time he walked into my office, he'd give me a big hug and several hearty pats on the back. "How are things going for you?" he'd ask, and then listen attentively to everything I said. It was obvious why he was such a successful psychotherapist and marriage counselor: He made you feel that every word you said was important and that he was absolutely fascinated by your insights and intelligence.

Joseph's private practice was thriving, and he was working twelve to fifteen hours six (and sometimes seven) days a week to keep up with his caseload. I noticed that his breathing was shallow and focused in his chest rather than his belly. When I commented on the fact that he seemed to hold his breath, particularly when he was deep in thought, he admitted that he sometimes became so lost in his work that he actually forgot to breathe. His voice was often hoarse from stress and had a quavery quality that was aggravated when he didn't get enough sleep.

We worked out a simple treatment strategy. Joseph's immune system was obviously suffering from an overload of stress, lack of exercise, insufficient sleep, and inattention to personal relationships. "I need to slow down and smell the roses," Joseph admitted. To accomplish that goal, he agreed to go through his appointment book and block out "personal time," leaving most evenings free after seven o'clock and working only five hours on Saturdays. On the weekends he took long walks with his wife, and three evenings every week he worked out on a stationary bike for half an hour as he watched the news. Bimonthly acupuncture sessions, breathing exercises, nutritional supplements, and Chinese and Western herbal remedies helped relieve his stress and support his immune system.

When Joseph occasionally slips back into his stressful, workaholic ways, he claims that he immediately notices his throat muscles tighten up. "All I have to do is listen to myself on the tape recorder," Joseph said. "If my voice trembles, I know it's time to breathe deep, take some herbs and extra vitamins, and go for a walk with my wife."

WESTERN INTERPRETATION

Western medicine defines a cold as an acute, highly contagious viral infection of the upper respiratory tract—also called acute rhinitis. Thousands of different viruses and rhinoviruses can cause the common cold; individuals with lowered resistance due to disease, age, or inadequate diet and nutrition are most susceptible. The symptoms, which vary with the particular virus and the individual's reaction to that virus, include a runny nose, sneezing, watery eyes, "stuffy" head, minor headaches, general achiness, sore throat, cough, and in some cases fever. The average cold lasts seven to fourteen days, with symptoms subsiding after three to four days.

Influenza (flu) is an acute infectious epidemic disease caused by several related viruses, with new strains appearing every year. After a brief incubation period, the symptoms appear suddenly, as the virus enters the respiratory tract and spreads through the body, causing fever, chills, headache, sore throat, cough, diarrhea and other gastrointestinal disturbances, and muscle aches and pains.

WESTERN TREATMENT

If you have a cold, your doctor will probably suggest that you get plenty of sleep, drinks lots of fluids, keep warm, avoid abrupt changes in temperature, eat moderately, and use over-the-counter pain relievers, decongestants, and antihistamines to relieve the symptoms. Although antibiotics are useless against viral infections, they are sometimes prescribed to prevent or treat complications of colds, which include sinusitis, middle ear infections, and lower respiratory tract infections.

For the flu, doctors will suggest the same general treatment strategies with some modifications. Because of the nausea and vomiting that accompany the flu, you may be advised to avoid eating or restrict yourself to liquid foods. Antibiotics are also useless against flu viruses but may be prescribed to avoid complications associated with secondary bacterial infections such as pneumonia.

Many doctors are becoming increasingly sensitive to the effects of nutrition, exercise, and general stress on immune function and offer their patients advice on dietary changes, nutritional supplements, exercise programs, healthy sleep patterns, and stress-reduction techniques. Increasing numbers of doctors are also becoming aware of the dangers associated with excessive antibiotic use—including the destruction of friendly bacteria, the creation of antibiotic-resistant bacteria, and generalized immune suppression—and prescribe these powerful drugs only when absolutely necessary.

If you are elderly, if you have chronic lung, heart, or kidney disease, if you are "immune compromised" by chronic immune disorders such as cancer or AIDS, or if you catch every flu that comes around, your doctor might suggest a yearly flu shot. Flu shots contain vaccines against three of the most common or expected strains of viral infections for a particular season, and they are administered *before* flu season begins. Unfortunately, flu shots offer no guarantee that you will be completely protected against all strains of flu.

Colds and flus can be extremely frustrating for both patients and doctors, because in the absence of a cure the basic advice remains: "Grit your teeth and get through it."

TRADITIONAL CHINESE INTERPRETATION

The doctor trained in traditional Chinese medicine would interpret recurring colds and flus as indications of deficient *wei chi,* which in turn reflects deficient Lung and Kidney energies. The Kidneys provide fuel for the Lungs, which are responsible for creating *wei chi* from *jing chi* (inherited energy stored in the kidneys), *gu chi* (energy derived from food and drink and stored in the Spleen/

Pancreas), *shen chi* (energy obtained from our interpersonal relationships and stored in the Heart), and *da chi* (energy synthesized from the air we breathe and stored in the Lungs). If the Kidney fires are depleted, the Lungs don't have enough energy available to produce sufficient amounts of *wei chi.* When the *wei chi* is weakened or depleted, the Five Devils have an easier time finding their way into the body, where they can wreak havoc in the form of colds and flus.

The symptoms of colds and flus often reflect our affinity with a particular element. If the sinuses, throat, and upper respiratory tract are affected whenever you get a cold or flu, you might have a Metal imbalance, because these are the areas Metal governs. If the symptoms concentrate in your joints and muscles—areas ruled by Wood energy—an imbalance in Wood is suspected. A flu accompanied by digestive ailments suggests an Earth imbalance; heart palpitations, thought dysfunctions, and anxiety indicate a Fire disharmony, while lower back pain, stiffness in the knees, lethargy, and recurrent urinary infections point to a Water imbalance.

The symptoms will also vary depending on which Devil penetrates the system. For colds and flus, Wind/Cold and Wind/Heat are the most common manifestations of external invasion:

Wind/Cold: Wind/Cold invasions begin suddenly (Wind) and include chills (Cold), an aversion to cold (Cold), and body aches and pains (Cold) that tend to migrate and move around (Wind). A runny nose is a Wind symptom, while clear or white mucus, a stiff neck, and headaches in the back of the head where the neck and skull join (the occipital area) are considered Cold symptoms.

Wind/Heat: Wind/Heat invasions begin suddenly (Wind) with fever and sore throat (Heat), runny nose (Wind) with yellow or green mucus (Heat), possible skin eruptions such as fever blisters, rashes, or hives (Heat and Wind), agitation, irritability, and dark urine (Heat).

The severity of the cold and/or flu symptoms depends on the virulence of the invading pathogen and the strength of the *wei chi.* Practitioners of traditional Chinese medicine believe that periodic colds or flus are actually beneficial because they challenge the *wei chi,* which, like most living organisms, can become lazy when untested and unprepared. All competitive athletes "test" their skills repeatedly before a major event, even to the point of straining muscles. The immune system also thrives on competition, and minor colds and flus are considered an important way to keep the *wei chi* on its toes.

However, if you catch every cold or flu that comes around, if your symptoms include severe fatigue or generalized weakness, and if your recovery time stretches into weeks or months, you are receiving strong signals that your immune system is weak and unable to meet the challenge. Numerous complementary treatments are available to help you restore health and vigor.

COMPLEMENTARY TREATMENTS

Diet

To prevent colds and flus, follow the dietary suggestions for your specific constitutional type as detailed in Part I.

To ease the symptoms and speed up recovery from colds and flus, try these specific dietary strategies:

Whenever you have a cold or flu, restrict your diet to *easy-to-digest foods* such as chicken broth, vegetable juice, apple juice, dry toast, and bananas.

Garlic contains a potent antibiotic called allicin, which is released when the raw cloves are chopped, crushed, or chewed. (Cooking destroys the volatile oils.) To get rid of a cold or flu, crush one clove of raw garlic in a teaspoon of honey and swallow. Garlic is most potent when raw; in garlic supplements the herb's volatile oils, which are responsible for its characteristic strong odor (and many of its infection-fighting agents), are often removed. Nevertheless, if raw garlic is too strong for you, garlic supplements are still effective in combating colds and flus. Take one capsule one to three times daily. Be sure to buy the enteric-coated capsules, which are easier to digest.

You can also make garlic oil by chopping four to six cloves of garlic and heating them (don't boil or fry them) in a pint of olive oil. Put one teaspoon of the oil in lemon juice or water, and drink it, repeating every hour as needed. (Garlic oil is also extremely effective for relieving the pain and inflammation of middle ear infections; use an eyedropper to put a few drops in the affected ear.)

Grapefruit's sour, bitter qualities support the Liver in its efforts to remove toxins from the blood. Grapefruit is also loaded with vitamin C, an extremely effective immune-supporting nutrient. Eat one or more grapefruits daily, with the pulp, to build immunity and fight off colds or flus.

Drink hot lemon water throughout the day to replace lost fluids, break down mucus in the respiratory system, and provide extra vitamin C for your immune system. To make lemon water, squeeze a fresh lemon into a cup of hot water; if you want, add honey as a sweetener. Drink four to six glasses of lemon water daily.

A *diaphoretic (sweat-inducing) tea* will help your body break a fever by inducing sweat. Garlic, ginger, yarrow, and mint are wonderful herbs for both colds and flus; use any combination of these herbs that tastes (and feels) good to you. Boneset is particularly effective in breaking fevers and relieving the muscle aches and pains that accompany the flu; the name comes from the herb's early use for relieving symptoms of breakbone fever (dengue) and has nothing to do with bones. These herbs and herbal teas are available in many health food stores.

Be sure to *drink plenty of water* to replace fluids lost through perspiration and vomiting. Sip water regularly if you have the flu; when your stomach settles down, drink vitamin-rich beverages such as apple juice and vegetable juice. *Chicken broth* is always good for replacing fluids and making you feel nourished.

Whenever you drink hot beverages (lemon water, teas, or broth), breathe deeply of the vapors to warm up your respiratory tract and make it less hospitable to rhinoviruses, which like a cooler environment.

Exercise

For chronic and recurrent colds and flus, we recommend that you avoid strenuous exercise and follow your doctor's advice to get plenty of rest and drink lots of fluids. When you start to feel better, try gentle exercises like walking, swimming, or bicycling (twenty to thirty minutes daily) until you have regained your energy and can engage in more vigorous activities. Refer back to Chapters 2 to 6, and choose the exercises that match your constitutional type.

Nutritional Supplements

For acute flare-ups of colds or flus accompanied by chills, sore throat, stuffy head and chest, sinus congestion, headache, and/or fever, take the following supplements for five days:

Multivitamin and mineral supplement: To make sure you get sufficient micronutrients, take a multivitamin and mineral supplement every day. Ask your health care practitioner or health food store owner to recommend a balanced, easily absorbed formula providing between 100 and 200 percent of the Recommended Daily Allowances for vitamins and minerals.

Vitamin C: Numerous studies support claims that vitamin C boosts immune function and can prevent and treat the common cold; if you're interested in learning more about this amazing vitamin, read *Vitamin C and the Common Cold* by two-time Nobel laureate Linus Pauling.

Take 1,000–2,000 mg. (1–2 grams) every two hours, up to 16–20 grams daily; if you experience diarrhea or loose stools, cut back on the dosage until the symptoms disappear. When your symptoms have subsided, return to a maintenance dose of 2,000–4,000 mg. (2–4 grams) daily.

Beta-carotene (vitamin A): Beta-carotene is converted into vitamin A in the intestines, but unlike vitamin A it is not toxic even in large doses. Vitamin A plays a vital role in maintaining the integrity of the body's mucous membranes and helping the cells and tissues establish a natural impermeability to external pathogens. Vitamin A also supports antibody response, enhances natural-killer-cell functions, supports monocyte functions, and strengthens the activities of the thymus gland, which produces the immune system's T-cells. Like vitamin C, vitamin E, and selenium, beta-carotene is a powerful antioxidant, protecting your cells and tissues against the irritating, potentially damaging effects of pollutants in the air, food, and water. Take 25,000 I.U. daily. *Note:* If you have liver damage or disease, do not exceed 5,000 I.U. of vitamin A without consulting with your health care practitioner.

Garlic: Crush one clove of garlic in a teaspoon of honey and swallow. Repeat every four or five hours. You can substitute garlic capsules for the raw garlic; take two capsules three times daily.

Zinc: Zinc enhances thymus gland function, supports the production of antibodies, and enhances white-blood-cell activities. Take 30 mg. as a preventive, and up to 60 mg. daily when actively fighting a cold or flu. Chelated forms of zinc—zinc gluconate, zinc citrate, and zinc monomethionine—are more easily absorbed than other forms; we prefer zinc gluconate because it is less irritating to the digestive tract. If you have a sore throat, try zinc lozenges instead of the capsules; follow the instructions on the package.

Chinese Patent Remedies

To strengthen your immune system and prevent colds and flus, we recommend:

Gejie Ta Bu Wan ("Gecko Great Tonifying Pills"): This favorite tonic is used for many different conditions to strengthen the *chi, yang,* and blood, replenish the Kidney and Lung energies, and offer general support to the Spleen and Heart. With desiccated gecko lizard reigning as the Emperor herb, supported by seventeen attending herbs, this excellent long-term tonic promotes health and strengthens your immune system. Take three to five capsules three times daily.

If you experience chronic "Heat" symptoms (fevers, irritability, yellow coating on the tongue), this formula might be too warming. In that case, you can substitute the following patent remedy (which does not contain animal parts):

Bu Zhong Yi Qi Wan ("Support the Center, Benefit Energy Pills"): This formula features ginseng and astragalus as the Emperor herbs, supported by eight attending herbs that work together to aid digestion, support the Kidneys, and balance Liver and Spleen energies. Take eight to ten pills (tiny pellets) three times daily or as directed on the product label.

For acute flare-ups of colds or flus:

Gan Mao Ling Pian ("Common Cold Effective Tablets"): Herbalists in China and throughout the world rely on this formula to prevent or combat the symptoms of colds and flus. The Emperor herb in this formula is isatis, which is famous for its antiviral qualities. Attending herbs (ilex root, evodia fruit, chrysanthemum flower, vitex fruit, lonicera flower, and menthol crystals) help the immune system neutralize and eliminate the invading pathogens. They relieve acute flare-ups of Wind/Cold (chills, aching muscles, nasal congestion, stuffy nose, sore throat, stiff neck and shoulders) and/or Wind/Heat (fever, swollen glands, headache). Take four pills three times daily, and continue until the symptoms have abated.

Yin Chaio Chieh Tu Pian ("Lonicera [honeysuckle] and Forsythia Dispel Heat Tablets"): Honeysuckle flower and forsythia fruit share Emperor status in this formula, working with eight attending herbs (burdock, platycodon, mint, soja seed, licorice, lophatherum leaf, and schizonepeta) to dispel Wind/Heat conditions, which cause fever, chills, swollen glands, headache, and, in some cases, hives or rashes. Because the herbs in this remedy are stronger than those used in the "Common Cold Effective Tablets" (described above), restrict your use to the first three days of a cold or flu. Take four to six pills three or four times daily.

Po Chai Pills ("Pill Curing Pills"): More than twenty herbs in this formula, which has been called "Chinese Alka-Seltzer," work gently and effectively to combat the symptoms of acute stomach flu and dispel Wind/Damp conditions in the Spleen and Stomach, including gas, bloating, constipation, and diarrhea. The pills are actually tiny pellets, with approximately seventy pellets contained in a small plastic vial. Take one vial every three to four hours as needed for relief of symptoms. This formula is considered safe enough for small children.

These gentle Chinese patent remedies can safely be combined with any of the following Western herbs. If you need help choosing the most effective formula or combination of herbs for your symptoms, consult an experienced herbalist.

Herbal Allies
To strengthen the immune system and prevent colds and flus:

Echinacea (*Echinacea angustifolia* or *Echinacea purpura*): Herbalists recommend taking echinacea as soon as you feel the first symptoms of a cold or flu—as many people have discovered, the symptoms often disappear thereafter. Recent research conducted in Germany and England showed that people taking low doses of echinacea every day for periods as long as two to three years had significantly fewer colds, flus, and other infections than a control group of the general population as a whole. (Low-level doses are often recommended for people with cancer, lupus, chronic fatigue syndrome, and HIV/AIDS.)

If you decide to try low-level doses, take ten to fifteen drops of the tincture daily, or two capsules every morning. If you use echinacea only when you feel a cold or flu coming on, take a teaspoon of the tincture every two hours, or two to three capsules three or four times (for a total of six to twelve capsules), daily.

Astragalus: This extremely safe, supportive herb has been used for thousands of years to increase energy and strengthen resistance to disease. A combination of equal parts echinacea and astragalus will help prevent colds and flus or relieve the symptoms of the illness.

For acute flare-ups of the upper respiratory tract, a potent yet balanced formula would include equal amounts of the following herbs:

- **Echinacea,** an immune-boosting herb with antimicrobial, antibiotic, antiviral and antifungal qualities
- **Goldenseal** (*Hydrastis canadensis*), a natural antibiotic and immune booster
- **Osha root** (*Ligusticum porteri*), an anti-infective agent that has powerful healing effects on the entire respiratory system
- **Licorice root** (*Glycyrrhiza glabra*), a gentle expectorant and antimicrobial agent that the Chinese call "the Great Unifier" because of its ability to bring out the best qualities of all the herbs in the formula.

For acute flare-ups affecting the stomach and bowels:

- **Ginger** (*Zingiber officinalis*) is the best herb available for the stomach and digestive tract. For colds and flus, ginger helps to reduce fevers by inducing sweating, and it generally soothes and heals the entire digestive tract.

A good tonic for stomach or intestinal flus would include equal parts:

- **Ginger,** a digestive herb that alleviates nausea and promotes sweating
- **Echinacea,** an immune-supporting, antimicrobial herb
- **Goldenseal,** a natural antibiotic and immune system enhancer

Dosage: If you purchase your herbs in a health food store (either in tincture form or, as dried herbs, in capsule or pill form), follow the dosage instructions on the label. Because herbs in dried form tend to lose their potency rather quickly, be sure to check the label for the expiration date.

For information on preparing your own herbs from the root, bark, leaves, flowers, or seeds of a plant, see Appendix II.

In the Resources section, we offer a list of mail-order sources for high-quality herbs and herbal preparations. For advice on ordering specially made herbal formulas, see Appendix I.

Acupoints

LUNG 9 ("Great Abyss"): The Chinese believe this acupoint offers a direct line to the Lungs. It is frequently used to activate and energize the Lung *chi,* helping to treat colds, bronchitis, asthma, and sinus infections; strengthen the *wei chi* (which originates in the Lungs); regulate the blood vessels, moving the blood through its channels to remove obstructions; support the *yin* (fluid) energy, helping to resolve anxiety, palpitations, and irritability; and balance Metal energies.

Location: Lung 9 is located on the crease on the palm side of the wrist in the depression at the base of the thumb (about half an inch in from the side of the wrist).

CONCEPTION VESSEL 17 ("Sea of Tranquillity"): This powerful immune-stimulating point provides strong support for the Lungs, which, in turn, produce the *wei chi.* It also nourishes the Heart, which houses the *shen* (spirit), thus relieving the anxiety and depression that so often accompany serious chronic illnesses.

Location: Conception Vessel 17 is located between the nipples on the center of the breastbone, directly above the thymus gland (the originating source of the T-cells). Gently massage this point with your fingers, using circular, clockwise motions.

Questions to Ask Yourself

Recurrent colds and flus are a sign that the *wei chi* is weak and needs support. In a very real sense, they signal that the *wei chi* is languishing from neglect. Have you ignored your body's cries for help, believing, perhaps, that your immune system is completely self-sufficient and doesn't require your active support?

The following questions will help you focus on the ways in which you can build up your defenses to prevent recurring illnesses. Focus on one or two questions that relate most directly to your particular situation:

- How do I neglect myself?
- In what areas of my life do I feel defenseless?
- How do my recurrent illnesses prevent me from dealing with certain conflicts in my life?
- How do my continual illnesses prevent me from achieving my goals in life?
- Is my illness asking me to take time off and think about the pressures and stresses that make me sick?
- What needs to be cleansed and eliminated from my life?
- Do I have a plan to maintain my health with diet, exercise, stress-reduction techniques, and other healing strategies?
- Do I have a plan to heal myself when I first begin to feel sick?

A STARTING POINT

Picking and choosing among the many and diverse remedies recommended for recurrent colds and flus may seem like an overwhelming task. Where should you begin?

The following supplements, herbal remedies, and healing strategies will give you a solid foundation to build upon. Use the other remedies suggested in this section when and if you need additional support.

For Prevention:

1. *Diet:* Follow the dietary suggestions on pages 188 to 189.
2. *Exercise:* Exercise twenty to thirty minutes every day.
3. *Nutritional supplements:* Follow the general formula for Maximum Immunity on page 37.

If Your Energy Is Low, Add:

1. *Bu Zhong Yi Qi Wan:* Take eight to ten pills three times daily.
2. *Echinacea:* Take ten to fifteen drops of the tincture or two capsules daily.

For Acute Flare-ups of Respiratory Colds and Flus (Head Colds, Sore Throat, Sinus Congestion, etc.), Add:

1. *Vitamin C:* Increase the dose to 1,000–2,000 mg. every few hours; if you experience diarrhea cut back on the dosage.

2. *Garlic:* Crush a clove of garlic in a teaspoon, add honey to sweeten it, and swallow; repeat two or three times daily.

3. *Echinacea and goldenseal:* Take half a teaspoon (approximately twenty drops) of the tincture every hour or two, or three capsules of the dried herbs three or four times daily.

4. *Gao Mao Ling Pian:* Take four tablets three times daily.

For Acute Flare-ups of Intestinal Viruses, Add:

1. *Ginger tea:* Take as much as you can drink throughout the day.

2. *Po Chai Pills:* Take one vial every four or five hours.

Allergies and Food Sensitivities

Stan, thirty-three years old, suffered from severe allergies. A woodworker and house builder, he seemed allergic to just about everything he encountered in his daily life, from sawdust, to wood additives, paint, animal hair, pollen, and mold spores. "I've tried every drug on the market, including antihistamines, nasal sprays, nasal douches, and desensitization shots," he told me. "You name it, I've tried it. You're my last resort."

Thin and tall, with dark circles under his eyes and a shy demeanor, Stan described himself as a loner who fiercely protected his privacy. Although he had a large circle of friends and acquaintances, he was extremely wary of intimate relationships, and he particularly resented the constant demands his girlfriend made on his time. While Stan's physical appearance, antisocial tendencies, and fears of intimacy indicated a strong affinity to Water, he was also clearly influenced by Metal, evident in his allergic sensitivities, his need for structure and discipline, and his strong desire to work on projects that required creative skill rather than simply "pounding nails for a living."

Stan's treatment consisted of several different approaches. Dietary changes included eliminating dairy products (the number-one food allergen) and eating only organic (nonchemically treated) meat and poultry. To support his immune system, strengthen his Liver, and help him cope with the physical and emotional stress caused by his allergies, he took an herbal tonic consisting of *ma huang* (ephedra), dandelion root, elecampane, licorice, and osha root; the Chinese

Liver-supporting remedy Hsiao Yao Wan ("Relaxed Wanderer Pills"); and nutritional supplements including vitamin C, vitamin E, beta-carotene, B-50 complex, selenium, and magnesium.

Stan particularly enjoyed the bimonthly acupuncture sessions, for this was one place where he felt free to let down his guard and talk openly about his grief over the tragic death of his father, when Stan was only fifteen years old. When I explained that unresolved grief injures the Lungs, Stan seemed to immediately understand the connection between emotions and physical illness. "I need to let go," he admitted. "Not only of the past but of all the parts of my life that I can't control."

Three months after starting treatment, Stan's symptoms were significantly improved. He continues to take his herbs and nutritional supplements, and he faithfully attends seasonal acupuncture sessions.

WESTERN INTERPRETATION

According to conservative estimates, more than one in five Americans has allergies, and the number rises every year. Although the vast majority of allergy sufferers consider their symptoms a major annoyance rather than a chronic disease, allergic reactions to insect venom, antibiotics, and other allergens take the lives of thousands of Americans every year.

Allergies are defined as an exaggerated immune response to an otherwise nonirritating or mildly irritating substance such as pollen, dust, mold, or insect venom, or to a "man-made allergen" such as synthetic fabric, various building materials, and food additives. The most common allergy is hay fever, an inflammatory reaction caused by hypersensitivities to pollens and mold spores. Symptoms of hay fever include sneezing, itchy and watery eyes, runny nose, and burning sensations in the throat and palate. Complications include lack of sleep, loss of appetite, inflammation of the ears, sinus, throat, and bronchi, asthma, and general immune system depletion.

In this section we focus on common allergies and food sensitivities.

WESTERN TREATMENT

The first step in treatment is to identify the allergy-causing substance. Diagnostic skin tests can be performed in which a miniscule amount of a suspected allergen is applied to the skin of the forearm, either through injection, an adhesive patch saturated with the allergen (patch test), or an application of the allergen to a small scratch on the skin (scratch test). Localized redness, swelling, and/or itching indicates an allergic reaction to the substance. Blood tests are now available to accurately identify allergic sensitivities.

Numerous prescription and over-the-counter drugs are available to provide symptomatic relief, including antihistamines, decongestants, and immunosuppressive corticosteroids. The side effects of antihistamines and decongestants—drowsiness, dizziness, fatigue, insomnia, digestive problems, mental confusion, and irritability—are relatively common and can be serious. Most doctors today offer nonsedating antihistamines and steroid sprays to avoid these side effects; however, antihistamines also create tolerance in regular users, so that you have to take ever higher doses of the drug in order to achieve the desired effect.

The newer, longer-lasting antihistamines like Seldane have become popular because you only have to use them once a day. Incidents of side effects and negative, even life-threatening, interactions with other drugs are becoming more and more prevalent, however. In fact, Seldane was recently taken off the market for these reasons.

Side effects associated with oral corticosteroids include swelling of the face ("moon face" or swollen cheeks), abdominal bloating, weight gain, increased vulnerability to infection, disturbances of the menstrual cycle, heartburn, fatigue, insomnia, and mood swings with anxiety and/or depression. Topical steroidal creams can have significant side effects as well, including thinning of the skin, a condition that can be permanent and lead to easy bruising; permanent lightening of the skin; and suppression of adrenal gland functioning, especially in children. Long-term use of inhaled steroidal sprays may cause thrush (yeast overgrowth) in the respiratory system; a deterioration of the mucosal lining of the airways, particularly the vocal cords; and systemic absorption of these drugs, increasing the possibility of the side affects associated with oral corticosteroids. With steroidal nasal sprays, most of these side effects can be minimized or eliminated.

The fourth step in treatment is desensitization. This is the treatment of choice for allergic reactions to bee stings or penicillin because no drugs are used and a complete cure is possible. The patient receives a series of gradually increasing amounts of the allergic substance until the system becomes desensitized and therefore less reactive to the offending allergen. Desensitization can be a life-saving procedure for anyone who has experienced anaphylactic shock, a serious, sometimes life-threatening state of shock brought about by hypersensitivity to drugs, foreign proteins, or insect venom.

Treatment for food allergies and sensitivities generally consists of eliminating suspected allergy-causing foods from the diet. Food allergies can also be detected through blood tests, diagnostic skin tests, or the Elimination Provocation Diet, in which various foods are eliminated from the diet and reintroduced with careful attention paid to recurring symptoms.

TRADITIONAL CHINESE INTERPRETATION

The Chinese believe that hay fever and other allergies are caused by two related factors:

1. *A deficiency in Lung (Metal) energy.* The Lungs synthesize *wei chi* (the body's defensive energy) and rule the quality, quantity, and circulation of *wei chi.* When Lung *chi* is deficient, the *wei chi* weakens and begins to react inappropriately to external irritants (allergens).

2. *Constrained Liver chi.* When the Liver is exhausted by stress, inadequate diet, insufficient exercise, lack of sleep, or emotional strain, toxins build up in the blood, and the body's vital energy (*chi*) slows down. "Constrained Liver *chi*" inevitably leads to a state of chronic irritability and emotional overreactivity, which contributes to allergic reactions and symptoms. A vicious cycle ensues as anxiety, fear, anger, and overexcitement create additional stress on an already overstressed system.

In the case of food allergies, the Liver deficiency is joined by Spleen/Pancreas and Stomach imbalances, which contribute to the inadequate digestion of proteins. (Other factors contributing to incomplete digestion include low hydrochloric acid levels, insufficient pancreatic enzymes or bile, and improper chewing of food.) These partially digested proteins (sometimes called "renegade" proteins) are absorbed through the intestinal walls into the body fluids, which carry them to various sites throughout the body, causing the immune system to overreact and resulting in such diverse and seemingly unrelated symptoms as muscle aches, joint pain, chronic sinusitis, itchy, irritated eyes, skin disorders, headaches, indigestion, and multiple food sensitivities.

Treatment is aimed at strengthening and nourishing the Lung energies and supporting the Liver to help restore the free flow of energy and blood. Treatments for food allergies or sensitivities with digestive symptoms focus on supporting the Spleen/Pancreas by paying special attention to diet, reducing or eliminating refined carbohydrates and refined sugars, and using various herbs to restore balance.

COMPLEMENTARY TREATMENTS

Diet

The *wei chi* is always on the lookout for marauding chemicals and proteins, immediately recognizing these substances as foreigners that it must evict from the body's kingdom before they stir up trouble. The *wei chi*'s job was much easier forty or fifty years ago, for our food was not uniformly sprayed with toxic chemicals, laced with food additives, or injected with hormones. Today, most of the animals we eat receive antibiotics in their feed (every year twenty million pounds of antibiotics are given to animals in the United States); our drinking water is contaminated with more than two thousand toxic chemicals (yet our public water systems test for fewer than thirty of these chemicals); and the average American citizen consumes *nine pounds* of chemical food additives every year.

Whether or not a given allergy has a direct dietary cause, you can safely assume that your diet—specifically, the fast-food, processed-and-refined-food, high-sugar, and high-fat diet that most Americans enjoy—plays a significant role in all allergic reactions. If you suffer from allergies of any kind, if you have a family history of allergies, or if you simply want to clean up your diet to strengthen your immune system, follow these general dietary guidelines:

• Eliminate or drastically reduce your consumption of dairy products, the number-one food allergen; if you use dairy products, always use the nonfat varieties, and limit your consumption to no more than two or three servings a week.

• Eliminate or drastically reduce your intake of wheat products (cereals, gravies, breads), the number-two food allergen. Substitute nonallergenic grains like white and brown rice. If you use wheat products, limit your consumption to one serving daily, and use *whole* (unprocessed and unrefined) forms of the grain (whole-grain cereals, breads, pastas). To avoid overconsumption of one particular grain, try adding other grains to your diet such as millet, buckwheat, quinoa, and amaranth (actually a seed but used as a grain).

• Reduce your consumption of meats, which are high in saturated fats and have been treated with numerous chemical additives, including estrogen and antibiotics. If possible, buy organic (nonchemically treated) meat and dairy products. If you can't afford to buy organic products (which are significantly more expensive than nonorganic products), substitute protein-rich grains, beans, nuts, seeds, and vegetables (the standard vegetarian fare) for red and white meat.

• Eat "whole" foods—foods that have not been processed, refined, treated with chemical preservatives, or loaded with artificial ingredients to enhance flavor or retard spoilage—whenever possible. Whole foods include whole-grain breads and pastas, fresh fruits and vegetables, beans, legumes, organic meats, nuts, and seeds (raw or baked without salt, hydrogenated oils, or additives).

• Eat plenty of vegetables and fruit, but watch out for corn, tomatoes, and oranges, which can trigger food allergies or sensitivities.

• If you have a sensitivity to yeast or have yeast infections, avoid baked goods, sugar, vinegar, mayonnaise made with vinegar, fermented foods, and "moldy" foods (mushrooms, alcohol, cheeses, dried fruits).

• Diversify your diet, choosing foods from many different food groups to help control preexisting food allergies and sensitivities and to prevent the formation of new allergies. When a particular food allergen is repeatedly present in the body, the immune system is on constant alert. Rotating different foods and food groups gives the immune system a much-needed rest.

• Pay special attention to your food cravings; many physicians and naturopaths who specialize in food allergies believe that food cravings are actually symptoms of an allergic reaction to a particular food or foods.

• If you continue to feel drained of energy, irritable, and hypersensitive, or if you experience any of the following symptoms—fatigue, headaches, mood swings, depression, muscle aches and pains, muscle weakness, digestive problems (gas, bloating, bowel irregularities), arthritis, chronic sore throat, chronic sinusitis, skin problems (hives, eczema, psoriasis), hay fever, or asthma—consider having your blood tested for allergic sensitivities or try the Elimination Provocation Diet.

• Drink eight to ten 8-ounce glasses of fresh, filtered water every day. For information on various water-filtering systems, see Appendix I.

Nutritional Supplements

Vitamin C: This vitamin is essential for a strong immune system and a powerful ally if you have allergies. In large doses vitamin C works as a natural antihistamine, relieving many of the symptoms associated with hay fever and food allergies. Take 1,000 mg. every one or two hours, up to 12,000 mg. (12 grams). If you experience loose bowels or diarrhea, cut back on the dosage until the symptoms subside.

Quercetin: This bioflavonoid reduces inflammatory and histamine levels, providing significant relief for allergy sufferers. Take 250 mg. thirty minutes before eating, two to three times daily.

Quercetin is often combined with a digestive enzyme such as bromelain, which increases its effectiveness. Be sure to look for a formula that includes bromelain or other pancreatic enzymes.

B-50 or B-100 complex: The B vitamins provide the spark for numerous physiological and neurological processes, helping your body cope with everyday stress as well as the additional strain of chronic illness. Take a B-50 or B-100 complex vitamin daily.

Vitamin A: This vitamin improves the immune system's antibody response and has a powerful effect on the *wei chi,* strengthening and supporting virtually every cell in the immune system. You can substitute beta-carotene, but vitamin A is slightly more effective for allergies. Take 20,000 to 25,000 I.U. daily.

Vitamin E: This vitamin supports the mucous membranes and promotes healing; take 400 to 800 I.U. daily.

Gamma linoleic acid (GLA): This essential fatty acid works as a natural anti-inflammatory agent, inhibiting the release of inflammatory prostaglandins and reducing the body's allergic response. Oil of evening primrose, borage seed oil, and black currant seed oil are all excellent sources of GLA. Take three to four 500-mg. capsules (each capsule contains 35 to 40 mg. GLA), for a total of 1,500–2,000 mg. daily.

Hydrochloric acid tablets: These tablets support the stomach acids to help you thoroughly metabolize your food, thereby reducing the "renegade" proteins that result from incomplete digestion and that contribute to allergic reactions. If you are prone to ulcers or hyperacidity, consult with your doctor or health care professional before taking this supplement.

Take one 5-to-10-grain tablet with each meal. (Some people with low stomach acid may require significantly more than this amount; check with your health care provider if you suspect your problems might be related to low levels of hydrochloric acid.)

Fiber: Fiber promotes regular bowel movements and helps propel the digestive contents through the intestines. When undigested food particles become bound or tied to fiber, the digestive process works more efficiently to move food quickly through the system and thereby reduce the risk of "renegade" proteins (undigested protein particles) leaking into body fluids and creating allergic reactions.

We recommend Yerba Prima's Daily Fiber Formula, a completely organic (nonchemically treated) fiber supplement available in most health food stores. Mix one tablespoon of the powder into a glass of room-temperature water (or you can use half apple juice, half water); mix thoroughly and drink quickly, as the fiber tends to gel quickly in water. Follow with a glass of fresh water, and be sure to drink plenty of water throughout the day. Yerba Prima also comes in capsule form; take three or four capsules with at least one 8-ounce glass of water. Repeat daily.

Fiber has many additional benefits, which we will discuss at length in the section on irritable bowel syndrome, pages 242 to 251.

Exercise

If you have allergies, try to exercise regularly to help the Liver maintain a free flow of energy and blood, thus preventing stagnation and "stuckness." Don't go overboard, however; when Kidney and Spleen energies are deficient, as they often are in allergy victims, strenuous exercise can further drain these vital reserves. Try to exercise at least twenty to thirty minutes every day; brisk walking, tai chi, yoga, or swimming are excellent choices. If you don't suffer from symptoms of deficient energy—lethargy, heavy limbs, aching muscles or joints—you can safely engage in more strenuous exercises. Start slow, and don't push yourself. Refer to Chapters 2 through 6, and choose the forms of exercise that match your constitutional type.

Chinese Patent Remedies

For hay fever symptoms, combine the following remedies:

Hsiao Yao Wan ("Relaxed Wanderer Pills"): This is considered the archetypal remedy for constrained Liver *chi,* which interferes with proper digestion and can lead to many allergies, including food allergies and sensitivities. Take eight to ten pellets three times daily.

Bi Yan Pian ("Benefit the Nose Tablets"): These pills dispel Wind/Heat or Wind/Cold from the nose, sinuses, and bronchioles. Traditionally used for acute and chronic sinusitis, Bi Yan Pian also works wonders for allergies, especially hay fever. Magnolia flower and xanthium fruit, the Emperor and Empress herbs, are assisted by phellodendrom, licorice, platycodon, schisandra, forsythia, angelica, anemarrhena, chrysanthemum, siler, and schizonepeta. Take five tablets up to five times daily.

For food sensitivities, the following remedies work well together:

Hsiao Yao Wan (see description above).

Bu Zhong Yi Qi Wan ("Support the Center, Benefit Energy Pills"): Considered the archetypal Spleen tonic, these pills support Kidney and Spleen energies. Ginseng and astragalus are the Emperor herbs, supported by eight attending herbs that work together to aid digestion, support the Kidneys, and balance Liver and Spleen energies. This quick and effective formula relieves such symptoms as abdominal bloating, gas, pain, and irregular bowel habits. Take eight to ten pellets three times daily.

These Chinese patent remedies are extremely gentle and can be safely combined with any of the following Western herbs. If you need help choosing the most effective formula or combination of herbs for your symptoms, consult an experienced herbalist.

Herbal Allies

For allergies caused by pollens, mold spores, or animal dander, an effective formula would include the following herbs:

Ephedra or *ma huang (Ephedra sinica*): In recent years ephedra has received a bad reputation due to its inappropriate (and excessive) use as a stimulant and dietary aid. In China herbalists have been using *ma huang* for more than five thousand years to treat asthma, and modern herbalists frequently rely on this powerfully effective herb for treating respiratory illnesses. When used in small amounts for upper respiratory infections or inflammatory conditions such as asthma and allergies, ephedra quickly and effectively soothes an overagitated system. Consult with your health care practitioner before using ephedra if you have a medical condition (such as high blood pressure) that could be aggravated by a gentle stimulant.

Licorice (*Glycyrrhiza glabra*): An incredibly versatile herb, licorice's expectorant actions work to eliminate excess mucus from the lungs and bronchial system, while its natural anti-inflammatory effects help to subdue the fires of allergies and such symptoms as inflamed nasal passages or sinuses; red, inflamed, or irritated eyes; and skin reactions with burning and itching. Licorice also has a balancing effect on the adrenal glands, easing the effects of stress on all body systems.

Dandelion root (*Taraxacum officinalis*): This herb supports the Liver, helps the digestive system work more efficiently, promotes a healthy flow of bile, and generally works to "unconstrain" constrained Liver *chi.*

Echinacea (*Echinacea angustifolium*): This herb provides a powerful boost to the immune system.

Osha root (*Ligusticum porteri*): This potent antimicrobial herb works to prevent infections and relieve the symptoms associated with allergies. Although osha root was used extensively and with great success by Native American tribes in the mountains and high deserts of the United States, it was never incorporated into the European herbal tradition, and even today the wonders of this amazing plant remain relatively unknown. If you can't find osha in your health food store, a good substitute is goldenseal, another antimicrobial herb with powerful effects on Liver functions.

You can have these five herbs mixed in equal parts by a qualified herbalist, or you can buy a premixed allergy formula that includes several of these popular herbs at your health food store. A simpler formula, wonderful for preventing allergies and/or treating allergic symptoms, consists of one part ephedra to two parts licorice and two parts dandelion root.

Dosage: If you purchase your herbs in a health food store (either in tincture form or, as dried herbs, in capsule or pill form), follow the dosage instructions on the label. Because herbs in dried form tend to lose their potency rather quickly, be sure to check the label for the expiration date.

For information on preparing your own herbs from the root, bark, leaves, flowers, or seeds of the plant, see Appendix II.

In Appendix I, Resources, we offer a list of mail-order sources for high-quality herbs and herbal preparations. For advice on ordering specially made herbal formulas, see pages 394–396.

Acupoints

LIVER 3 ("Great Rushing"): This point helps the Liver in its job of circulating and distributing blood and *chi* throughout the body. It is often used when Liver energy is constrained or deficient. It also helps to expel "Wind" conditions caused by an imbalance in Liver *chi,* including tremors, muscle twitches, migrating pains in the joints or muscles, dizziness, and headaches.

Location: Liver 3 is located on the upper part of the foot in the depression in the webbing between the big toe and the second toe.

LARGE INTESTINE 4 ("Great Eliminator"): This point is used for draining or dispersing energy "stuck" in the upper part of the body, especially the head and neck areas, and for relieving headaches, irritated or swollen eyes, sinus congestion, stuffy nose, sore throat, swollen glands, and neck or shoulder tightness with pain and spasm. It is also used to soothe the digestive system, alleviating gas, diarrhea, and constipation.

Location: Large Intestine 4 is located on the top of the hand, in the webbing between the thumb and index finger.

Questions to Ask Yourself

Allergies indicate an immune system overreacting to otherwise harmless irritants (pollen, dander, dust, food proteins, and additives). Recognizing an enemy intruder, the *wei chi* engages in all-out war when a well-organized skirmish would suffice. Stress and emotions play an important role in allergic reactions; most of my clients report that their symptoms flare up when they're physically or emotionally stressed.

The following questions will help you understand and appreciate the role your emotions play in your allergic sensitivities and guide you to potential solutions. Focus on one or two questions that relate most directly to your particular situation.

- How can I bring more balance into my life and respond, rather than simply react, to situations that arise?
- How do I suppress my emotions?
- How are my allergies working for me? What are they allowing me to do? What are they preventing me from doing?

Allergies are often associated with Lung (Metal) imbalances, which makes sense since Metal energy rules the Lungs, Skin, bronchial passages, and sinuses. The Chinese believe grief, the emotion associated with Metal, can cause or exacerbate allergic reactions. If unresolved or unexpressed grief is a factor in your life, ask yourself:

- What am I grieving for?
- What do I need to let go of before I can move ahead with my life, my goals, my relationships?

Liver (Wood) imbalances are also associated with allergies. If Wood is deficient, friction builds up in the system, and you become more irritable and hyperreactive. Stifled creativity (a symptom of "stuck" Wood energy) is also connected with allergies. Ask yourself:

- What irritates me these days?
- Why do I feel frustrated or discontented?
- Is something interfering with my ability to move forward and express myself creatively?

A STARTING POINT

Picking and choosing among the many and diverse remedies recommended for allergies may seem like an overwhelming task. Where should you begin?

The following supplements, herbal remedies, and healing strategies will give you a solid foundation that you can build upon. Use the other remedies suggested in this section when, and if, you need additional support.

1. *Diet:* Follow the dietary suggestions on pages 200–202.
2. *Exercise:* Exercise for twenty to thirty minutes every day.
3. *Nutritional supplements:* Take the general formula for Maximum Immunity.
4. *Vitamin C:* When allergies flare up, increase the dose to 1,000 mg. every hour or two, up to bowel tolerance.
5. *Quercetin:* One 250-mg. tablet half an hour before each meal.
6. *GLA:* Take 1,500 mg. daily.
7. *Hsiao Yao Wan:* Take eight tablets three times daily during allergy season.
8. *Western herbal tonic:* For prevention during allergy season, take a formula consisting of one third licorice, one third dandelion root, one sixth echinacea, and one sixth osha root.

9. LEVEL TWO: THE *CHI*

When you look for it, there is nothing to see.
When you listen for it, there is nothing to hear.
When you use it, it is inexhaustible.

—Tao Te Ching

When the *wei chi* is weakened and disease is able to penetrate deeper into the system, symptoms of distress intensify. Digestive disturbances, chills, fevers, migrating aches and pains, lack of energy, and chronic fatigue signal that the immune system is on constant alert. As the weeks and months go by and the symptoms stubbornly persist, you begin to wonder if something serious might be wrong. Doctor visits increase. You take over-the-counter and prescription medications to allay chronic pain, induce sleep, and boost your flagging energy. Inevitably your emotional health is affected, and you begin to feel anxious, irritable, and depressed.

These wide-ranging physical and emotional symptoms arise when the body's second level of defense—the *chi*—is under siege. The relationship between *chi* and *wei chi* is complex and deeply intertwined. In truth, they are not separate entities at all but different manifestations of the same basic force. The *wei chi* is the visible manifestation of an invisible but massive inner force: *chi*.

In traditional Chinese medicine, *chi* is synonymous with life itself. In the world around us, *chi* is the energy that allows night to become day and day to become night, the force that keeps the earth rotating on its axis, and the power that radiates the sun's warmth through space. Inside your body, *chi* is the vital energy that begets all movement, generates all heat, produces all moisture, and protects every cell in your body from harm. *Chi* gives you the energy to walk, talk, think, reason, feel hunger and thirst, and experience emotions such as passion, empathy, desire, and love.

Because you can't see *chi,* you may find it difficult to believe that it really exists. Yet *chi* is not the only form of vital energy that is ethereal and impalpable. Life depends on the involuntary act of inhalation and exhalation, for example, but the life-giving essence of breath is intangible and invisible.

The wind offers another example of a powerful but invisible energy source. When the wind circles through the aspen tree, the leaves quiver and shake. When the curtains rise and fall, seemingly of their own volition, you know the wind is a guest in your house. Although you can't see the wind, you know it exists because you have witnessed its effects on the visible world.

Like breath and wind, *chi* is beyond your grasp and control. You can't hold it in your hands, feel its rounded or squared edges, mold it, bend it, divide it, or clone it. You can't measure it in meters or decibels; nor can you analyze its properties under a microscope. When you reach for it, it disappears.

This story may help you to understand the nature of *chi,* the dynamic energizing force underlying all movement—even the movement of your mind.

> Two monks were arguing about a flag. One said, "The flag is moving."
>
> The other said, "The wind is moving."
>
> The Master overheard them and said, "It is not the wind nor the flag, but your mind that moves."
>
> The monks were speechless.

What is *chi? Chi* is the energy in the atmosphere that moved the flag. *Chi* is the force that enabled the monks to perceive that the flag moved. *Chi* is the power that prompted the observers to ask whether it was the flag or the wind that moved. *Chi* is the wisdom that understood that the flag and the wind moved only when the mind moved.

Chi is the spark that infuses matter with energy; it is the dynamic principle underlying all life.

The Five Functions of *Chi*

In the human body *chi* has five basic life-giving functions: movement, warmth, protection, transformation, and support.

MOVEMENT

Our hearts beat and our lungs involuntarily expand and contract because of *chi*. *Chi* gives us the energy and the motivation to move, and when we move, we replenish the *chi*.

At this point the question arises: Does *chi* generate movement, or does movement generate *chi*? Does life create *chi,* or does *chi* create life? The Chinese wouldn't bother themselves with such chicken-and-egg questions, because they don't think of life in linear terms. The living world is not represented by a straight line beginning with birth and ending with death, but by a circle with each point on the curve depicting both the beginning and the ending. *Chi* and movement are synonymous, as are life and movement; *chi* is life.

WARMTH

When you're alive, you're warm; when you're dead, you're cold. *Chi* moves the blood, which generates the warmth that nurtures life. When *chi* is abundant and vigorous, your internal temperature remains steady at 98.6 degrees, no matter how cold or hot your surroundings may be. When it is 20 degrees below zero outside, circulating *chi* keeps you warm on the inside; when it is 110 degrees in the shade, *chi* cools the blood and dissipates internal heat. If your internal temperature rises or drops by just one degree, you know that the *chi* is somehow obstructed and unable to circulate freely.

PROTECTION

Chi is the defensive energy that moves through a complex series of invisible channels or meridians (see Appendix III for illustrations of the major meridians) to protect the body's inner kingdom. *Wei chi,* the immune energy, travels in the tendinomuscular vessels and represents the surface power of *chi*; *chi* also flows in the meridians, nourishing and enriching the blood and extending its influence deep into the heart of the kingdom to protect the vital organs.

Your natural resistance to disease and disorder depends upon the invigorating energy of *chi*. When the *chi* flows effortlessly and smoothly through the meridians, you are able to evict unwelcome invaders; when the *chi* is blocked or impeded, your body's defensive energy is weakened.

TRANSFORMATION

Chi is the alchemist's flame, the magical spark that converts one type of energy into another. *Chi* transforms energy on four levels: physical, mental, emotional, and spiritual.

Physical: At the most basic, tangible level, *chi* transforms the food you eat and the beverages you drink into vital energy and blood.

Mental: *Chi* transmutes facts, memories, thoughts, and perceptions into creative energy. When the formula "$E = mc^2$" suddenly materialized in Einstein's mind, he cried out "Eureka!" because he knew that something astonishing had just happened. The Chinese would credit *chi* as the transforming energy responsible for turning years of accumulated knowledge into unexpected wisdom.

Emotional: *Chi* "moves" the emotions, preventing them from getting "stuck," dispersing their energy, and instantaneously converting one emotion into another. When a child chases a ball across the street and is almost hit by a car, her watching parents experience intense fear, which in a moment is transformed into anger, which is instantaneously changed into grief (the painful acknowledgment of life's transient nature), and finally to joyous relief.

This energy that allows one emotion to flow into another is *chi*.

Spiritual: The ultimate alchemy generated by *chi* occurs at the spiritual level, where ordinary consciousness is transformed into sudden awareness. Taoist philosopher Lieh-tzu, writing more than two thousand years ago, tells of his experience of awareness, a state of sudden enlightenment that merged his soul with the spirit of the wind:

When I had come to the end of everything inside and outside me, my eyes became like my ears, my ears like my nose, my nose like my mouth. . . . My mind concentrated and my body relaxed, bones and flesh fused completely, I did not notice what my body leaned against and my feet trod, I drifted with the wind East and West, like a leaf from a tree or a dry husk, and never knew whether it was the wind that rode me or I that rode the wind.

Chi is the energy that creates the space for self-realization and enlightenment, moving the inside to the outside and the outside to the inside, fusing bones and flesh so that the separation of mind and matter no longer exists and the individual soul becomes one with the world.

SUPPORT

Chi is the indispensable "stuff" that gives living things a shape and an identity, creating from the building blocks of water, proteins, and genetic codes an identifiable creature who can stand straight and tall, run, walk, think, feel, and react. The ability to withstand the forces of gravity without collapsing in a heap is called "upright *chi*."

Newton's Third Law of Motion states that whenever one object exerts a force on a second object, the second exerts an equal and opposite force on the first; in other words, for every action there is an equal and opposite reaction. Upright *chi* is the equal and opposite reaction to gravity; it is the antigravity energy that gives us buoyancy, a sense of weightlessness, the ability to run with the wind, to feel weightless, to be graceful, to be open to grace.

The Flow of Chi

Chi circulates continuously throughout the body in a series of invisible channels called meridians, which can be compared to an underground irrigation system that feeds, nourishes, and supports the body's "earth." For hundreds of years Western scientists have scoffed at this theoretical construct, calling the meridians a figment of the mysterious Eastern imagination. In recent decades, however, researchers using sophisticated electromagnetic technology have been able to map the electrical potential of the skin; over ninety percent of the skin points with high electrical conductivity correspond precisely to the acupoints first described in ancient China over five thousand years ago.

While the Western scientific community continues to regard the concepts of *chi* and the meridian system with skepticism, increasing numbers of physicians are incorporating acupuncture into their medical practices for one simple reason: It works. The Mayo Clinic has offered acupuncture since 1975, and the World Health Organization lists forty-seven different illnesses that respond to acupuncture treatments, including digestive, respiratory, neurological, muscular, urinary, menstrual, and reproductive disorders. "The modern scientific explanation is that needling the acupuncture points stimulates the nervous system to release chemicals in the muscles, spinal cord, and brain," notes the American Academy of Medical Acupuncture. "These chemicals will either change the experience of pain or trigger the release of other chemicals and hormones which influence the body's own internal regulating system."

Fourteen major meridians traverse the body from head to toe. Two "extraordinary meridians" run vertically up the midline of the body: *Du Mo* (the "Governing Vessel" that connects to the central nervous system) unites the six *yang* meridians on the back of the body—Small Intestine, Urinary Bladder, Triple Heater, Gallbladder, Colon, and Stomach—while *Ren Mo* (the "Conception Vessel," which is considered central to reproduction and digestion) joins the six *yin* meridians on the front of the body—Lung, Spleen, Heart, Liver, Kidney, and Pericardium.

Located along the meridians, like dams erected at various points along a river, are a series of hollows or holes through which you can access the *chi,* redirect its flow, break through blockages, and strengthen its vital essence. The Chinese compare the acupoints to "gates" that can be opened or shut to influence the direction and flow of energy in the body.

Chi's journey through the body is said to begin in the Lungs, because the Lungs are responsible for creating *wei chi* and *chi* from the food we eat (*gu chi*), the air we breathe (*da chi*), and the inherited energy passed from generation to generation (*jing chi*). Beginning at Lung 1, an acupoint located on the chest about two inches above the armpit, you can follow *chi*'s journey as it travels from the Lung to the Large Intestine, Stomach, Spleen, Heart, Small Intestine, Urinary Bladder, Kidney, Pericardium, Triple Heater, Gallbladder, and Liver meridians.

Disturbances of Chi

The symptoms of disturbance at the *chi* level are characterized by their stubborn chronicity—they simply won't go away. When the *wei chi* is under siege, short periods of illness are replaced by longer stretches of good health. When the *chi* is blocked or disturbed, the ratio between illness and health begins to change, with intervals of good health becoming shorter and less predictable and periods of illness lasting longer and adversely affecting the patient's quality of life.

At the *chi* level the symptoms are still relatively minor—a dry cough, constipation or diarrhea, a bright red tongue often covered with a yellow coating, a rapid pulse, persistent fever or chills, lack of energy and motivation—and the diseases associated with this stage are not considered life-threatening. Nevertheless, the constant drain on your system inevitably affects your emotional stability, contributing to chronic irritability, anxiety, mood swings, and periodic depression.

Diseases and disorders associated with a breakdown at the *chi* level include:

- Chronic sinusitis
- Chronic intestinal problems, including irritable bowel syndrome (IBS) and Crohn's disease
- Asthma
- Skin disorders, including eczema and psoriasis

We'll examine each of these disorders in detail, offering Western interpretations and treatment strategies followed by Chinese interpretations and complementary healing techniques. The gentle, safe remedies offered in this and other chapters can be used in conjunction with standard medical care to strengthen your immune system to prevent and combat disease.

Chronic Sinusitis

Tom, forty-five, has suffered from recurrent sinus infections for ten years. His brother, a physician specializing in internal medicine, diagnosed his condition and prescribed broad-spectrum antibiotics, decongestants, and antihistamines. During acute flare-ups, which occurred every month or two, Tom renewed his prescription for antibiotics, using over-the-counter nasal sprays for congestion and ibuprofen for pain.

When it became clear that Tom's symptoms were becoming worse, not better, a friend suggested that he try nutritional supplements and herbal therapy. After consulting with his brother, who assured him that the alternative healing methods he was considering wouldn't hurt him, Tom began taking megadoses of vitamins A, C, and E on a preventive basis and, at the first signs of an infection, a combination of echinacea and goldenseal. A steam inhaler cleared up his blocked sinuses, and saline nasal sprays helped lubricate his nasal passages.

Although Tom still suffers from periodic (two to three times yearly) sinus infections, the symptoms are not nearly as debilitating as they once were. When he does get an infection, he relies on herbs to relieve his symptoms; he hasn't taken an antibiotic for more than two years. Amazed at the change in his physical and emotional health, he claims that he has more energy in his forties than he did in his twenties.

WESTERN INTERPRETATION

Chronic sinusitis, defined as an inflammation of one or more of the paranasal sinuses, is one of the most common chronic illnesses in the United States. One of every seven Americans suffers from sinusitis, which is caused by multiple factors, including structural defects of the nose that interfere with breathing (most commonly a deviated septum), upper respiratory infections that spread to the sinuses (excessively strong nose blowing is often implicated), allergies, infectious diseases such as pneumonia and measles, air pollution, diving or swimming underwater, sudden extremes of temperature, and complications from tooth infections.

People who suffer from chronic allergies are particularly susceptible to sinusitis, because allergies create hyperreactions in the nasal membranes, leading to postnasal drip, which, in turn, irritates and inflames the sinuses. (For allergies, see Chapter 8.)

Indoor pollution, caused by a lack of circulating fresh air in the home (the most common culprits are air conditioning and certain types of heating systems, as well as energy-saving devices such as double-paned windows that keep the air locked in the house), can also contribute to irritation and hypersecretion of the sinus cavities. If you are like most people, you spend much, if not most, of the day inside your home, school, or office, where the air contains varying amounts of toxic substances such as carbon monoxide, nitric oxide, and nitrogen dioxide. Older buildings may be insulated with asbestos, or the walls may be covered with lead-based paint. In newer homes carpeting, plastics, glue, textiles, and foam insulation release toxic formaldehyde vapors.

Formaldehyde is also found in antiperspirants, mouthwashes, germicidals, dentifrices, shampoos, air deodorizers, hair-setting gels, nail polish, oils, polishes, waxes, adhesives, and detergent soaps. Numerous house-cleaning products, including bleaches, laundry soaps, toilet cleaners, disinfectants, floor waxes, mildew removers, and oven cleaners, contain toxic chemicals that can damage your health, impair your immune system, and contribute to chronic allergies and sinus infections.

Symptoms: Sinusitus causes the mucous membranes to become inflamed and swollen, which leads to partially or wholly blocked nasal passages. Mucus accumulates in the nose and sinuses, putting pressure on the sinus walls, which, in turn, creates discomfort, pain, and difficulty breathing. Consequently, your entire head feels congested, and you find it difficult to think clearly. Extreme fatigue, general weakness, and chronic pain concentrated around the nose and behind the eyes make you cranky and irritable. Symptoms tend to be worse in the morning, and many people with sinusitis claim that they can't find the energy to drag themselves out of bed. Moving around helps stimulate nasal drainage (which often has a yellow or greenish tint to the mucus), and you generally feel better as the day goes on.

While these symptoms occur with both chronic and acute sinusitis, chronic infections can also cause persistent low-grade fevers (especially at night), daytime cough, generalized achiness, chronic headaches (often behind the eyes), and dizziness when you stand up, lie down, or change position.

WESTERN TREATMENT

Doctors often prescribe antibiotics for sinus infections, usually for a three- or four-week course. The most commonly prescribed antibiotics are in the "broad-spectrum" category, because they are capable of destroying many different kinds of bacteria. While broad-spectrum antibiotics typically offer fast relief from symptoms, in most cases the underlying disorder remains, and the symptoms simply reappear after the antibiotic is discontinued. Increasing numbers of doctors are sensitive to the dangers associated with repeated doses of broad-spectrum antibiotics—specifically, the destruction of large populations of friendly bacteria and the creation of antibiotic-resistant bacteria—and encourage their patients to take nutritional supplements, change their diet, and reduce stress to help prevent recurrent infections.

Both prescription and over-the-counter decongestants and expectorants (Dristan, Allerest, Drixoral, Actifed, Afrin) are available to relieve the symptoms of congestion. Decongestant nasal sprays work quickly to clear blocked nasal passages, but as you build up tolerance to these drugs, you have to use more and more of them to attain the desired effect. These decongestants also cause side effects. One common side effect is "rhinitis medicamentosis," in which the symptoms are exacerbated when you stop using the medication. People often interpret this flare-up as evidence of how well the medication worked and immediately begin using it again. For these reasons physicians caution patients to use over-the-counter decongestants only when absolutely necessary and only for short periods of time.

Aspirin and other over-the-counter pain relievers offer some relief from symptoms. Humidifiers often help break up congestion, and air purifiers may improve the quality of the air in your home and reduce the risk of allergies, which in many cases also reduces the risk of sinusitis.

When sinusitis continues for months or years and other methods fail to prevent recurrences, your physician may suggest surgery to enlarge the sinus openings and create adequate drainage and ventilation. While surgery often provides short-term relief, there is no guarantee of a long-term cure, and many surgery patients continue to suffer from chronic and acute attacks within weeks or months after the operation.

TRADITIONAL CHINESE INTERPRETATION

The Chinese interpret sinusitis as a continuous or repeated invasion by the Wind/Heat Devil or the Wind/Cold Devil (indicating a general depletion of *wei chi),* which interferes with the Lungs' ability to disperse and spread *chi.* One of *chi*'s main functions is to keep the blood and fluids moving throughout the body, and when *chi* becomes blocked or inhibited, the fluids accumulate and thicken into a mucuslike substance called *tan.* With insufficient *wei chi* and *chi* available to combat the invading Devils, Heat or Cold lodges in the nose and sinuses and over time the *tan* begins to stagnate and become infected.

If the source of the infection isn't eliminated, the Lung energy weakens, and infections become chronic and difficult to uproot. Repeated invasions of the nasal passages by Wind, Heat, or Cold gradually weaken the Kidney *chi,* interfering with the Kidneys' ability to "grasp" and distribute the Lung *chi,* which leads to "stuck" energy in the head and general fatigue, weakness, and lethargy.

General treatment strategies involve using acupuncture points and appropriate herbs to drain the "stuck" Wind/Heat or Wind/Cold from the head and support the functions of the Lungs and Kidneys. Taking an individual's constitutional strengths and weaknesses into account is an essential part of treatment. Because the constant fatigue, congestion, foggy thinking, headaches, and general discomfort inevitably create emotional stress, attention is paid to the individual's ability to withstand stress, and various stress-reduction techniques are suggested on an individual basis.

If you suffer from sinusitis, be sure to look back at the specific stress-reducing strategies in Chapters 2 through 6.

COMPLEMENTARY TREATMENTS

Diet

Diet plays a major role in susceptibility to chronic sinusitis. Dairy products, the primary food allergen, are particularly troublesome because they cause allergic reactions in susceptible individuals *and* create additional mucus in the system. If you suffer from sinusitis, your first step should be to eliminate milk and other dairy products from your diet for three weeks. Keep careful track of your symptoms, noting any improvements. After three weeks, gradually reintroduce these foods, and again carefully note any recurring symptoms. If your symptoms return, stay off dairy products for six months; at that point, if you want to try reintroducing dairy products into your diet, you can do so very gradually, but be on the lookout for any returning symptoms.

In addition to reducing or eliminating dairy products, try to cut down on your sugar and caffeine intake. Many sinus sufferers are addicted to their caffeine drinks because caffeine temporarily relieves symptoms such as foggy thinking, headaches, and fatigue. Counteracting these beneficial effects, however, are caffeine's negative impact on numerous bodily functions. Caffeine interferes with digestion and the assimilation of nutrients; overstimulates the adrenal glands, which over time can lead to exhaustion, chronic fatigue, anxiety, and panic attacks; and burdens the Liver, which is responsible for detoxifying drugs and other chemicals.

Like caffeine, sugar is an antinutrient—a substance that takes more from the body than it gives. Calorie rich, nutrient poor, heavily refined and processed, sugar exhausts the Spleen/Pancreas, stresses the Liver, and overstimulates the adrenal glands. Avoid sugar and sugar-rich foods whenever possible.

In addition to these dietary changes, be sure to drink at least eight to ten 8-ounce glasses of water daily to help the Liver and Kidney perform their functions and to thin the mucus in the sinus and nasal passages, allowing for easier drainage. Unsweetened apple juice or dark grape juice will also help thin and drain the mucus.

Exercise

Exercise helps to move *chi* through the body, stimulating healing, combating physical fatigue, and relieving emotional stress. If you feel achy and depleted of energy, try a gentle exercise like brisk walking. If your energy remains fairly strong and is drained only during acute infections or flare-ups, feel free to exercise more vigorously in between flare-ups.

Consult Chapters 2 to 6 for specific advice regarding exercise for your constitutional type.

Nutritional Supplements

Vitamin C: This crucial immune-enhancing vitamin and natural antihistamine plays a significant role in keeping your sinuses healthy. When you are feeling healthy and asymptomatic, take 2,000–4,000 mg. (2–4 grams) daily as a general preventive measure. If you suffer from chronic allergies and/or chronic sinusitis, take 1,000 mg. every hour or two, up to 20 grams daily (or to bowel tolerance).

The sicker you are, the more vitamin C your body can tolerate. If you take megadoses of vitamin C and experience diarrhea or loose bowels, cut back about ten percent or until the symptoms disappear, maintaining that dose until the infection is gone. At that point, return to the suggested "maintenance dose" of 2–4 grams daily.

Vitamin A or beta-carotene: Vitamin A helps produce mucopolysaccharide, a vital component of the mucous membranes, and helps maintain the integrity of the skin and mucous membranes, fortifying the body's protective barriers against infectious organisms. With its powerful antioxidant and immune-stimulating qualities, vitamin A is extremely important for preventing and curing sinusitis.

It is important to remember that because vitamin A is fat soluble, it can accumulate in the body's tissues. To avoid any danger of toxicity, we recommend that you take beta-carotene or mixed carotenes, which are converted in the intestines into vitamin A. Even in large amounts, beta-carotene is nontoxic. The only side effect of megadoses is a slight yellowing of the skin, which disappears when large doses are discontinued. Take 25,000 I.U. of beta-carotene twice daily (50,000 I.U. total); if you take vitamin A, do not exceed 25,000 I.U. daily without professional supervision. *Note:* If you have liver damage or disease, do not exceed 5,000 I.U. of vitamin A without consulting with your health care practitioner.

Vitamin E: A powerful antioxidant, vitamin E prevents free radicals from forming, protects the body's cells from free radical damage, and stimulates the immune system to fight infections. Take 400 I.U. daily as a general preventive measure and 800 I.U. daily during acute flare-ups.

Zinc: Zinc increases T-cell production, stimulating the immune system and specifically helping the body fight viral infections and promote healing of cells and tissues; zinc also reduces the incidence and severity of colds and infections. Take 30–50 mg. daily on a preventive basis, and up to 60 mg. daily during active infections; zinc gluconate is particularly well tolerated and easy to absorb.

Whenever you supplement zinc, you should take extra copper to maintain a healthy balance between the two minerals. The ratio of zinc to copper should be fifteen to one; thus, if you take 30 mg. of zinc, take 2 mg. of copper.

Caution: Because zinc can be toxic in large doses, do not exceed 100 mg. daily.

Selenium: Selenium works synergistically with vitamin E, multiplying its protective effects. Like vitamin E, selenium protects macrophages from destruction by free radicals and protects the body against carcinogens (cancer-causing substances). Selenium has also been proven to be useful in treating a variety of inflammatory and autoimmune disorders, including chronic sinusitis, asthma, arthritis, and lupus. Take 200 mcg. daily.

Note: The antioxidant effects of selenium and vitamin E are synergistic, so take these supplements together. Because vitamin C can hinder the absorption of selenium, you might want to take these vitamins at different times.

Caution: Selenium can be toxic in large doses; do not exceed 600 mcg. daily unless you are under professional supervision.

Sinus Cleanse

If you have chronic sinusitis, you've undoubtedly heard about nasal washes and sinus cleansing. Warm saltwater washes are commonly recommended, while more exotic cleanses (which involve using an eyedropper to insert fresh-squeezed garlic directly into the nasal passages or sniffing ginger) are becoming increasingly popular.

For preventing and curing sinus infections, we recommend a variation of a cleanse suggested by Japanese acupuncturist Kiiko Matsumoto. Put a teaspoon of sea salt and a pinch of baking soda in a cup of lukewarm water, mix well, and pour a small amount of this solution into the cupped palm of your hand. *Gently* inhale through each nostril, moving your head around to circulate the saltwater solution. Let the water drain out of your nose, or spit it out of your mouth; gargle with the remaining solution, and spit it out. Repeat daily.

For acute flare-ups, repeat this procedure three to five times daily.

Chinese Patent Remedies

For acute sinus infections, we recommend:

Bi Yan Pian ("Benefit the Nose Tablets"): This formula contains twelve herbs (Magnolia Flower is the Emperor herb) to help eliminate the Wind/Heat or Wind/Cold from the nasal areas. Take five pills two to three times a day for symptomatic relief of sinus congestion.

To prevent chronic recurrences, take five pills daily of Bi Yan Pian along with ten pills taken twice daily of:

Hsiao Yao Wan ("Relaxed Wanderer Pills"): This famous remedy was specifically designed to keep the Liver *chi* moving and flowing. Hsiao Yao Wan also helps relieve the allergic response so often associated with chronic sinusitis. The formula, which consists of eight herbs, with bupleurum reigning as Emperor, is extremely gentle and can be used safely for long periods of time.

These Chinese patent remedies are gentle and can safely be combined with any of the following Western herbs. If you need help choosing the most effective formula or combination of herbs for your symptoms, consult an experienced herbalist.

Herbal Allies

An effective herbal remedy for chronic sinusitis would include three different kinds of herbs:

1. *Decongestant and expectorant herbs,* which work to break up the blockages in the sinus cavities
2. *Antimicrobial herbs,* to fight off bacterial or viral invaders
3. *Supportive (tonic) herbs,* to strengthen the system and enhance overall immune function

We highly recommend the following herbs, which can be mixed together in a formula. They may also be found in various remedies (usually combined with other herbs) in health food stores.

Ephedra (*Ephedra sinica*): Also known as *ma huang,* ephedra is the most effective *decongestant herb* available, helping to open the nasal and sinus passages. Its anti-allergic actions enhance its effectiveness for sinusitis.

Caution: Ephedra is a powerful herb and should be used only for short periods of time, in small amounts, and only for allergies, sinus infections, upper respiratory infections, and asthma. Do not exceed the recommended dose.

Licorice root (*Glycyrrhiza glabra*): This wonderful *expectorant* herb assists the respiratory system in eliminating excess mucus. Licorice also replenishes the mucous membranes, helps to clear the bronchial system, breaks up congestion in the head, and has both antimicrobial and anti-inflammatory qualities. Licorice is an excellent choice for children with sinus problems.

Mullein (*Verbascum thapsus*): Used for centuries by Native Americans to ease upper respiratory congestion, this *expectorant* herb soothes irritated mucous linings, relieves coughs, colds, and sore throats, and subdues the pain and discomfort associated with bronchial tissues that become inflamed due to postnasal drip.

Osha root (*Ligusticum porteri*): This extremely powerful *antimicrobial* herb offers fast and effective relief for sore throats and acute sinus infections.

Goldenseal (*Hydrastis canadensis*): This *antimicrobial,* antibiotic, and immune-boosting herb works to heal inflamed mucous membranes and generally supports the Liver's ability to detoxify allergens and other toxic substances.

Echinacea (*Echinacea angustifolia* or *Echinacea purpura*): This Native American tonic was adopted by European settlers and is now used worldwide. It is renowned for its immune-enhancing antibiotic and antimicrobial actions.

For acute flare-ups of sinusitis, try this effective herbal antibiotic treatment: Crush a clove of garlic, mix it with a teaspoon of honey, and swallow. Repeat every two or three hours (if your stomach doesn't rebel) until your symptoms relent.

Dosage: If you purchase your herbs in a health food store (either in tincture form or, as dried herbs, in capsule or pill form), follow the dosage instructions on the label. Because herbs in dried form tend to lose their potency rather quickly, be sure to check the label for the expiration date.

For information on preparing your own herbs from the root, bark, leaves, flowers, or seeds of a plant, see Appendix II.

In Appendix I, Resources, we offer a list of mail-order sources for high-quality herbs and herbal preparations. For advice on ordering specially made herbal formulas, see pages 394 to 396.

Herbal Inhalations

To relieve the stuffed-up congestion in your nose and sinuses and the headaches that often accompany these symptoms, add a handful of chamomile flowers or several chamomile tea bags to a pot of boiling water. Cover, remove it from the heat, and let it sit for a few minutes. After five or ten minutes, put a towel over your head, uncover the pot, and breathe deeply, inhaling the steam vapors. (Be careful not to burn yourself.) If you are still congested, you can add cinnamon and a drop of eucalyptus or peppermint oil to the hot water.

If you're in a hurry, try this strategy: Before you shower in the morning, put a few drops of eucalyptus or pine oil on a wet washcloth. Hang the washcloth over the shower head or shower door, turn the water on as hot as you can stand it, and breathe deeply of the sweet-smelling steam.

As a general preventive, use an over-the-counter saline (saltwater) nasal spray. These inexpensive sprays (Ocean is a popular brand) help lubricate the nasal passages and wash away allergens. When used on a daily basis, saline sprays can help prevent or alleviate the symptoms of allergies and sinus infections.

Acupoints

Two Large Intestine points will give you temporary relief from sinus pain and related congestion.

Large Intestine 4 ("Great Eliminator"): This is one of the most frequently used points in acupuncture. Traditionally used for draining or dispersing constrained ("stuck") energy in the upper part of the body, especially the head and neck areas, it relieves headaches, sinus congestion, stuffy nose, irritated eyes, sore throat, swollen glands, and chronic tension in the neck and shoulder regions. This point can be extremely sensitive, even painful to the touch.

Location: Large Intestine 4 is located on the top of the hand in the webbing between the thumb and index finger. Massage in circular, clockwise movements for one or two minutes.

Large Intestine 20 ("Receiving Fragrance"): This point opens the nasal passages and clears the sinuses, allowing you to "receive the fragrances" of the world around you. (It is commonly used to help people stop smoking.) This point is often painful in people who suffer from chronic or acute sinusitis.

Location: Large Intestine 20 is located on either sides of the nostrils, in the depression just beneath the cheekbone. Press firmly with your fingers using circular motions; continue massaging for one or two minutes. If one side is more sensitive than the other, spend an extra minute or so on that side.

Yin Tang ("Seal Hall"): This extra point is not located on any particular meridian. Yet it is one of the most important points to unblock the nasal passages and ease the symptoms of chronic sinusitis. It is also used to promote inner vision and create the space for meditation and enlightenment. It is sometimes called "the Third Eye."

Location: Yin Tang is located between the eyebrows in the center of the forehead. Massage in small clockwise circles with the tips of your fingers.

Questions to Ask Yourself

The Chinese believe that sinusitis is always related to "stuck" *chi* in either the Liver, Lungs, or Kidneys. These questions will help you "talk" to your illness and discover where your energy is blocked or deficient.

If you are a Wood (Liver) type, you will need to look at your ability to express anger:

- Who is the object of my anger?
- How can I effectively express my anger?
- Where do I typically store my anger?

If you are a Metal (Lung) type, excess or stored-up grief may be affecting your ability to resist disease. Ask yourself:

- How do I prevent myself from feeling grief?
- What do I need to let go of? Why am I holding on?
- Where do I tend to store my grief?

If you are a Water (Kidneys) type, fear often obstructs your energy. Ask yourself:

- How does my fear create blockages that prevent me from attaining my goals in life?

- Where do I tend to store my fear?
- How do I allow fear to rule my life?
- What exactly do I fear and why?

Fire and Earth types also suffer from periodic sinus infections. Fire types are prone to overexcitement and agitation, while Earth types are often adversely affected by excessive worrying. Ask yourself these questions:

- Why do I feel stuffed up emotionally?
- What can I do to "decongest" my life and give myself more time and space to pursue my goals and passions?
- Am I overreacting in any way? What can I do to calm myself down?

A STARTING POINT

Picking and choosing among the many and diverse remedies recommended for sinusitis may seem like an overwhelming task. Where should you begin?

The following supplements, herbal remedies, and healing strategies will give you a solid foundation that you can then build upon, using the other remedies suggested in this section when and if you need additional support:

1. *Diet:* Follow the dietary suggestions on pages 219 to 220.
2. *Exercise:* Exercise twenty to thirty minutes every day.
3. *Nutritional supplements:* Take the general formula for Maximum Immunity, with the following change: Increase vitamin C to 1,000 mg. every hour or two during active infections; cut back on the dosage if you experience diarrhea.
4. *Zinc:* Take 30 to 50 mg. daily preventively and up to 60 mg. daily during acute infections.
5. *Sinus cleanse:* Follow the instructions on page 222 for the Sinus Cleanse.
6. *Bi Yan Pian:* Take five of these pills two to three times daily.
7. *Western herbal tonic:* Take a tonic of licorice root (one third of the total), mixed with equal amounts of mullein, ephedra, osha root, and echinacea.

Asthma

When I asked Margaret how her asthma made her feel, she was momentarily taken aback. No one had ever asked her that question before. "I feel like I can't breathe," she said, her words nearly choked off by fear. "I feel as if I'm suffocating."

"How do you feel suffocated in your life?" I asked, and with that question Margaret began to explore the physical, psychological, and spiritual dimensions of her illness. She talked about the terror she experienced when she couldn't breathe, and she discussed her feelings of being smothered by her work. Recently promoted to nursing supervisor in the intensive care unit of a large hospital, she felt as if she were buried under a mountain of paperwork, with no breathing room and no time to spend with her friends and family.

"I feel stifled emotionally," she admitted as the tears ran freely down her cheeks. "Living with a chronic disease is like dying a little bit every day. Day after day, moment to moment, I live with the knowledge of my own mortality. I try to hide my fears from my husband and children because I don't want to upset them, but that only increases my sense of isolation."

Pulse and tongue diagnoses along with the physical examination and family history suggested an imbalance in Water energy; the blue-black hue around her eyes and temples, her strong, sturdy physique, the moaning sound of her voice, and the ever-present emotion of fear supported the diagnosis of deficient Water energy.

The Chinese believe that the power of Water nourishes and cleanses the body with energy called *chi*. Water is stored in the Kidneys, vital zones of activity that function as the pilot light of the entire system. Margaret's long history of allergies and prolonged doses of antibiotics in her childhood and teenage years had depleted her Kidney *chi,* creating an underlying imbalance and vulnerability to asthma. The deficient Kidney energy is unable to grasp and circulate the Lung *chi,* leading to congested, stagnating energy that manifests itself in symptoms such as wheezing, coughing, and choking sensations.

During the acupuncture sessions we talked about the power of Water and its emotional expression: fear. "Water is the element of self-empowerment," I explained as I inserted the ultrafine, stainless steel needles in Lung 7 ("Broken Sequence"), Kidney 6 ("Luminous Sea"), and *Ding Chuan* ("Benefit Asthma Point"). "Fear is not necessarily a negative emotion, for it teaches us to be ready and prepared. Water knows its limitations—it doesn't plunge recklessly ahead but gathers its energy, waiting for the right moment before proceeding along the path of least resistance. In the same way, you can learn how to prepare yourself, contain your energy, and use your fear appropriately to guide you through difficult situations in life."

A year after she began acupuncture and herbal treatments, Margaret was no longer taking any prescription medications, she was exercising daily, and she had switched to a new job that allowed her more freedom and "breathing space." "I feel as if my whole life has expanded," she told me. "I don't live in fear anymore, because I know that I have the inner resources to take care of myself. Whenever I get confused or afraid, I shut my eyes, breathe deep, and imagine that I am Water—endlessly adaptable, infinitely resourceful, filled with both power and potential."

WESTERN INTERPRETATION

A chronic disease of the bronchi, the large passages that convey air throughout the lungs, asthma (now referred to as reactive airway disease, or RAD) occurs periodically rather than constantly, and the symptoms vary in frequency, duration, and intensity.

The disease is caused by multiple triggers, which first induce bronchoconstriction and then swelling and inflammation, eventually leading to obstruction of the airways.

Allergic (atopic) *asthma* is triggered by an allergic reaction to hay, dust, mold, and other airborne allergies, as well as food and drugs; more than half of asthma cases are allergy related. Allergic asthma typically begins in childhood (approximately one third of allergic asthma victims are children) and tends to be hereditary; if your parents or grandparents had asthma, you have a greater likelihood to inherit a susceptibility to the disease. Allergy-induced asthma tends to be troublesome in the spring, summer, and fall, when flower and weed pollens abound.

Secondary asthma is caused by chronic and recurrent infections of the bronchi, sinuses, tonsils, or adenoids and may develop because of a hypersensitivity to the bacteria causing the infection.

Factors that contribute to the development of asthma include exposure to irritating chemicals inside and outside the home (pollen, dust, mold, chemical products, house-cleaning agents), cigarette smoke (including secondhand smoke), diets high in sugar and fat, emotional stress, and an inherited predisposition. House dust is a common cause, especially for people who live in cramped, crowded conditions with little fresh air to breathe.

Because stress, nervous tension, and emotional problems often contribute to the severity and frequency of the attacks, asthma has long been considered a psychosomatic (psychologically induced) disease. Strenuous exercise can also induce attacks (exercise-induced asthma, or EIA) in both allergy-induced and secondary asthma.

Asthma *symptoms* range from relatively mild to severe and even life-threatening—they include shortness of breath, labored or difficult breathing, coughing, wheezing, and feelings of tightness or constriction in the chest. At the end of an attack, the asthma victim may cough up thick, mucus-filled sputum from the lungs. When the airways are constricted, panic can occur, particularly in children who do not understand the nature of their illness.

More than 14 million Americans, including 5 million children, suffer from asthma—an increase of 61 percent since the early 1980s. Although Western medicine has worked miracles with asthma, prolonging the lives of severe asthmatics and offering quick, effective treatment for acute flare-ups of the disease, the incidence of asthma continues to rise. In the last two decades the death toll has nearly doubled, to 5,000 a year.

WESTERN TREATMENT

For allergic (atopic) asthma, treatment typically begins with attempts to isolate the allergen causing the attacks; the patient is then advised to make every effort to avoid the offending substance(s).

For both allergic and secondary asthma, various medications are used to relieve symptoms. The most common include:

• **Anti-inflammatory medications.** These drugs are used for routine maintenance of moderate to severe asthma. The most frequently prescribed are the anti-inflammatory steroids, which block the progression of bronchial inflammation and help prevent future flare-ups. To control an asthma attack, inhaled corticosteroids such as Azmacort, Beclovent, and Vanceril are most frequently used. Oral corticosteroids (prednisone, prednisolone, Medrol) can have dangerous side effects and are usually reserved for severe asthma cases and emergency situations.

• **Bronchodilators** (Ventolin, Alupent, Proventil, Metraprel). These drugs work by dilating (widening) the airways, which helps to alleviate acute attacks. Prolonged use of these products makes them less effective over time when inflammatory swelling is present; although the medications dilate the bronchi, the swelling caused by the inflammation is *not* affected. This often leads people to use more of these drugs with less effect. Patients are cautioned to use bronchodilators only when absolutely necessary.

• **Expectorants.** These medications help thin the mucus, which allows the patient to cough up any phlegm that might be obstructing the airways. Guaituss, Anti-Tuss, and Robitussin are popular over-the-counter varieties; Fenesin, Sinumist, and Humibid are prescription expectorants. Although expectorants are relatively harmless, beware of added ingredients such as antihistamines, which can actually thicken the mucus and aggravate the asthmatic condition.

• **Theophylline.** This potent stimulant is used to dilate bronchial passages. Side effects include fast or racing heart rate, elevated blood sugar levels, and nausea and vomiting. Medications that include theophylline are Bronkodyl, Dilor, Theo-Dur, and Theolair.

• **Cromolyn and Tilade.** These drugs act like Teflon to coat the bronchial mucosa, preventing allergens from attaching to the mast cells and instigating an asthmatic episode. Although these drugs can induce coughing, they are usually well tolerated and are considered the drugs of choice for exercise-induced asthma (EIA).

Other strategies are commonly recommended by Western medicine as well:

• *Special air filters* help remove dust, pollen, and other airborne allergens.
• Patients are often advised to *avoid overexcitement and excess stress.*
• *Psychotherapy* can sometimes help the patient resolve emotional problems that may be causative or contributory.

TRADITIONAL CHINESE INTERPRETATION

When an asthma attack occurs, you experience difficulty exhaling the air trapped in your Lungs, a process that in traditional Chinese medicine is described as "the Kidney *chi* unable to grasp the Lung *chi*." Asthma is considered a deficiency of both Lung and Kidney *chi*; the weakened Kidney *chi* doesn't have the strength to grab hold of the Lung *chi*, and the energy circulates without being replenished, eventually stagnating in the Lungs. In allergic asthmatic reactions the Chinese would look to an imbalance in Liver *chi*.

Wind is considered the most important pathogenic force in asthma. When the Lung and Kidney *chi* are deficient, Wind penetrates the surface through the Wind points on the neck and shoulders, causing colds, chills, fevers, migrating aches and pains, and sinusitis. If the weakened *wei chi* is unable to evict the intruder, Wind eventually penetrates deeper, infiltrating the Lungs and causing the wheezing, difficult breathing, coughing, fear, and panic associated with asthma.

According to traditional Chinese medicine, the emotions play an extremely important role in every disease and disorder, and the complex interconnections between emotional and physical factors are given careful attention. Metal energy, which is closely aligned with the emotion of grief, governs the Lungs, while the Kidneys (Water) are associated with Fear and the Liver (Wood) with anger. Extreme grief, fear, or anger is considered injurious to these vital organs, and treatment will always involve helping patients identify the underlying source of their emotional distress and discover ways to express their emotions, thus dissipating their negative effects.

Diet

Foods that restore the smooth and even flow of energy in the Lung, Kidney, and Liver are highly recommended. Because half of all asthma cases are allergy-induced, the first and most important dietary change you can make is to eliminate potential food allergens from your diet. Since dairy products (milk, butter, cheese, yogurt, cottage cheese, and ice cream), eggs, and wheat products (bread, cereal, gravies, crackers, cookies) are the most common food allergens, eliminate these foods first. Other common food allergens include egg products, chocolate, citrus fruits and juices (particularly oranges and orange juice), soy products, peanuts and other nuts, shellfish, and yeast.

One of the best methods of determining food sensitivities is the Elimination Provocation Diet, in which the patient eliminates the suspected food allergen for at least five days and then reintroduces the food back into his diet for three days. Blood tests such as the Radio Allergo Sorbent Test (RAST) can also detect immune reactions to food by measuring IgG or IgE antibodies to specific food allergens. If you suspect that you might have food allergies or sensitivities, ask your health care provider about these tests.

Even if you aren't allergic to dairy products, they should be restricted because they cause mucus to build up in the upper respiratory system, aggravating and intensifying the distressing symptoms of asthma. Drink water instead of milk, and avoid cheese, butter, yogurt, cream, and ice cream whenever possible.

Be sure to drink a minimum of eight to ten 8-ounce glasses of fresh, filtered water every day. Water will help thin the mucus and ease its elimination from the body.

Onions are a favorite folk remedy for asthma, which makes sense because onions contain various compounds that relax the bronchial muscles and help prevent spasms. Some naturopathic physicians suggest drinking onion juice; if you find that particular remedy hard to stomach, simply add extra onions to your sandwiches, salads, soups, and stews.

Exercise

Exercise is essential to strengthen the Lungs and Kidneys; however, the specific amount of exercise you can tolerate is highly individual. As always, moderation is the key. When asthma symptoms are not bothering you, feel free to exercise as much and as often as you want. Aerobic exercises that require you to breathe deeply and regularly are particularly beneficial for the Lungs. Brisk walking, swimming (unless chlorine irritates your skin or lungs), and bicycling are all excellent choices. Yoga and tai chi exercises will also increase your energy and resilience. In general, try to exercise for twenty to thirty minutes every day.

During asthma attacks, avoid exercise and take time to rest and relax.

Refer back to Chapters 2 through 6 for specific advice on exercises to match your affinity to Wood, Fire, Earth, Metal, or Water.

Environmental Strategies

If you suffer from asthma, creating a safe indoor environment free from chemical irritants should be one of your first priorities. Choose house-cleaning products that are natural and unperfumed. If you use air conditioning, have the vents cleaned and disinfected at least once a year. Carpets are great hiding places for all sorts of irritants such as molds, dust mites, pollen, and other microorganisms, so have them professionally cleaned on a yearly basis. Be sure to ask the carpet cleaners if they can steam-clean without using perfumes or toxic dry-cleaning chemicals. Green plants continually absorb toxins and release fresh oxygen into the air, so place plants in strategic areas of your house.

Whenever you use toxic chemicals, either at home or on the job, wear an OSHA-approved mask, which is guaranteed by the federal government to filter out various pathogens. If your asthma is allergy-induced, you might consider purchasing an air cleaner or purifier. The best brands combine an activated carbon filtration system with an air ionizer. Bionaire makes an excellent model, which is available at finer department and electronics stores. Whatever brand you buy, make sure it is OSHA-approved.

Nutritional Supplements

The following eight vitamins and minerals will help you prevent and/or treat asthma. While this is a fairly hefty number of supplements to take on a daily basis, rest assured that they are all safe, even in large doses, and can be used for long periods of time with no ill effects. Once your symptoms are under control, you can gradually cut back and return to maintenance levels.

Children over age fourteen can take the supplements recommended, while children between ages five and thirteen should take half the recommended dosages. For children under five years of age, it's best to consult with a qualified professional before administering nutritional supplements.

Vitamin C: Vitamin C stimulates immune activity and acts as a natural antihistamine to relieve sneezing, wheezing, and coughing. If your asthma attacks are allergy-induced, take 2,000 mg. every two hours, up to 20 grams daily, during allergy season. To determine the optimal dose for vitamin C for you, increase your dosage until you experience loose stools or diarrhea; then cut back approximately ten percent or until symptoms subside.

For atopic (nonallergic) asthma, take 2,000–4,000 mg. (2–4 grams) daily.

Vitamin A or beta-carotene: A powerful antioxidant and immune stimulant, vitamin A helps fortify the body's defense system against infectious organisms. Because vitamin A is fat soluble, it can accumulate in the body's tissues; to avoid any danger of toxicity, we recommend taking 25,000–50,000 I.U. of beta-carotene, which is converted in the intestines into vitamin A.

Vitamin E: Vitamin E is a powerful antioxidant with impressive healing effects on tissues and mucous membranes. Take 400–800 I.U. daily.

Selenium: Selenium works synergistically with vitamin E to multiply its protective effects. Take 200 mcg. daily with vitamin E. Because vitamin C can hinder the absorption of selenium, you might want to take these vitamins at different times.

Caution: Selenium can be toxic in large doses; do not exceed 600 mcg. unless you are under professional supervision.

Magnesium: Magnesium possesses both antihistamine actions (reducing the symptoms of stuffed-up or runny nose, itching or watery eyes, sneezing, and coughing) and bronchodilating effects (promoting the opening of the respiratory airways). It has been used successfully in asthma treatment since the 1930s. There are two additional reasons to use magnesium: (1) Many commonly used asthma drugs leach magnesium from the cells lining the airways, creating a deficiency that can contribute to bronchial constriction; and (2) the meats, soft drinks, and food additives and preservatives that make up the typical Western diet generate large amounts of dietary phosphorus, which binds to magnesium and makes it unavailable for digestion and distribution to body tissues.

Take 500–1,000 mg. of magnesium daily; use the higher amount if you are taking asthma medications. Magnesium citrate, aspartate, or gluconate are easier to absorb and better tolerated than magnesium oxide. Look for chelated forms of magnesium.

Omega-3 fatty acids: These effective anti-inflammatory agents work to prevent and treat asthma; they also work to thin the blood, lower blood pressure and triglycerides, raise high-density lipoproteins (good cholesterol), and protect you against heart attacks and strokes. Found naturally in deep sea fish such as salmon, mackerel, herring, anchovies, canned sardines, and tuna, omega-3's are also available in fish oil capsules, sometimes called EPA (eicosapentaenoic acid, the active ingredient in fish oil) capsules. If you suffer from dry skin, acne, eczema, dry mouth, excessive thirst, hair loss, and/or cracked heels or nails, you may have a deficiency of omega-3 fatty acids.

Take 1,500 mg. daily for three or four weeks; then cut back to 500 mg. daily. If you can't tolerate fish oil because of allergies or the fishy aftertaste, flaxseed oil is a good substitute; take one tablespoon daily. Because flaxseed oil can quickly go rancid, be sure to refrigerate it and store it in an amber, light-protective container.

Vitamin B complex: This complex of vitamins helps your body cope more efficiently with stress, which can play a major role in the frequency and severity of asthma attacks. Take a B-50 or B-100 complex daily.

Pycnogenol (proanthocyanidan): This powerful antioxidant, with anti-inflammatory, immune-enhancing, and antihistamine effects, is derived from the seeds of grapes or the bark of pine trees. Fifty times more powerful than vitamin E and twenty times more potent than vitamin C, pycnogenol has been used in Europe for decades with promising results in the treatment of asthma and hay fever. Extensive research is now being conducted on this herb's healing potential for other inflammatory diseases, including arthritis and lupus.

Because grape seed is the more potent source of pycnogenol, buy supplements derived from grape seed or a combination of pine bark and grape seed. Take 50–100 mg. daily.

Chinese Patent Remedies
Ping Chuan Pills ("Relieve Asthma Pills"): This remedy has been used with great success to prevent chronic asthma and chronic bronchitis, for it supports Kidney and Lung *chi,* breaks up phlegm, and stops coughing attacks. Armeniaca seed reigns as the Emperor herb and is attended by codonopsis root, licorice

root, eleagnus fruit, morus root-bark, ficus leaf, citrus peel, cynanchum root, gecko lizard, and cordyceps fungus.

Take ten pills three times daily, reducing to ten pills twice daily as symptoms resolve; after a few weeks of being symptom-free, gradually reduce the dosage until you stop completely.

Su Zi Jiang Qi Wan ("Perilla Seed Guiding *Chi* Downward Pills"): This effective tonic for preventing asthma helps "ground" the *chi* and bring it back to the Kidneys. The Emperor herb is perilla seeds, an effective expectorant traditionally used for asthma and chronic bronchitis; ten attending herbs (perilla fruit, pinellia root, magnolia bark, peucedanium root, citrus peel, aquilaria, dong quai, ginger, ziziphus fruit, and licorice root) support the Lungs, disperse mucus, and nurture the Kidney *yang* (fire).

The formula comes in small bags; each bag contains eighteen grams. Take three grams (one sixth of a bag) three times daily; after a month or two, you can reduce the dosage to three grams daily.

Caution: This formula contains herbs that tend to be warming; do not use it if you experience "hot" symptoms such as green mucus, fever, or a dry, irritated cough.

These Chinese patent remedies are gentle and can be safely combined with any of the following herbs. If you need help choosing the most effective formula or combination of herbs for your symptoms or if the patient is a child, consult an experienced herbalist.

Herbal Allies

The following herbs can be used alone or combined in a single formula. Popular formulas available at health food stores offer different combinations of these herbs. You can also contact a qualified herbalist, who will mix up a formula tailored to your specific needs.

Ephedra (*Ephedra sinica*): Ephedra, or *ma huang,* has been used for more than five thousand years to treat asthma, especially allergy-induced asthma. Western researchers extracted ephedra's active ingredient, the alkaloid compound called ephedrine, and for many years this was the drug of choice for asthma. Ephedra should be used only under professional guidance, for in large amounts it can raise blood pressure, and long-term use in large doses can weaken adrenal function.

Used in small amounts, however, ephedra doesn't have the adrenalinelike side effects typically associated with ephedrine.

Caution: Always take ephedra in the doses recommended on the label, and do not take this powerful herb for conditions other than those for which it is prescribed. For long-term use, take under the supervision of a herbal professional.

Licorice (*Glycyrrhiza glabra*): Licorice combines well with ephedra to support the adrenal glands, lubricate the mucous membranes, and reduce inflammation and swelling. A gentle expectorant, it also helps to break up congested mucus. If you are taking corticosteriod drugs such as prednisone, be sure to take licorice, which supports and balances the adrenal glands, encouraging your body to produce natural steroids.

Lobelia (*Lobelia inflata*): Also known as Indian tobacco, lobelia was used with great success by Native Americans to prevent asthma attacks. Today, herbalists use it in teas or tinctures to prevent a minor asthmatic episode from escalating into a full-fledged attack. Lobeline, the active ingredient in lobelia, is a powerful expectorant that relaxes the bronchioles and helps relieve spasms. In larger doses, however, lobeline can induce vomiting.

Mullein (*Verbascum thapsus*): This gentle expectorant has been used by Native Americans and Europeans alike to soothe the entire respiratory system and heal various respiratory ailments.

Ginkgo (*Ginkgo biloba*): This potent circulatory stimulant helps reduce inflammation and counteract allergic reactions.

Dosage: If you purchase your herbs in a health food store (either in tincture form or, as dried herbs, in capsule or pill form), follow the dosage instructions on the label. Because herbs in dried form tend to lose their potency rather quickly, be sure to check the label for the expiration date.

For information on preparing your own herbs from the root, bark, leaves, flowers, or seeds of a plant, see Appendix II.

In Appendix I, Resources, we offer a list of mail-order sources for high-quality herbs and herbal preparations. For advice on ordering specially made herbal formulas, see pages 394 to 396.

Acupoints

Kidney 3 ("Great Mountain Stream"): This point supports and nourishes every aspect of Kidney function, including the *yin, yang, chi,* and *jing,* relieving conditions characterized by depleted energy such as asthma. Pressing or massaging this point can also work as a preventive for asthma.

Location: Kidney 3 is located in the depression between the inside ankle bone and the Achilles tendon. Use your fingers to poke around in the valley until you feel the tender spot.

Lung 9 ("Great Abyss"): This point is used to support the *wei chi* (immune energy) and activate and energize the Lung *chi,* helping to remedy asthma as well as colds, bronchitis, and sinus infections. A *yin* (Water)-supporting point, Lung 9 is also helpful for anxiety, heart palpitations, and general irritability.

Location: Lung 9 is located on the crease on the palm side of the wrist in the depression at the base of the thumb, about half an inch in from the side of the wrist.

Ding Chuan ("Benefit Asthma Point"): This "extraordinary" point—that is, a point with special powers not located on any particular meridian—is specifically used to prevent and treat asthma.

Location: Find the prominent vertebra at the base of your neck (the seventh cervical vertebra) and move your fingers outward one half-inch on either side of the spinal column. Gently massage with your fingertips for one or two minutes; repeat several times a day.

Questions to Ask Yourself

The Lungs are governed by Metal energy, which is closely aligned with the experience of grief. Practitioners of traditional Chinese medicine believe that extreme grief is damaging to the Lungs. Treatment often includes questions and exercises designed to help the patient express grief and thus dissipate its negative influence on the Lungs.

If you suffer from asthma, ask yourself:

- What have I lost that I continue to grieve over?
- How can I mourn my loss and then let it go?
- Why do I choke off my emotions?
- What do my symptoms prevent me from doing or accomplishing?

Fear is the emotion connected with the Kidneys. Excess fear can weaken the Kidneys to the point that they are unable to "grasp the Lung *chi*" and replenish it, which can lead to asthma. These questions may help you to identify the source and nature of your fears:

- How do my symptoms contribute to my fears of being closed in, choked off, and unable to breathe?
- Does my disease in some sense represent a fear of dying?
- What can I do to take control of my fear and my life?
- How can I expand my horizons, express my fears, and move beyond them?

A STARTING POINT

Picking and choosing among the many and diverse remedies recommended for asthma may seem like an overwhelming task. Where should you begin?

The following supplements, herbal remedies, and healing strategies will give you a solid foundation that you can then build upon. Use the other remedies suggested in this section when, and if, you need additional support:

1. *Diet:* Follow the dietary suggestions on pages 232–233.
2. *Exercise:* Exercise for twenty to thirty minutes every day.
3. *Nutritional supplements:* Take the general formula for Maximum Immunity, with the following changes: *Increase vitamin C* to 1,000 mg. every hour or two when feeling symptomatic; and *increase magnesium* to 1,000 mg. daily.
4. *Omega-3 and GLA oils:* Take 1,500 units of each or 3,000 units combined daily.
5. *Ping Chuan pills:* These pills, safe and effective for mild cases of asthma, can be used for long periods of time.

6. *Western herbal tonic:* Licorice (one third of formula), mullein (one third), and ephedra and lobelia (remaining third).

Irritable Bowel Syndrome

"My senior year in high school was a disaster," twenty-seven-year-old Alison told me. "During midyear exams I had attacks of diarrhea that came on so suddenly I couldn't make it to the bathroom. You can't imagine how embarrassed and humiliated I felt."

After ruling out ulcers, Crohn's disease, and cancer, Alison's doctor diagnosed her disorder as irritable bowel syndrome and prescribed medication to control the symptoms. The medications helped, but whenever she was under stress, the sudden attacks of diarrhea and acute abdominal pain intensified. By the time Alison came to me for complementary treatments, her stress level had skyrocketed. Recently divorced, she was working two shifts as a sales clerk in order to make the mortgage payments for the house she had once shared with her husband.

"I can't seem to control anything in my life," she said, breaking into tears. "It's just a losing battle."

Slightly overweight, with broad hips and shoulders and soft, smooth skin, Alison tended to obsess about her physical problems, which included chronic indigestion, water retention, and a constant desire to eat. Her physical problems, her tendency to worry and fret, and her persistent self-doubt confirmed a strong affinity to Earth energies. In the acupuncture sessions we talked about her feelings of loss of control over her life and discussed various strategies she could take to regain control. Changes in her diet, herbal remedies, and stress-reduction techniques gradually gave her the feeling that she was capable of controlling her disease and managing the stress in her life.

One day Alison announced that she had decided to give up her beautiful old house and move into a smaller, less expensive home. Within a few months of the move, her symptoms basically disappeared. Now when she's stressed or anxious, she occasionally feels the familiar "twinges" and cramping sensations, but rather than give in to the feeling of losing control, she takes her herbs and nutritional supplements, schedules an acupuncture appointment, practices her breathing techniques, and takes whatever steps are necessary to "hold it all together."

WESTERN INTERPRETATION

Irritable bowel syndrome (IBS) is a catchall term for any dysfunction of the large or small intestine for which there is no apparent physiological cause. Often associated with stress, IBS has also been called "nervous dyspepsia," "spastic colon," "irritable colitis," "nervous colitis," or "intestinal neurosis."

Twenty-five years ago, medical and nursing dictionaries didn't even list IBS; today, thirty to fifty percent of all physician referrals to gastroenterologists are eventually diagnosed with IBS. Twenty to thirty percent of people in the United States have been diagnosed with this syndrome, and more than one third of the people in the Western world have experienced, at least temporarily, the full collection of symptoms known as IBS.

Women are three times more likely to experience chronic symptoms of IBS; however, since men are much less likely to go to a doctor when they are sick, the incidence among men may be significantly higher than it appears. The average age of onset occurs in the early adult years, between twenty and forty, although many people diagnosed with IBS recall suffering from IBS-type symptoms during childhood and/or adolescence.

Anxious and tense individuals are the most likely victims of IBS, and a clear connection has been established between the severity of symptoms and the level of stress in a person's life. Sudden bouts of IBS can be triggered by eating unusual, exotic, or extremely rich foods, or simply by eating too much food at once ("holiday tummy"). Antibiotics can also inflame the stomach and intestines, upsetting the delicate balance of beneficial bacteria in the digestive tract and triggering an attack of IBS.

Symptoms: The most common symptoms include a combination of diarrhea and constipation, intestinal spasms, and acute abdominal pain. Other gastrointestinal symptoms include heartburn, regurgitating acid (acid burp), flatulence, nausea, loss of appetite, watery diarrhea (usually in the morning), and thick, pasty stools that are difficult to eliminate and have a foul odor. Fatigue, headaches, and general feelings of weakness and lack of energy are also common.

With any chronic digestive disturbance, your doctor will conduct a series of tests to rule out more serious conditions like ulcers, Crohn's disease, ulcerative colitis, diverticulitis, gallbladder disease, bowel parasites (bacteria, amebic, or worms), or cancer. Specific diagnostic tests include a rectal exam; barium enema (GI series); various blood tests to check for infection, anemia, liver disease, or gallbladder disease; and a sigmoidoscopy, a procedure that uses an instrument for direct visual examination of the lower (sigmoid) colon. If all tests come back negative, the diagnosis will most likely be irritable bowel syndrome.

WESTERN TREATMENT

Because IBS has no obvious, easily identifiable cause and therefore defies the magic-bullet approach to healing, the doctor's job is basically limited to offering symptom relief. Treatment varies according to the symptoms. If you appear extremely nervous, anxious, or tense, your doctor may consider the disease psychosomatic and offer a palliative drug such as a tranquilizer, muscle relaxant, or pain-killer, as well as an antacid drug like Tagamet or Zantac to reduce stomach acid levels. When the pain is extreme, antispasmodics (muscle-relaxing drugs with specific actions on smooth muscles like the bowels) may be prescribed, along with bulking laxatives to help restore normal conditions in the digestive tract.

Increasing numbers of doctors are including complementary treatments in their practices and offering their patients advice about dietary changes (particularly the need to test for food allergies or sensitivities and consume adequate dietary fiber) and various stress-reduction techniques. Acupuncture is increasingly recognized as a valuable treatment for numerous gastrointestinal problems.

TRADITIONAL CHINESE INTERPRETATION

In traditional Chinese medicine the constellation of symptoms included under the diagnostic label IBS are described as "constrained Liver *chi* invading Spleen and Stomach." The Liver is the main organ responsible for processing and eliminating stress, and any obstruction in the free flow of energy and blood immediately affects the Liver. When the Liver *chi* begins to stagnate, a common symptom is acute abdominal pain (colic).

Deficient Spleen *chi* leads to problems with the absorption and assimilation of nutrients, causing loose bowels and lack of energy. The Liver controls the Spleen, and when the Spleen *chi* is weak, the Liver becomes domineering. "Liver Invading Spleen" symptoms include constipation and/or diarrhea, and acute pain in the upper and lower abdomen.

When the Liver is domineering, it also interferes with the natural descending actions of the digestive system, causing the Stomach to rebel and move food upward, which creates the nausea, belching, and acid-reflux burps so commonly associated with irritable bowel syndrome.

COMPLEMENTARY TREATMENTS

Diet

Test for food allergies: The first step in treatment is to search for possible food allergies or sensitivities. *We cannot state this too strongly: If you have been diagnosed with IBS or suffer from chronic intestinal symptoms, your problems may be caused by food allergies or sensitivities.* Blood tests such as the Radio Allergo Sorbent Test (RAST) can detect immune reactions to food by measuring IgG or IgE antibodies to specific food allergens. If you suspect that you have a food allergy or sensitivity, ask your health care provider about these tests or try the Elimination Provocation Diet. Because people are generally more allergic to dairy products (milk, butter, cheese, cream, ice cream, yogurt) than to any other food, try eliminating these foods first.

Take dietary fiber: Adding dietary fiber to your daily menu is essential in the treatment of any bowel dysfunction. The typical American fast-food, refined-carbohydrate diet does not provide us with sufficient roughage, which in itself may be a significant contributing factor to the epidemic rise in chronic intestinal disorders. Mucilaginous (slippery or viscous) fibers like psyllium, pectin, guar gum, and oat bran work in two basic ways: First, they coat the bowel, which supports the healing process; and second, they bulk the stools, making them lighter and easier to eliminate.

Psyllium is the main bulking agent in commercial laxatives like Metamucil and Fiberall, but it's best to avoid these products because they are treated with artificial colors and flavors and are sweetened with sugar or artificial sweeteners. Furthermore, most commercially grown psyllium is heavily sprayed with pesticides. For a completely organic (nonchemically treated) source of psyllium, we recommend Yerba Prima Daily Fiber Formula, which is equally effective for diarrhea and constipation. If you can't find Yerba Prima Formula at your health food store, ask the store owner for another organic brand of psyllium.

Bran (wheat bran), which is found in many cereals, is a hard fiber and can be abrasive to the intestinal lining, so use it with caution. *Do not use bran products if you are allergic or suspect you might be allergic to wheat.*

Whenever you take dietary fiber, be sure to drink a full glass of water immediately afterward to expand and soften the fiber. If you don't have enough water available in your system to "bulk" the fiber, it can thicken, harden, and actually obstruct your colon. A good general rule is to drink eight to ten 8-ounce glasses of fresh, filtered water daily.

Steam your vegetables: The Chinese believe that raw foods stress the Spleen, making it difficult to extract the essential nutrients from the plant. To help break down the tough cellulose coating that surrounds most vegetables, steam your vegetables before you eat them.

Eat plenty of complex carbohydrates: Complex carbohydrates—including whole-grain breads, cereals, and pastas, potatoes, brown rice, barley, oatmeal, millet, beans, and the like—are rich in natural dietary fiber and essential nutrients. Simple or refined carbohydrates (found in cakes, cookies, pastries, pretzels, chips, white bread, white flour, and refined pasta products) are stripped of bran, fiber, and virtually all nutrients.

Eat plenty of starchy vegetables: Winter squash, parsnips, turnips, yams, and butternut squash are all easily digested, nonallergenic foods.

Eat simply: Avoid eating too many different food groups at one sitting; different kinds of food stimulate the digestive system to release various and assorted enzymes, which may compete with each other and contribute to the distress of IBS. Try to stick to one or two food groups at each meal.

Avoid spicy foods: Spicy, exotic, and highly seasoned foods are difficult to digest, so avoid them whenever possible.

Stress Reduction Techniques

Stress plays a major role in IBS. A healthy, optimally functioning Liver is able to neutralize stress and minimize its effects on the body, but when stress is excessive or prolonged (and IBS, like all chronic illnesses, creates significant physical and emotional stress), the Liver becomes agitated and "invades" the Spleen and Stomach, interfering with digestion and contributing to acid buildup, gas, bloating, and abdominal pain.

Stress is indigestible—you can't swallow it and expect it to pass through your system without causing at least minor damage. To relieve the symptoms associated with IBS, practice stress-reduction techniques like deep breathing exercises, meditation, or massage therapy. Refer back to the advice on lifestyle changes in Chapters 2 to 6, and follow the suggestions for your constitutional type.

Exercise

Regular exercise helps the Liver create a free flow of energy and blood; when the Liver works efficiently, you will feel less stressed, both physically and emotionally. Since irritable bowel syndrome is exacerbated by stress (or in Chinese terms, "constrained Liver *chi*"), exercise is extremely important for restoring balance and harmony.

During acute flare-ups of the disease, try gentle stretching exercises such as yoga or tai chi. In between flare-ups, feel free to exercise strenuously. Refer back to Chapters 2 to 6 for advice on specific exercises geared to your constitutional type.

Nutritional Supplements

Beta-carotene: This is a powerful antioxidant and immune stimulant. Take 25,000–50,000 I.U. daily.

Vitamin C: This vitamin supports immune function, protects your cells from oxidative damage, and is vitally important in the repair and maintenance of the intestinal lining. Take 1,000 mg. three to six times (for a total of 3–6g) daily.

Vitamin E: This vitamin strengthens the *wei chi* and *chi* to fight off infection, protect the body from damage by free radicals, and shield the body systems from stress. Take 400–800 I.U. daily; the natural d-alpha tocopherol form is best.

B complex: These vitamins calm the body and mind, protecting you against stress. Vitamin B$_6$ (pyridoxine), PABA (para-aminobenzoic acid), and folic acid are all actively involved in stimulating the metabolism of carbohydrates, fats, and proteins. Both pyridoxine and folic acid help regulate hydrochloric acid production. Take one B-50 or B-100 complex daily.

Alfalfa: Rich in chlorophyll, vitamins, and minerals, these tablets contain all eight essential amino acids. Alfalfa is a safe, nutritious supplement that will gently support your digestion and metabolism. Take one or two tablets with each meal. (Follow the directions on the product label.)

Quercetin: This important bioflavonoid will help your body digest food more efficiently, reducing or eliminating allergic reactions. Quercetin is most effective when mixed with a pancreatic enzyme like bromelain; take one 250-mg. tablet three times daily, preferably a half hour before meals.

Acidophilus (*Lactobacillus acidophilus* and/or *Lactobacillus bifidus*): These friendly bacteria work to nourish and heal the entire digestive system. Healthy gut flora is vital to good health and supports bowel functions in general. *Always* take acidophilus if you have a yeast infection or if you are taking antibiotics, for it reintroduces friendly bacteria into the colon to restore normal bodily functions. We recommend enteric-coated capsules, which are coated to survive the acid bath in the stomach and release in the intestines where they are needed. In general we prefer a combination of *Lactobacillus acidophilus* and *Lactobacillus bifidus.*

Magnesium: This antistress mineral relaxes the smooth muscles of the intestinal tract as well as the skeletal muscles, promoting relaxation both internally and externally. (Calcium tends to foster contraction, while magnesium encourages relaxation.) Magnesium also stimulates the enzyme activity necessary for metabolizing proteins and carbohydrates, assists in the absorption of nutrients from food, and relieves fatigue, anxiety, and insomnia.

Take 500–1,000 mg. of magnesium daily; magnesium citrate, aspartate, or gluconate are easiest to absorb and better tolerated than magnesium oxide. If you take calcium, make sure your magnesium is at least equal to (and preferably double) the amount of calcium you take.

Zinc: Zinc enhances immune function and fights free radical damage. Take 30 mg. daily preventively; zinc gluconate is particularly well tolerated and easy to absorb.

Whenever you supplement zinc, you should take extra copper to maintain a healthy balance between the two minerals. The ratio of zinc to copper should be fifteen to one; thus, if you take 30 mg. zinc, take 2 mg. copper.

Caution: Because zinc can be toxic in large doses, do not exceed 100 mg. daily.

Chinese Patent Remedy

Shu Kan Wan ("Soothe Liver Pills"): This remedy invigorates and replenishes the *chi,* breaking up stagnation and relieving the pain that always accompanies obstructed energy. It is specifically formulated to restore the free and easy flow of Liver *chi,* resolving the adverse effects of energy blockage on the Stomach and Spleen. Peony root, which soothes and supports the Liver, reigns as Emperor and is assisted by the attending herbs cyperus root, peony root, aurantium fruit, amomum fruit, citrus peel, corydalis root, bupleurum root, moutan root-bark, inula flower, citrus *qing pi,* licorice, curcuma root, aquilaria wood, cardamom fruit, and santalum wood.

Take eight pills three times daily or twelve pills twice daily.

Caution: This is a strong combination of herbs, used to break up stagnation in the digestive tract and restore the free flow of blood and *chi.* Do not use during pregnancy.

Herbal Allies

The following herbs can be used alone or combined in a single formula. Popular formulas available at health food stores offer different combinations of these herbs, or you can contact a qualified herbalist, who will mix up a formula tailored to your specific needs. If you need help choosing the most effective formula or combination of herbs for your symptoms, consult an experienced herbalist.

Lemon balm (*Melissa officinalis*): This herb has a generalized relaxing effect on the entire digestive system.

Chamomile (*Matricaria chamomilla*): This herb helps relax the stomach and intestines and has a natural ability to reduce intestinal spasms and associated pain.

Ginger (*Zingiber officinalis*): This herb has been used extensively for intestinal problems in virtually every country of the world. A warming herb, ginger relaxes the gut, helps expel gas, and supports the natural movements of the intestines.

Licorice (*Glycyrrhiza glabra*): This herb lubricates the walls of the intestines and has natural anti-inflammatory actions.

Marshmallow root (*Althaea officinalis*): This herb can also be used for its lubricating effects.

In addition to the herbs described above, I often recommend the following herbal capsules for IBS:

Slippery elm (*Ulmus rubra*): This herb contains a gentle, nutritive substance called mucilage that helps ease the irritation and soothe the inflammation associated with digestive problems ranging from diarrhea to colitis, gastritis, and duodenal ulcers. Always take this herb in enteric-coated capsules before meals to ensure that it is released in the intestines rather than in the stomach.

Peppermint capsules: Used in Europe for IBS with considerable success, peppermint oil calms the intestines, relaxes the smooth muscles to relieve spasms, reduces gas, and alleviates abdominal pain. The oil must be in capsule form in order to release in the intestines rather than in the stomach. Take one capsule twice daily or as directed.

Herbal teas: To soothe your stomach, put two or three drops of peppermint oil in a cup of warm water; this comforting tea can be sipped throughout the day. *Wintergreen, catnip,* or *lemon balm* can be substituted for peppermint, or you can safely combine all four herbs in a soothing, relaxing tea.

Dosage: If you purchase your herbs in a health food store (either in tincture form or, as dried herbs, in capsule or pill form), follow the dosage instructions on the label. Because herbs in dried form tend to lose their potency rather quickly, be sure to check the label for the expiration date.

For information on preparing your own herbs from the root, bark, leaves, flowers, or seeds of a plant, see Appendix II.

In Appendix I, Resources, we offer a list of mail-order sources for high-quality herbs and herbal preparations. For advice on ordering specially made herbal formulas, see pages 394 to 396.

Acupoints

Stomach 25 ("Heavenly Axis"): This point is used to regulate digestive and intestinal functions, strengthen Earth's organs (the Spleen/Pancreas and Stomach), and resolve stagnation or "stuck" energy in the Stomach. Its balancing effects are thought to extend to the mind and spirit as well.

Location: Stomach 25 is located approximately two inches from the belly button on either side. Gently massage each point in clockwise circles for two or three minutes.

Liver 3 ("Great Rushing"): This point is often used when the Liver energy is constrained or deficient. Stimulating it helps to promote the free flow of *chi* and blood and expel Wind conditions, including tremors, muscle twitches, migrating aches and pains, dizziness, and headaches.

Location: Liver 3 is located on the upper part of the foot, in the depression in the webbing between the big toe and the second toe; massage in clockwise circles for two or three minutes.

Stomach 36 ("Walks Three Miles"): This point assists the Stomach and the Spleen in their task of transforming nutrients into usable energy. A powerfully energizing point, Stomach 36 supports the assimilation of food and fluids, regulates digestive problems, and rids the body of excess dampness.

Location: Stomach 36 is located three inches below the dimple or depression on the outside (pinky side) of the knee, in a groove or depression in the muscle. Massage in clockwise circles for two or three minutes.

Questions to Ask Yourself

Metaphors can be powerful agents in healing, helping you to imagine your illness and "talk" to it, asking the symptoms what they want from you. Overcoming fear and feelings of loss of control can significantly influence your ability to cope with IBS. These questions can help you identify the sources of your distress and guide you to potential solutions:

- Why am I afraid to open up to new possibilities in my relationships, career, and life in general?
- What am I afraid of losing?
- I feel as if too much is happening right now, and I'm losing control. Why am I so afraid to lose control?
- I feel stuck, particularly regarding my emotions. How can I learn to express my emotions rather than let them eat away at my insides?
- What am I unwilling to swallow and digest?
- What's eating me up inside?

Inflammatory Bowel Disease (Crohn's Disease and Colitis)

Before twenty-four-year-old Monica started acupuncture and herbal treatments for Crohn's disease, she had been taking steroids for more than a year. Concerned about the long-term effects of the drugs, her doctor had suggested she try complementary medicine.

Tall, thin, and impeccably dressed, with deep-set eyes, sculptured features, and a voice that sounded as if she were constantly on the verge of tears, Monica was clearly influenced by Metal energies. Chronic bowel problems, a long history of acne and skin-related disorders, perfectionist tendencies, and rigid adherence to schedules and routines confirmed Monica's natural affinity to Metal. Wood was also a dominant force in her life, apparent in her fiercely competitive nature and her desire to be the best at everything she attempted. An advertising executive in a large firm, Monica had gained a reputation as a highly efficient but difficult and demanding supervisor. In a recent meeting with her boss, she had been reprimanded for her lack of tact and insensitivity to her subordinates.

Monica's health problems began with intermittent episodes of bowel problems and abdominal pain, which evolved over a period of several years into chronic, debilitating diarrhea. After several hospitalizations, she was forced to take a medical leave from her job and move in with her parents. Of all the changes brought about by her illness, being forced to live with her parents caused her the most distress. "I struggled my whole life to get away from my parents and become self-sufficient," she said, "but this disease took away my independence."

After six months of acupuncture treatments and herbal therapy, Monica felt strong enough to move out of her parents' home and into an apartment in New York City, where she now lives with a female roommate and works at an advertising agency. Every few months she returns for an acupuncture session and "a good long talk"; she claims to love her herbal brew, which she credits for her renewed strength and vigor, but the acupuncture sessions seem to have made the biggest difference in her physical health and emotional well-being. "Every time I get stuck with those little needles, I feel stronger and more powerful," she explained. "I'm not exactly sure why it works—but it does."

WESTERN INTERPRETATION

Crohn's disease (also called "regional ileitis," "regional enteritis," "granulomatous ileitis," and "ileocolitis") is characterized by inflammation of the portion of the small intestine called the ileum. The disease can begin slowly or develop quite suddenly; some people experience mild discomfort, while others have severe and disabling symptoms. The cause—and therefore the cure—is unknown.

Diagnosis begins with various tests to rule out other bowel disorders. A gastrointestinal (GI) series will show whether the intestines have thickened, causing a narrowing of the channel within the bowel; a narrowed bowel channel is considered typical of Crohn's disease. Stool samples are tested for the presence of intestinal parasites, which are increasingly prevalent in the United States and can cause symptoms similar to Crohn's disease. Another test involves using a flexible endoscope to search for granulomas, or microscopic lesions on the intestinal walls caused by masses of inflammatory cells; approximately half of Crohn's cases feature granulomas, generally in the large intestine but also in the small intestine, stomach, and esophagus.

Symptoms of Crohn's disease include diarrhea, abdominal pain, rectal bleeding, fever, decreased appetite, and weight loss. The symptoms of ulcerative colitis are similar to those of Crohn's disease, and the two diseases are often grouped together under the name inflammatory bowel disease (IBD). In ulcerative colitis, however, the rectum is typically inflamed, whereas in Crohn's the rectum is generally not affected, and while granulomas are common in Crohn's, they are rare in ulcerative colitis.

Every year, approximately thirty thousand new IBD patients are admitted to American hospitals. Conservative estimates indicate that half a million people in this country suffer from Crohn's disease and ulcerative colitis; the Crohn's and Colitis Foundation of America calculates the number at more than two million. IBD tends to strike people at an early age, most frequently between twelve and twenty-eight.

Both Crohn's and ulcerative colitis are diseases of the Western world, with the United States, England, Scotland, the Scandinavian countries, Europe, and Israel reporting the majority of cases. Both diseases are rare in Asian countries and Africa. Many physicians consider the Western diet, which is high in fat, animal protein, sugar, and refined carbohydrates, and low in whole grains, fresh fruits and vegetables, to be a major causative or contributory factor in IBD.

Although extensive research has been conducted to discover a virus, bacterium, or parasite that might cause IBD, at this point a pathogenic cause remains elusive. Increasing numbers of physicians and researchers theorize that IBD may involve a hyperimmune response to some irritant in the digestive tract; one of the most likely suspects causing the irritation and abnormal immune response is a food allergy or sensitivity. A genetic predisposition is definitely implicated in the disease.

WESTERN TREATMENT

Medical treatment for both Crohn's and ulcerative colitis generally consists of managing the symptoms with various medications. The most commonly prescribed medications include sulfasalazines and corticosteroids, both anti-inflammatory drugs. The sulfasalazines blend sulfa drugs and an aspirinlike drug to reduce the inflammatory symptoms and provide relief; as the symptoms subside, the dosage is reduced. The corticosteroids work by suppressing the immune system's overreaction to the unknown digestive irritant, thus reducing the inflammation and its associated pain.

When these drugs are first used, the results are often quite dramatic, and the patient may experience complete relief from all symptoms. With repeated use of these drugs, however, the patient builds up tolerance and the original dosage becomes increasingly less effective. Side effects, particularly with larger doses over prolonged periods of time, can be severe and include weight gain, puffing and swelling of the face and neck, increased body and facial hair, thinning of the bones, peptic ulcers, diabetes, hypertension, and personality changes.

When the wall of the intestines becomes so thick and narrow that the stools cannot pass through, or when the colon is perforated by inflammation or ulcers, surgery may be necessary. In most surgeries for Crohn's disease, a bowel resection is performed, in which the diseased portion of the intestine or bowel is removed and the healthy ends are reattached. Approximately two thirds of people suffering from Crohn's disease are candidates for surgery; a second operation is required for forty percent of surgery patients.

TRADITIONAL CHINESE INTERPRETATION

In Chinese theory Crohn's disease and ulcerative colitis always involve a combination of deficient Spleen/Pancreas *chi* and stagnant Liver *chi*. In a typical case, the individual has a congenitally weak digestive system (indicating deficient Earth functions). Exposure to chronic physical or emotional stress creates obstructions in the Liver, and the constrained Liver *chi* begins to back up, creating stress on the already-vulnerable digestive system. Lethargy, diarrhea, a sallow complexion, a swollen, pale tongue, and a weak pulse are considered symptoms of deficient Spleen/Pancreas and Stomach *chi,* while pain and bloating are regarded as manifestations of stagnant Liver *chi.*

In acute flare-ups of Crohn's disease and ulcerative colitis, patients experience extreme pain, diarrhea, and fevers, which are interpreted as false *yang* symptoms caused by a buildup of heat and stagnation in the Liver, that eventually ignite small brushfires (false *yang*) in the digestive tract and colon. The perpetual brush fires drain the body's *yin* (fluid) supplies, eventually creating chronic inflammation in the digestive system. Although all types of people are diagnosed with Crohn's disease and ulcerative colitis, Wood and Earth types seem to be most susceptible.

Treatment strategies are selected to strengthen the Spleen and Stomach energies, break up the stagnating Liver *chi,* and drain the Liver fire, which is flaring up in the digestive tract. Herbal and acupuncture treatments focus on strengthening Earth (Stomach/Spleen) energies; when the power of Earth is strong, the Wood energy is grounded, its roots properly nourished. See Chapter 4 for more information on Earth-supporting treatment strategies.

COMPLEMENTARY TREATMENTS

Diet

Numerous studies show a distinct correlation between diet and the incidence of Crohn's disease and ulcerative colitis. The fact that these diseases are common in Western countries, where the diet is high in fat and sugar, and uncommon in Africa and Asia, where the diet is high in whole grains, fruits, and vegetables, confirms the influence of diet on these diseases.

Dietary treatment strategies generally follow those for irritable bowel syndrome (see pages 244 to 246). The Elimination Provocation test for food allergies or sensitivities is critical; research involving patients with Crohn's disease and ulcerative colitis point to dairy products and wheat as the most common food allergens.

Keep in Mind

- Avoid simple (refined) carbohydrates, which are found in sugar-rich, white-flour foods such as pastries, cakes, cookies, white breads, Italian or French breads, and white pasta products.
- Increase your daily intake of fiber and whole grains.
- Eat plenty of vegetables; to ease stress on your digestive system, gently steam them before eating.
- Avoid exotic or overspiced foods.

- Eat simple, nourishing, nonallergenic foods like broths, cooked carrots, rice, potatoes, winter squash, and bananas.
- Eat smaller, more frequent meals.
- Eat slowly—sit down, relax, take your time. Never eat on the run.

Exercise

Follow the general recommendations for irritable bowel syndrome, page 246.

Nutritional Supplements

If you are taking corticosteroid or sulfasalazine drugs for Crohn's disease or ulcerative colitis, you will need to take nutritional supplements to replace essential nutrients depleted by these drugs. The corticosteroids (prednisone, prednisolone, Medrol) interfere with protein metabolism, decrease the absorption of calcium and phosphorus, increase the urinary excretion of vitamin C, calcium, potassium, and zinc, and increase the body's requirements for vitamin B_6, ascorbic acid, folate, and vitamin D. The sulfasalazine drugs (Salazopyrin, for example) inhibit the absorption of folic acid, decrease the body's supply of iron, and increase the urinary excretion of vitamin C.

For Crohn's disease and ulcerative colitis, we recommend the same nutritional supplements (described on pages 246 to 248) for irritable bowel syndrome. One more supplement may offer additional benefits:

Essential fatty acids: EFAs are essential to the health and integrity of every cell in the body; their anti-inflammatory effects make them particularly important for Crohn's disease and ulcerative colitis. EFAs are available in the form of omega-3 oils (fish oils) derived from cold-water fish such as salmon, herring, mackerel, and sardines; you can eat these fish three times a week or take EPA (eicosapentaenoic acid) capsules, which contain the essential oils. The other source of EFAs is gamma linoleic acid (GLA), a powerful anti-inflammatory agent and immune stimulator that can be found in oil of evening primrose, borage seed oil, or black currant seed oil.

Omega-3 fish oils and GLAs are available in combined capsules. Whether you take the supplements separately or in a combined formula, make sure you get 1,500 mg. *each* of omega-3's and GLAs daily.

Chinese Patent Remedy

Shen Ling Bai Zhu Pian ("Codonopsis, Atractylodes, and Poria Pills"): This extremely gentle remedy is formulated to build Spleen *chi* and *yang,* thus helping to relieve the chronic diarrhea associated with Crohn's disease and ulcerative colitis. It is also used to treat fatigue, nausea, and indigestion. Atractylodes, the Emperor herb, is attended by codonopsis (or ginseng) root, dioscorea root, poria fungus, platycodon root, amomum fruit, and citrus peel to combat fatigue, nausea, and indigestion.

Take twelve pills twice daily before meals. Children ages five to twelve can take half the adult dosage; the pills can be crushed into powder and eaten with applesauce or apple juice.

This Chinese patent remedy can safely be combined with any of the following Western herbs. If you need help choosing the most effective formula or combination of herbs for your symptoms, consult an experienced herbalist.

Herbal Allies

The same herbs and dosages recommended for irritable bowel syndrome (pages 244 to 246) work well for Crohn's disease or IBD. For their anti-inflammatory effects, you may add the following herbs to the herbal formula:

Echinacea (*Echinacea angustifolia* or *Echinacea purpura*): This antiviral, antimicrobial herb has a general balancing effect on the immune system. It prevents the spread of infection, preserves the integrity of the body's cells and tissues, and heals inflamed tissues.

Comfrey (*Symphytum officinale*): This herb has been used since ancient times for its great healing powers. Modern herbalists consider it particularly useful in ulcerative or inflamed intestinal conditions because of its anti-inflammatory and tissue-healing actions. Caution: In large quantities comfrey can overburden the Liver; medicinal amounts should be taken only after careful consultation with a trained professional.

Dosage: If you purchase your herbs in a health food store (either in tincture form or, as dried herbs, in capsule or pill form), follow the dosage instructions on the label. Because herbs in dried form tend to lose their potency rather quickly, be sure to check the label for the expiration date.

For information on preparing your own herbs from the root, bark, leaves, flowers, or seeds of a plant, see Appendix II.

In Appendix I, Resources, we offer a list of mail-order sources for high-quality herbs and herbal preparations. For advice on ordering specially made herbal formulas, see pages 394 to 396.

Acupoints

Stomach 25 ("Heavenly Axis"), Stomach 36 ("Walks Three Miles"), and Liver 3 ("Great Rushing") work well for Crohn's disease as well as irritable bowel syndrome; see page 250.

Questions to Ask Yourself

In Crohn's disease, as in irritable bowel syndrome, Earth and Wood energies are typically out of balance. Earth is associated with constant fretting and an inability to care for yourself or receive emotional nourishment from others, while imbalances in Wood energy are closely connected to anger and rash decision making.

Use these questions to "talk" to your disease. Let the answers guide you to a deeper understanding of your needs, desires, and fears.

- What conflict in my life is eating away at me, and how can I deal with it?
- How am I not allowing myself to be nourished and mothered?
- Why do I deserve to be loved and supported?
- How am I internalizing my fire—my passion, energy, drive, and ambition?
- How do I turn my anger and passion against myself?
- What is my disease preventing me from doing?
- What benefits do I get from my disease?

A STARTING POINT

Picking and choosing among the many and diverse remedies recommended for chronic intestinal problems (IBS and IBD) may seem like an overwhelming task. Where should you begin?

The following supplements, herbal remedies, and healing strategies will give you a solid foundation that you can then build upon. Use the other remedies suggested in this section when, and if, you need additional support:

1. *Diet:* Follow the dietary suggestions on pages 244 to 246.
2. *Exercise:* Exercise for twenty to thirty minutes every day.
3. *Nutritional supplements:* Take the general formula for Maximum Immunity.
4. *Zinc:* Take 30 mg. each day.
5. *Quercetin:* Take a 250-mg. tablet three times daily, preferably a half hour before meals.
6. *Acidophilus:* Take one capsule with each meal.
7. *Chinese patent remedies:* For abdominal pain, gas, flatulence, belching, and/or acid reflux, take *Shu Kan Wan,* eight pills three times daily or twelve pills twice daily. For loose bowels, bloating, poor appetite, and/or sluggish digestion, take *Shen Ling Bai Zhu Pian,* twelve pills twice daily before meals.
8. *Western herbal formula:* Use equal parts licorice, lemon balm, chamomile, and approximately half that amount of ginger.

Chronic Skin Disorders (Eczema and Psoriasis)

ECZEMA (ATOPIC DERMATITIS)

Three years ago, William, a forty-six-year-old certified public accountant, suddenly developed a red, itchy rash that covered every inch of his skin from the top of his feet to his scalp, with only his groin area free from the inflamed lesions. For eight months the pain and itching worsened, to the point that he slept for only two or three hours at night. Rather than lie in bed with no hope of sleep, he would work on carpentry projects or office work until collapsing into a restless sleep, only to awaken a few hours later from the intense itching. It became necessary for him to sleep with his clothes on because the constant itching made his skin bleed, staining the sofa or bed sheets. In the winter, when the temperature dropped below freezing, William had a favorite strategy that offered him temporary relief from the itching—he rolled down all the windows in his car and drove at breakneck speed, the cold air providing soothing relief for his hot, inflamed body.

Over a period of two and a half years, William consulted with six dermatologists, two nutritionists, a Chinese doctor specializing in Chinese herbal remedies, and a Russian doctor who recommended colon irrigations. He tried macrobiotic diets, liver cleanses, Kombucha mushroom tea (he kept the mushroom cultures in his closet), Chinese herbs, and dozens of nutritional supplements. The only remedy that seemed to work was the prescription corticosteroid drug prednisone; unfortunately, it caused his skin to thin and bruise easily, and whenever he stopped taking it, the rash came back worse than ever.

I first met William two years after his first outbreak. I noted an affinity to Metal because of his dry skin, dry hair, shallow breathing, and long history of allergies and asthma. His pride in being efficient and methodical in his work habits and his impatience with clutter confirmed a strong Metal constitution. A dual affinity to Wood was evident in his strong, muscular body type, his love of competitive sports, and his anger and frustration with his disease. "If I don't get over this soon, I don't know what I'll do," he told me. "I've been so miserable for so long that I sometimes think about suicide."

Treatment consisted of bimonthly acupuncture sessions, nutritional supplements, an herbal formula consisting of burdock, yellow dock, dandelion, licorice, and dong quai, and periodic applications of Skin Cap, a newly marketed zinc spray used to control the itching and inflammation. Although William enjoyed the relaxation he experienced in the acupuncture sessions and felt they gave him some relief from his symptoms, he was frustrated by the gradual nature of the treatments. When tax season came and his workload increased, he decided to stop the acupuncture sessions, although he continued to use the Skin Cap spray and herbal formula.

Several months later I called William to see how he was doing. "I feel like I have it under control," he told me. "The Skin Cap spray and lukewarm baths every other night help control the itching, and I stopped drinking alcohol and taking showers because they seemed to cause flare-ups. I've actually been sleeping eight or nine hours every night without waking up!"

For the first time in three years, William felt there was reason for hope.

WESTERN INTERPRETATION

Between three and seven percent of Americans suffer from eczema, a skin rash characterized by itching, swelling, blistering, oozing, and scaling. The connection between allergies and eczema is strong: Many people with eczema also suffer from hay fever, sinusitis, and/or asthma, and approximately eighty percent have elevated levels of IgE (antibodies involved in allergic reactions). The genetic link is also undeniable—sixty to seventy percent of people with eczema have at least one family member with the disease.

Eczema is characterized by four criteria:

1. Dry skin. As the disease progresses, the patient's noticeably dry skin begins to crack open, most often around the joints, where the skin is constantly stretched. For some unknown reason, the sebaceous glands, which naturally secrete sebum to lubricate the skin and hair, don't work properly, and the skin dries and cracks.

2. Itching. The unrelenting urge to itch and scratch the inflamed areas is the cruelest symptom of all; for some people, the itching never goes away, and a good night's sleep is a distant memory.

3. Rash. *Eczema* is derived from a Greek word that means "to boil," and the inflamed lesions literally seethe and bubble, causing severe itching and pain. The rash may be limited to small patches behind the elbows or knees or on the hands, feet, or neck, but for some unfortunate individuals, the lesions literally cover the entire body.

4. Thickening skin. Over time the dry patches thicken to form crusty layers of skin.

The causes of eczema remain elusive, but many factors appear to be involved including:

• **Allergies.** Numerous research studies point to a strong connection between eczema and allergies in general, and specifically to certain food allergies or intolerances. People with eczema typically suffer from seasonal allergies, and many are asthma victims as well. (The allergic connection with asthma is well established; see pages 229 to 230.)

• **Weakened immune response.** The white blood cells in the skin itself seem to have a reduced ability to destroy bacteria, which leads to chronic bacterial infections that can aggravate and prolong the disease.

• **Nutritional deficiencies.** The typical Western diet—high in fat and refined carbohydrates, low in complex carbohydrates and fresh fruits and vegetables—appears to aggravate eczema. Dietary changes can significantly reduce the inflammation and itching of eczema.

• **Stress.** Emotional, mental, and physical stress often trigger flare-ups of eczema.

WESTERN TREATMENT

Contact dermatitis (also called allergic eczema) is an allergic reaction to a topical irritant such as poison ivy or a seemingly benign substance such as a cosmetic, laundry detergent, polyester fabric, or nickel or chromium button or jewelry. Hydrocortisone creams and oral steroids such as prednisone help to cool down the inflammation. Skin infections, usually caused by excessive itching, are often treated with antibiotic creams and lotions.

The more insidious type of eczema, and the one that we cover in this chapter, is called atopic eczema (or atopic dermatitis), an intensely itchy, inflammatory disease of the skin with no known single causal factor. Treatment usually involves the use of topical creams and lotions; the most effective creams are steroidal, but these medications can create dependence, requiring more frequent application to achieve the desired relief. If the creams don't work, oral corticosteroidal drugs may be used for short periods of time.

If the skin lesions become infected (either from itching, which introduces bacteria into the open sores, or as a natural consequence of severe eczema), topical and oral antibiotics may be prescribed.

Baking soda baths (one cup of baking soda in a tub of lukewarm water) and oatmeal baths offer temporary relief of symptoms.

Psychotherapy is often suggested to help the patient deal with the emotional stress associated with eczema.

Vaccinations should be avoided during eczema flare-ups. In all autoimmune diseases the body generates large amounts of autoantibodies; vaccinations intensify the activities of these antibodies, which can overstimulate the immune system and cause an acute flare-up of the disease.

PSORIASIS

Silvery patches of flaky, scaly skin covered Norma's entire body; underneath the "dragon scales," as she called them, bacteria collected, causing frequent infections and chronic inflammation. "I feel as if I'm burning alive," Norma told me. For five years she had been using a full-spectrum light, taking tar baths every night, and using every lotion and salve on the market to relieve the symptoms of psoriasis, but nothing worked.

"Although I'm hoping for a miracle, I don't expect acupuncture or herbs to get rid of my disease," she told me. "I'm really here to figure out why I feel so stuck, as if I'm riding a bicycle in sand. If I can get through this stage, I know I'll be able to live with this disease."

Fifty-eight years old, Norma was a professor of archaeology at a private liberal arts college. She wore no makeup, dressed in jeans and T-shirts, and kept her gray hair cropped short. ("I like to play racquetball on my lunch hour," she explained. "Who has time to mess with a fancy hairdo?") Chronic headaches, a tendency to develop muscle cramps and spasms, an impulsive, somewhat headstrong personality style, and an underlying fear of helplessness and dependence on others confirmed Norma's strong affinity to Wood.

Her chronic digestive problems—bloating, diarrhea, and indigestion—indicated that Norma's Liver was overburdened and unable to keep the energy and blood moving smoothly through her body, which contributed to a buildup of toxins and wastes in her digestive system. I explained that both Eastern and Western medicine consider psoriasis a manifestation of stagnant energy and toxicity in the Liver. Treatment is aimed at stimulating the energy flow in the Liver, which would resolve her digestive problems and over time alleviate her skin disorder.

I mixed two separate herbal formulas for Norma. The first formula included the herbs dandelion and dong quai and the remedy Shou Wu Chih; it was designed to support her Liver and digestive system. The herbs in the second formula—burdock, yellow dock, and red clover—helped cleanse her blood by removing toxins and enhancing general circulation. Weekly acupuncture sessions, stress-reduction techniques, and vitamin and mineral supplements completed the treatment program. Norma's diet was basically faultless: A strict vegetarian, her only dietary weakness (if it could be called that) was a fondness for white wine, which she limited to one glass before dinner.

After two months Norma's digestive symptoms disappeared, her energy increased, and she claimed that the stress of exams and grading papers no longer made her so irritable. Although her psoriasis did not immediately respond to treatment, she continued the weekly acupuncture sessions. After eighteen months she began to notice a slight improvement in her skin condition—the "dragon scales" seemed to be shrinking, and she no longer felt that she was burning up from the inside out.

Slow but steady improvement continued over the next two years, with only occasional flare-ups. Norma continues to take her herbs and comes in every month for an acupuncture treatment.

WESTERN INTERPRETATION

Three percent of the U.S. population suffers from psoriasis, a chronic, recurring skin condition characterized by bright red patches covered with silvery scales. While most people's skin cells grow, mature, and die every month or so, with psoriasis the skin cells divide at a greatly accelerated rate—up to one thousand times faster than normal. The dead and dying cells pile up on top of each other, creating the silvery scales that are the tell-tale sign of psoriasis.

The areas underneath the scales are often red and inflamed and may become infected when the skin is scratched or rubbed. Lesions appear most often on the knees, elbows, and scalp, but other commonly affected areas include the chest, abdomen, backs of the arms and legs, palms of the hands, and soles of the feet. In acute flare-ups, the red patches and silvery scales can cover more than half of the body surface.

The cause of psoriasis is unknown, although a strong genetic predisposition exists: Fifty percent of people with psoriasis have a family member who also suffers from the disease. The disease strikes early; most people experience the first symptoms before the age of twenty. Psoriasis often occurs with rheumatoid arthritis, although the connection between the two diseases remains unclear.

While a precise cause continues to elude medical science, many clinicians and researchers believe the disease is connected to a combination of the following:

- **Food allergies and/or sensitivities.** A particular food causes an allergic reaction, which directly affects the skin.
- **Faulty protein metabolism.** Undigested proteins leak into the body fluids, creating an allergic reaction.

- **Intestinal toxins.** Harmful bacteria are absorbed through the intestinal walls into the bloodstream, causing an immune reaction that can exacerbate psoriasis.
- **Stress.** Psoriasis flare-ups occur during periods of intense stress, although stress is considered contributory rather than causative.

WESTERN TREATMENT

Just as the cause of psoriasis remains elusive, so does the cure. Treatments are basically geared to symptom relief and may include:

- Topical creams and ointments (often steroidal), to help relieve pain and inflammation
- Sleeping pills, if insomnia is a problem
- Anti-depressant drugs, to elevate mood and treat depression
- Warm salt baths, to soothe the inflamed lesions
- Sunlight and ultraviolet light therapy, to reduce the replication of skin cells, relieving many of the symptoms
- Stress-reduction techniques, to alleviate anxiety and tension
- Psychotherapy, to help the patient cope with the stress of chronic illness

TRADITIONAL CHINESE INTERPRETATION
(ECZEMA AND PSORIASIS)

According to traditional Chinese medicine, the most likely cause of chronic atopic eczema and psoriasis is a deficiency of Liver *chi* and blood, which allows Heat to build up in the blood. As the Heat accumulates, the body tries to eliminate it through the skin, which leads to inflammation, skin rashes, pain, and itching. To further complicate the situation, deficient Lung and Kidney *chi* inevitably weakens the *wei chi,* leaving you more vulnerable to attack.

The Chinese also interpret contact dermatitis (contact eczema) as an invasion of the Wind and Damp Devils as well as Heat; they penetrate the Skin and create numerous problems. The Wind Devil causes itching, while the burning and inflammation are attributed to the Heat Devil, and the "weeping" (oozing) skin results from the Damp Devil. If the external Devils get "under the skin" and penetrate deeper into the system, they can cause or exacerbate eczema or psoriasis.

If asthma is involved in either eczema or psoriasis, the Lung/Kidney deficiency is addressed first, with acupuncture and herbal therapies selected to strengthen and support those organs. If the individual is hypersensitive or experiences arthritic symptoms, the Liver is given prompt and immediate attention.

COMPLEMENTARY TREATMENTS

Diet

For both psoriasis and eczema, nutrition is the key to treatment. Once again, as with so many chronic illnesses, the possibility of food allergies or sensitivities should be immediately addressed. The foods most likely to cause problems include dairy products, wheat products, citrus fruits, nuts, and corn. If you avoid these common food allergens, the chances are good that your symptoms will be significantly reduced or eliminated. *Most people who suffer from eczema and psoriasis experience dramatic improvement when they eliminate common food allergens from their diet.* (For more information on food allergies and sensitivities and the Elimination/Provocation Diet, refer to pages 105 to 107.)

Most allergies are caused or aggravated by incomplete digestion of food. If your digestive system is not working properly, "renegade" (incompletely digested) proteins are assimilated into body fluids. The immune system recognizes these "renegade" proteins as enemies and initiates a full-scale campaign to get rid of them. The frenzied activities of the immune system create an allergic reaction.

Saturated fatty acids in meat and dairy products tend to stimulate a general inflammatory response that manifests in the skin, giving you one more reason to avoid these problematic foods. Polyunsaturated fats, which are chemically altered to behave like saturated fats, can also aggravate eczema and psoriasis and should be strictly avoided; these fats, also known as trans-fatty acids or TFAs, are found in margarines, vegetable shortening, and all foods labeled "partially hydrogenated vegetable oils."

Avoid cooking with polyunsaturated vegetable oils, which become highly unstable when heated; use olive oil instead. Olive oil is high in monounsaturated fats, which have an anti-inflammatory effect and can dramatically reduce the symptoms of inflammatory diseases such as eczema and psoriasis. (People who regularly use olive oil also have lower rates of cancer and heart disease.) Buy extra-virgin olive oil, which is extracted without the use of high heat or chemical solvents.

Strictly avoid stimulants like sugar, caffeine, alcohol, and tobacco products, which can exacerbate skin conditions.

Concentrate on a well-balanced diet with plenty of whole grains, vegetables, fruits, and fiber-rich foods. Meat, chicken, turkey, and lamb are much less likely to cause you problems than beef and pork; whenever possible, choose organic meats that are completely uncontaminated with chemicals or hormones. Rice, potatoes, pears, apples, and most vegetables are generally nonallergenic, highly nutritious foods. Beware of citrus fruits, which can exacerbate both eczema and psoriasis.

Drink at least eight to ten 8-ounce glasses of water daily, to support the Liver and Kidney in their detoxification and elimination duties.

EXERCISE

The Chinese believe that both eczema and psoriasis are caused by constrained Liver *chi* and a buildup of Heat (toxins) in the blood. Because regular movement stimulates Liver *chi* and helps to "move" the blood, supporting and increasing its circulation to all areas of the body, exercise is considered an important part of prevention and treatment for both eczema and psoriasis. Exercise also promotes perspiration, which assists the body in its efforts to eliminate toxins through the skin.

Both yoga and tai chi exercises stimulate the flow of energy and blood; these ancient healing methods also help "still" the mind, removing distracting thoughts and emotions. Regular strenuous exercise may offer long-term benefits; refer back to Chapters 2 through 6 for advice on specific exercises geared to your constitutional type.

NUTRITIONAL SUPPLEMENTS

Beta-carotene: This substance, once it is converted in the intestines into vitamin A, supports and nourishes the skin and maintains the structural integrity of the cells and membranes of the body, particularly the skin and mucous linings. Take 25,000 I.U. daily.

Vitamin C: This amazing all-purpose vitamin has antioxidant and antihistamine actions that make it an essential part of treatment for eczema and psoriasis. In double-blind studies vitamin C significantly improved the symptoms of people suffering from severe eczema. If you are taking antibiotics for skin infections, vitamin C will boost your immune response so that you need a lower dosage of the drug for a shorter period of time. Take 2,000–4,000 mg. daily.

Quercetin: This bioflavonoid has strong anti-inflammatory and antihistamine actions. Take 150–250 mg. three times daily. Quercetin is often combined with bromelain, a digestive enzyme, to aid absorption.

Zinc: Zinc helps the body heal from wounds and lesions and is useful in any kind of skin disease, but it seems particularly effective in treating eczema and psoriasis. Take 20–40 mg. daily preventively and up to 60 mg. daily during acute flare-ups. Zinc gluconate is particularly well tolerated and easy to absorb.

Whenever you supplement zinc, you should take extra copper to maintain a healthy balance between the two minerals. The ratio of zinc to copper should be fifteen to one; thus, if you take 30 mg. zinc, take 2 mg. copper.

Caution: Because zinc can be toxic in large doses, do not exceed 100 mg. daily.

Hydrochloric acid (HCl): This supplement aids digestion and can help eliminate the "renegade" proteins that leak into the body's fluids and provoke allergic responses. Studies show that the majority of people with eczema and psoriasis have a deficiency of hydrochloric acid in their stomachs. Furthermore, as Melvyn Werbach, M.D., states in his book *Healing Through Nutrition,* "the lower the acid level, the worse their skin problems, and the more likely they are to complain of gastrointestinal symptoms." Take one five-gram tablet of betaine HCl before each meal, or as directed on the product label.

Caution: Because hydrochloric acid can be irritating to the digestive tract, take it only with food or just after eating, and always use it under the supervision of a qualified professional. Don't use hydrochloric acid if you have a history of ulcers.

Omega-3 fatty acids (eicosapentaenoic acid or EPA): These fatty acids promote the health and integrity of the immune system and have significant anti-inflammatory effects. Numerous studies show that people with skin diseases experience significantly less itching and scaling when they use EPAs. The best food source of omega-3 fatty acids is certain oily fish—salmon, sardines, herring, mackerel, bluefish, and albacore tuna. Eat fish rich in omega-3's three times a week, or supplement your diet with 1,500 mg. daily.

If you can't tolerate fish oil because of allergies or a general intolerance for the fishy aftertaste, flaxseed oil is a good substitute; take one tablespoon daily. Because flaxseed oil can quickly go rancid, be sure to refrigerate it and store it in an amber, light-protective container.

Gamma linoleic acid (GLA): GLA is a valuable ally in protecting your cells from degenerative changes and reducing inflammation throughout the body. Numerous research studies support claims that GLA reduces the symptoms of arthritis, lupus, inflammatory skin conditions (eczema and psoriasis), premenstrual syndrome, and bowel disease (Crohn's and ulcerative colitis). GLA is found in oil of evening primrose, borage seed oil, and black currant seed oil. Take 1,500 mg. daily.

Chinese Patent Remedies

For general support, we recommend the following:

Shou Wu Chih ("Polygonum Multiflorum Juice"): This wonderful tonic is traditionally used to help people "age gracefully." Used widely throughout China, it nourishes the *yin* (Water) reserves throughout the body, supports the blood, increases circulation, nourishes the Liver and Kidneys, relaxes the muscles and tendons, improves vision, keeps the skin moist and the hair lustrous and healthy, and strengthens the bones. Although this formula was not created specifically for the skin, its ability to nourish the *yin* and strengthen the blood helps keep the skin moist and healthy.

The Emperor herb in this formula is polygonum, which nourishes the Kidneys and is said to promote longevity; eight attending herbs support the digestion, cleanse the blood, and provide general support. Take 1–2 tablespoons three times daily.

For symptomatic relief of itching, we recommend:

Chuan Shan Jia Qu Shi Qing Du Wan ("Armadillo Counter Poison Pill"): This famous formula consists of twenty herbs to cool the heat and dispel the chronic itch of eczema. Although the constant need to itch and scratch is less common in psoriasis, this remedy is recommended for both diseases. The animal parts in the formula—armadillo scales (the "Emperor" ingredient) and tortoise shell—are credited with relieving the itching and inflammation; the attending herbs (codonopsis root, rehmannia root, ox gallstone, euphorbia leaf, hydnocarpus seed, astragalus, dictamnus root, smilax root, chrysanthemum flower, xanthium fruit, ligusticum root, fritillaria bulb, forsythia fruit, arctium fruit, cnidium fruit, scutellaria root, peony root, and lonicera flower) work together to nourish and "move" the blood, support the immune system, and strengthen Kidney and Liver *chi*.

During severe flare-ups take four pills three times daily for one or two weeks. This formula is not appropriate for long-term use.

Caution: Because this is a blood-moving formula, it should not be used during pregnancy.

These Chinese patent remedies can safely be combined with any of the following herbs:

Herbal Allies

The following herbs can be used alone or combined in a single formula. Popular formulas available at health food stores offer different combinations of these herbs, or you can contact a qualified herbalist, who will mix up a formula tailored to your specific needs. If you need help choosing the most effective formula or combination of herbs for your symptoms, consult an experienced herbalist.

Licorice (*Glycyrrhiza glabra*): Licorice suppresses inflammation and has been used with great success in the topical treatment of eczema and psoriasis. Its adaptogenic effects on the adrenal glands and its anti-allergic actions make it doubly effective for skin diseases.

Burdock (*Arctium lappa*): This blood-cleansing herb, which helps the cells eliminate toxins, has been used for thousands of years to treat skin conditions. Its gentle diuretic and laxative qualities and supportive actions in the Liver help encourage the elimination of toxins. Burdock also has anti-inflammatory and antimicrobial actions.

Yellow dock (*Rumex crispus*): This liver-tonifying herb and gentle blood cleanser has a mild laxative action. Yellow dock combines well with burdock—it helps stimulate the removal of toxins that burdock works to dislodge.

Red clover (*Trifolium pratense*): A gentle blood cleanser, red clover has been used extensively with great success for skin diseases and cancer.

Dandelion (*Taraxacum officinalis*): Dandelion is the archetypal Liver tonic. An extremely nourishing herb, rich in vitamins and minerals, it offers general support to the Liver, encouraging the removal of toxins from the blood and allowing the skin to heal.

Dong quai (*Angelica sinensis*): Dong quai is the most important blood tonic in Chinese medicine and is now used extensively in the United States and Europe. It invigorates and "moves" the blood, helping to eliminate Damp/Heat or Wind/Heat from the blood, which relieves many of the symptoms of eczema and psoriasis.

Caution: Because dong quai is a blood mover, it should never be used during pregnancy.

Shou Wu Chih (see page 269) can be substituted for dong quai, or you can combine the two remedies for enhanced effectiveness.

Dosage: If you purchase your herbs in a health food store (either in tincture form or, as dried herbs, in capsule or pill form), follow the dosage instructions on the label. Because herbs in dried form tend to lose their potency rather quickly, be sure to check the label for the expiration date.

For information on preparing your own herbs from the root, bark, leaves, flowers, or seeds of a plant, see Appendix II.

In Appendix I, Resources, we offer a list of mail-order sources for high-quality herbs and herbal preparations. For advice on ordering specially made herbal formulas, see pages 394 to 396.

ACUPOINTS

Spleen 6 ("Three Yin Meeting Point"): This is one of the most popular points in acupuncture because of its many and diverse functions. Primarily used to support the *yin* essence (it is located at the point where three *yin* channels intersect), Spleen 6 strengthens Spleen and Stomach energies, aids digestion and metabolism, and helps to resolve damp conditions, particularly Damp/Heat. When this point is stimulated, obstructions in the blood are removed, and heat is dispelled.

Location: Spleen 6 is located on the inner lower leg, approximately three inches above the inside ankle bone, in the depression just on the inside of the bone.

Spleen 10 ("Sea of Blood"): This point is used to move and invigorate the blood, harmonize the Spleen energies, support menstruation, facilitate blood flow, and remove Heat from the blood. It offers fast and effective relief for virtually any skin disease or inflammation, including eczema, psoriasis, hives, and herpes zoster (shingles).

Location: With your knee flexed, move your fingers along the inner ridge of the kneecap, stopping about two inches above the upper part of the kneecap in the bulge. This point is universally painful to the touch.

Large Intestine 4 ("Great Eliminator"): This point is used to disperse "stuck" energy, heat, or wind from the upper part of the body and helps to relieve the Wind/Heat symptoms of eczema and psoriasis. Famous for draining toxins and breaking through obstructions, it is also used to relieve headaches and/or congestion in the head and neck.

Location: Large Intestine 4 is located on the top of the hand, in the webbing between the thumb and index finger.

Other Complementary Strategies

Zinc spray: Relatively new on the market, the zinc spray called Skin Cap has been studied extensively in clinical trials in Spain and has recently been imported to this country. I've used this spray, which consists of only one active ingredient, zinc pyrithione, with severe cases of eczema and psoriasis and achieved impressive results. After only a few weeks of daily treatments, the skin lesions and associated inflammation, itching, and pain are significantly improved.

Moisturizing baths: Excessive dryness is a symptom of both eczema and psoriasis. Soaking in a bath treated with a natural emulsifier, which locks the water into the skin, temporarily relieves the itching and discomfort of these diseases. Eucerin, Alpha Keri, Aquaphor, and Unguentum lotions and creams are common store brands; mix two tablespoons into a pot of boiling water, stir until mixed, and then add to your bathwater.

Oatmeal baths can help relieve the itching and moisturize the skin.

Tar baths have been used for psoriasis with excellent results; tar, a derivative of coal tar, is available from health food stores and pharmacies.

A ten-to-fifteen-minute warm-water *salt bath* (use a pound or more of sea salts, mineral salts, or table salt) may also help people with psoriasis. (After you take a salt bath, be sure to rinse off with a quick, cold shower.)

For eczema, *baking soda baths* are soothing; put one cup of baking soda in your bathtub, and soak for as long as you want.

For both psoriasis and eczema, try adding five drops of German (high-quality) *chamomile oil* to warm bathwater, and soak for at least ten minutes.

Creams and ointments: While numerous commercial brands of moisturizing creams are available, natural creams and ointments may offer you better results in the long run. For fast, effective relief for the itching of eczema, nothing comes close to chickweed (*Stellaria media*) cream or ointment. Other gentle yet effective herbal creams include calendula ointment, Self-Heal Salve (a combination of prunella, burdock, St. John's wort oil, and calendula), vitamin E and aloe ointment, and Purple Gold Ointment, a Chinese herbal preparation. These products are available in many health food stores, or they can be ordered (see Appendix I).

Many eczema and psoriasis patients find *zinc oxide ointment* effective in healing their skin lesions. Zinc oxide is available without a prescription.

In Europe the main topical herb for psoriasis is cleavers (*Galium aparine*), which is also an excellent herb for internal use in skin conditions of all kinds; a topical cream or ointment for psoriasis might include both chickweed and cleavers.

Although these ointments are not curative, they can provide significant temporary relief.

Sunlight: Sunlight and ultraviolet light stop the skin cells from replicating at such a furious pace, relieving the symptoms of psoriasis. People with eczema also often find that their problems are alleviated during the summer months, when they spend more time in the sun.

Try to spend a few minutes every day in the sun, but remember to avoid prolonged exposure to sunlight, and use sunscreen whenever appropriate. You might also consider purchasing a special light box that creates a full-spectrum light, to use in your home to help relieve the symptoms of psoriasis and eczema. Research indicates that you will get as much benefit and significantly less radiation from an ultraviolet B (UVB) lamp.

Hypoallergenic products: Chemicals added to laundry detergents, cosmetics, soaps, shampoos, underarm deodorants, and virtually every cleaning substance we use in the home can cause irritation and allergic reactions. Switch to hypoallergenic products for all your personal hygiene needs, and use mild detergents such as Ivory Snow for washing your clothes. Avoid perfumed products like scented toilet paper and fabric softeners.

Questions to Ask Yourself

On a metaphorical level, you can conceive of skin irritations and diseases with a strong itching component as the body's way of saying, "I need to let something out." The disease might also be asking you to look at your relationships and your need—or, conversely, lack of desire—for contact with others.

The following questions will help you to look at your disease as a constructive process that seeks change and redirection, rather than a completely evil force to be eliminated as soon as possible.

- I'm itching to let people know what I'm thinking or feeling: How can I express myself clearly and forcefully?
- I'm burning up inside: How can I cool things down?
- I tend to hide inside myself: What am I afraid of? What will happen to me if I "expose" my thoughts and feelings?

- Why do I prevent myself from making contact with other people?
- How can I let people under my skin and into my heart without letting them irritate me?
- How do my symptoms support me? What do they give me that is positive and enlightening? What are they asking me to do, to say, to become?

Skin conditions are often associated with Metal and Wood imbalances. Metal types might benefit by asking questions that focus on grief, loss, and the need for order and control:

- What past loss am I still grieving over?
- Can I find a way to let go of my grief?
- How can I bring some sense of order and routine back into my life?
- What can I control in my life? What can't I control?

For Wood types, feelings of being stuck, blocked, or impeded often lead to physical and emotional problems. Ask yourself:

- How am I holding myself back?
- Where do I feel stuck physically, mentally, emotionally, and spiritually?
- What can I do to break through the obstacles confronting me?
- How can I use my creativity to move forward in my life?

A STARTING POINT

Picking and choosing among the many and diverse remedies recommended for chronic skin disorders (eczema and psoriasis) may seem like an overwhelming task. Where should you begin?

The following supplements, herbal remedies, and healing strategies will give you a solid foundation that you can then build upon. Use the other remedies suggested in this section when and if you need additional support.

1. *Diet:* Follow the dietary suggestions on pages 266 to 267.
2. *Exercise:* Exercise twenty to thirty minutes every day.
3. *Nutritional supplements:* Take the general formula for Maximum Immunity.

4. *Zinc:* Take 30–50 mg. daily
5. *GLA and EPA oils:* Take 1,500 mg. of each daily or 3,000 mg. of the combined formulas.
6. *Shou Wu Chih:* Take one tablespoon twice daily.
7. *Western herbal formula:* Take a tonic of licorice, burdock, yellow dock, and red clover, mixed in equal parts.

10. LEVEL THREE: THE BLOOD

Men are born soft and supple;
dead, they are stiff and hard.
Plants are born tender and pliant;
dead, they are brittle and dry.

Thus whoever is stiff and inflexible
is a disciple of death.
Whoever is soft and yielding
is a disciple of life.

The hard and stiff will be broken.
The soft and supple will prevail.

—Tao Te Ching

For some people at some point in their lives, illness is no longer a weekend guest but becomes a permanent resident. No matter how hard you try to kick the unwelcome visitor out, it won't budge. For weeks, months, or even years, you're stuck with it, every hour of every day, wearily adjusting yourself to its presence while bitterly resenting the loss of freedom and control over your life.

When disease penetrates deeper into the body's kingdom, overwhelming the *wei chi* sentries and gradually draining the body's vital energy (*chi*) reserves, it threatens the next level of defense: the blood. We all know what blood is—the life-giving fluid consisting of red blood cells, white blood cells, platelets, and plasma that courses through our veins and arteries. In both Western and Chinese medicine, blood is considered the chief transportation system of the body, responsible for the following functions:

- Transporting oxygen from the lungs to the body's tissues
- Transporting carbon dioxide from the tissues to the lungs
- Carrying food from the digestive system to the tissues
- Carrying fluids to and from the tissues
- Removing waste products from the kidneys
- Distributing hormones from the endocrine glands to the organs they influence

The Chinese, however, think of blood as more than just a material substance; in the most basic sense, blood is the mother of life, the great nourisher and provider who cares for each and every cell, suffusing the body with warmth, sensation, and consciousness. The blood is said to house the mind and the spirit, providing a safe home for thoughts and perceptions as well as a dwelling place for compassion, generosity, and love.

When the blood is disturbed, the spirit becomes unsettled. If the condition remains unresolved, the spirit is dislodged from its stable dwelling place in the blood and wanders aimlessly through the body. A disembodied spirit leads to feelings of restlessness and agitation. Thoughts, perceptions, and sensations are disrupted. Warmth and light fade. Memory falters. Sleep is disturbed. The ability to communicate with others or to understand your own needs and desires is affected.

We can only understand the vast impact of these disturbances on the body, mind, and spirit by considering the relationship between *chi* and blood. In Chinese theory blood is imagined as the mother impregnated with the child of *chi*: The blood nourishes the *chi,* and the *chi* gives the blood energy, direction, and vitality. Without *chi,* the blood would stagnate, like a pond of water with no revitalizing spring to give it new life. Without blood, the *chi* would have no form to inhabit, and the vital energy would dry up and evaporate.

The relationship between *chi* and blood illustrates beautifully the inseparable nature of the two primal powers, *yin* and *yang. Chi* (which is the aggressive *yang* force) is said to command the *blood,* strengthening and nourishing it as it circulates throughout the body. Blood (which is the submissive *yin* force) is considered the mother of *chi,* because its fluid, yielding nature provides nourishment to every cell in the body. If these two life-giving substances were for some reason separated, the blood would not be able to circulate throughout the body, the *chi* would have no medium through which to exert its power, and life itself would cease to exist.

Yin and *yang* are not opposites or contradictions, for the Chinese believe that everything in life—literally and figuratively—contains its opposite. Over time, each half is transformed into the other in a continuous cycle of change. According to Taoist philosophy, which forms the philosophical foundation of traditional Chinese medicine, we cannot say that something is solely good or evil, dark or light, night or day, heaven or earth, male or female. Such either-or categories do not exist, because all of reality encompasses both this *and* that, good *and* evil, black *and* white, night *and* day, heaven *and* earth, male *and* female.

In the human body, *yin* and *yang* are perfectly balanced when *chi* commands the blood with gentle authority, and the blood responds by circulating smoothly and effortlessly throughout the body to nourish and revitalize the cells. When the mother/child relationship between blood and *chi* is carefully nurtured through attention to diet, exercise, nutrition, sufficient sleep, and stable relationships, harmony reigns within the body's kingdom. But if the *chi* becomes rebellious or domineering, or if it gets "stuck" and cannot circulate freely, the blood will feel the effects, moving recklessly through its channels or becoming dense and sluggish like a stream polluted at its source.

The Chinese trace the origin of blood problems to three organ spheres: the Spleen/Pancreas, the Liver, and the Heart. The Spleen/Pancreas is responsible for creating blood from food and drink; a deficiency in this function will adversely affect the quality and/or quantity of blood. The Liver is said to "command" the blood; if its functions are impaired, the blood is like a field army cut off from headquarters, confused about how to proceed. The Liver also stores "quiescent blood," akin to reserve troops that can be released when needed to heal wounds, assist organs in need, and regulate the menstrual cycle. Finally, the Heart circulates the blood through the meridians and blood vessels; disturbances in the Heart affect the circulation and flow of blood to the organs, nervous system, and extremities.

When illness or disorder disturbs the blood, the symptoms are numerous and widespread. Deficient blood, which can be caused by deficient Spleen/Pancreas *chi* or loss of blood from an accident, internal bleeding, or excessive menstrual bleeding, causes fatigue, lethargy, listlessness, dizziness, aching muscles, and dry skin. Blood that is blocked from reaching its destination creates inflammation, fevers, and swollen or painful joints. Rebellious blood can lead to extreme fevers and "reckless bleeding," with symptoms such as bloody noses, blood in the urine or stools, or heavy menstrual flow. If the *chi* gets dammed up or "stuck," the blood will congeal, leading to many types of skin diseases, joint problems, and serious degenerative diseases.

While deficiencies or excesses of blood and *chi* create numerous and diverse problems, one symptom is universal: pain. The pain at this level is qualitatively and quantitatively different from the pain experienced at the *wei chi* and *chi* levels. Colds, flus, allergies, and asthma cause pain, but the discomfort is usually short-lived and eventually disappears. Sinusitis, irritable bowel syndrome, Crohn's disease, eczema, and psoriasis can be extremely painful, but once again, the pain tends to be localized and comes and goes with the illness.

At the blood level, however, the pain ebbs and flows but never entirely recedes. The ocean of pain is too deep and broad to evaporate. It is not a stabbing or jolting pain that one experiences as much as a constant aching and a deep sense of discomfort or dis-ease. The pain itself makes you weary and exhausts your vital reserves of energy.

Physical distress, mental confusion, and spiritual anguish signal that something is wrong, but the pain tends to be so diffuse and widespread that you often don't know what it means, or why it is slowly draining away all your vital energy. You only know that something is wrong, and you fear the worst.

What is pain? Why do you experience it? What purpose does it fulfill? Somewhere along the way you may have learned to associate pain with debility and decay, a sure sign that you are sick, possibly diseased, and in danger of falling apart. But pain is your ally, not your enemy. A vital component of the body's early warning system, pain alerts you to the fact that something is wrong. Pain protects you—just as when you put your finger too close to the flame, you feel pain, and in pulling back, you protect your body from serious damage.

Any disruption of the pathways between mind and body can cause the pain signals to malfunction, leaving you vulnerable to serious injury. Dr. Paul Brand, an orthopedic surgeon who devoted his skills to helping the lepers of Vellore, India, tells of an encounter with a leprous twelve-year-old boy who offered to help him turn a key in a rusty lock. Using all his strength, Dr. Brand had been unable to turn the key, but the young boy accomplished the task in seconds. Mystified by what appeared to be uncommon strength, Dr. Brand inspected the boy's hand and discovered that the flesh had been cut to the bone. Leprosy had destroyed the nerve endings in his hand, leaving the pain impulses without a pathway to communicate their important message. Because he couldn't feel the pain that signaled damage to his body's tissues, the boy suffered serious injury.

Pain is not necessarily a symptom of disintegration or disease; as the story of the leprous boy teaches, pain is actually a sign that the body works precisely as it should. In traditional Chinese medicine, physical and emotional pain are interpreted as signs of obstruction within the inner kingdom. Something is blocking the vital energy within, and because the energy cannot perform its healing work, you experience the distress and discomfort known as pain. When you feel pain, the body is asking you to remove the obstacle and restore the smooth flow of energy.

Every disease that affects the blood involves some kind of obstruction or blockage, which in turn causes chronic physical pain. More important than the physical suffering, however, is the emotional and spiritual distress of disease at this level. Because the blood houses the mind and the spirit, your thoughts, emotions, enthusiasm for life, and will to live will be affected. Confusion, fear, despair, and depression drain your energy and vitality, further depleting the defensive energy of the blood and *chi*.

The Chinese view emotional and spiritual pain as more dangerous to longterm health than the actual process of physical disease. "Where there is spirit, the prognosis is positive," pronounced the Yellow Emperor more than three thousand years ago. "When the spirit is gone, the condition is very grave. . . .

> When patients lack the confidence to conquer illness, they allow their spirits to scatter and wither away. They let their emotions take control of their lives. They spend their days drowned in desire and worries, exhausting their jing/essence and qui and shen/spirit. Of course, then . . . the disease will not be cured.

While it is always possible to help the body fight infections and disease—even so-called "incurable" disease—once the mind starts working against the body, fear and panic create distinct biochemical changes that block the vital healing energy. Panic, with its accompanying states of helplessness and hopelessness, is an affliction as destructive to health and well-being as the illness that gives rise to it.

Chinese medicine considers patients' emotional balance and spiritual yearnings to be crucial to their health and their ability to recover from debilitating illnesses. Treatment consists of numerous strategies designed to help them confront their fears and revitalize hope, confidence, and the will to live.

Another vital component of treatment in Chinese medicine is teaching patients the importance of yielding to their illness and learning from it. "What is your illness saying to you?" the doctor of traditional Chinese medicine might ask. "What are your symptoms telling you about the deep disharmonies within? How can you become more attuned to the needs of your body, mind, and spirit?"

While the Western world views illness as an enemy to be defeated, Chinese medicine sees illness as an obstacle that can be overcome by "following the line of least resistance." In this sense, traditional Chinese medicine asks you to be like water: When a river encounters a tree or boulder blocking its pathway, it pauses until it increases, gathering strength and power until it can flow over or around the impediment. When you encounter obstacles in your healing journey, follow water's example as it proceeds along the line of least resistance. If you find yourself getting stuck, pause and take thought. As you stand still, collecting yourself, your energy will increase until it overflows. At that point, you are ready to proceed.

If you cannot remove the impediment that blocks your progress, be content to move around it, then continue on. If you are unable to find the strength or the energy to continue on, wait patiently for reinforcements to arrive. Do not be afraid to ask for help, and always remain open to good advice.

Whatever you do, don't give up the struggle, throwing up your hands in resignation because the difficulties appear too great for you to overcome. Use the struggle itself as an occasion to go into yourself to discover, in the words of poet Rainer Maria Rilke, "how deep the place is from which your life flows."

In the ancient Chinese book of wisdom *The I Ching*, this is known as the way of the "superior man":

> Difficulties and obstructions throw a man back upon himself. While
> the inferior man seeks to put the blame on other persons, bewailing

his fate, the superior man seeks the error within himself, and through this introspection the external obstacles become for him an occasion for inner enrichment and education.

In the remainder of this chapter, we'll look at the chronic illnesses that occur when the blood is disturbed, and we'll show you what you can do to restore balance and harmony.

Illnesses of the Blood
- Arthritis
- Chronic fatigue syndrome
- Lupus
- Diabetes

Arthritis (Rheumatoid Arthritis and Osteoarthritis)

Peter, thirty-nine years old, has osteoarthritis, otherwise known as degenerative joint disease. When the condition was first diagnosed five years ago, Peter felt like the Tin Man in *The Wizard of Oz,* desperate for some magic oil to lubricate his joints and release him from his painful imprisonment. Aspirin, Tylenol, and ibuprofen offered temporary relief, but as the pain gradually intensified, he began taking prescription pain-killers and anti-inflammatory drugs.

As the months went by and it became obvious that the pain and stiffness were not going to disappear miraculously, Peter decided to try herbal therapy and acupuncture. His pale skin, deep-set eyes, finely sculptured face, and strong "runner's physique," his reticent manner and his somewhat cynical attitude, and his complaints of sleep problems, weight loss, and poor appetite confirmed Peter's affinity to Water and suggested a deficiency of Water energy. I assured Peter that he possessed deep reserves of energy that could be tapped into like an underground spring to replenish the deficient blood and *chi.*

The piercing nature of the pain, which was localized in his knees and shoulders, supported a diagnosis of Cold Bi, a type of arthritis characterized by sharp, stabbing pains located in specific areas of the body. Treatment included eliminating dairy products and red meat from his diet; an herbal remedy consisting of licorice, dandelion root, and devil's claw; gentle, supportive exercises like swimming, yoga, and *tai chi;* breathing exercises; nutritional supplements; monthly acupuncture sessions to invigorate and replenish the *chi* and *blood;* and moxibustion, an ancient acupuncture technique designed to dispel cold and disperse warmth throughout the body.

Although X-rays recently confirmed the calcification in his joints, Peter's pain has completely disappeared. Now when he is physically or emotionally stressed, he notices the stiffness and pain in his joints, but he refuses to think of these symptoms as signs of a "degenerative disease." Instead, he views them as messages from within, signaling that it is time to pay more attention to himself and his basic needs.

WESTERN INTERPRETATION

A term that covers more than a hundred different joint diseases, arthritis is defined as inflammation of a joint or joints, with related symptoms such as redness, swelling, tenderness, and stiffness in the affected joints. Onset is usually very subtle and gradual. In the first stage of the disease, you may experience morning joint stiffness, which typically disappears as you begin to move around. Months or years later, the stiffness is more widespread, and throbbing or stabbing pains migrate from one affected joint to another.

Nearly forty million Americans (one in seven) experience symptoms of arthritis, one of the most widespread of all chronic illnesses. Every year they spend $25 billion on diagnostic tests, medications, doctor visits, and hospital stays; this figure does not include the many millions of dollars spent each year on complementary treatment strategies such as herbal therapy, acupuncture, and nutritional supplements.

The two most common types of arthritis are rheumatoid arthritis and osteoarthritis.

Rheumatoid arthritis: More than two million Americans suffer from this progressive joint disease, which is most common in people twenty to forty years old and afflicts more than twice as many women as men. Symptoms include stiff, sore joints, usually in the fingers, wrists, knees, ankles, or toes, and swelling, redness, and tenderness in the soft tissue surrounding the affected joints. Fatigue and low-grade fevers are also common.

Rheumatoid arthritis is considered an *autoimmune disease,* a term used to describe those conditions in which the body systematically attacks its own tissue, misidentifying "self" as enemy. Although the cause is unknown, food allergies, emotional disturbances, the accumulation of toxic chemicals in food and water, and lifestyle factors such as excessive exercise or a complete lack of exercise are thought to provoke or aggravate the disease. There is also a strong genetic predisposition involved in this disease.

The course of the disease is unpredictable, and symptoms often stop abruptly, only to recur again unexpectedly. Without proper care and early treatment, permanent deformity and immobility of joints may occur.

Osteoarthritis: Also called degenerative joint disease, osteoarthritis is most likely to strike the large, weight-bearing joints that receive the most use or stress over the years—the knees, shoulders, hips, joints of the big toes, joints of the lower part of the spine, and the distal joints of the fingers (most commonly in women). Characterized by disintegration of the cartilage covering the ends of the bones, osteoarthritis causes pain, stiffness, and in some cases, crippling deformities in nearly sixteen million Americans. Osteoarthritis is considered part of the normal aging process and occurs in approximately 80 percent of adults over the age of fifty.

WESTERN TREATMENTS

Medications: Anti-inflammatory drugs are taken to relieve pain and inflammation. Aspirin is the most commonly used, but since the amounts needed for symptom relief tend to be high, toxic reactions can occur, including gastric problems and tinnitus (ringing ears). Other medications include nonsteroidal anti-inflammatory drugs (NSAIDs) such as ibuprofen, indomethacin, and naproxen; but these drugs may produce unpleasant and potentially serious side effects such as headaches, fever, fatigue, allergic reactions, hypertension, blood count abnormalities, and liver disease. Side effects are most likely to occur with high dosages and long-term use.

Steroidal anti-inflammatory drugs (corticosteroids) may be used on a short-term basis for severe symptoms. Steroidal and nonsteroidal creams and ointments such as aspercreme or cortisone cream applied to the affected joints offer some relief from the pain, swelling, and tenderness. Ben-Gay, Tiger Balm, and other blood-circulating agents may help to increase circulation in the inflamed area.

Physical therapy: Applying cold or moist, warm compresses to the affected joints can help relieve the swelling and pain. In general, warm compresses seem to work well in relieving symptoms of stiffness and dull pain, while cold compresses or ice packs are preferred for sharp, stabbing pain and inflamed tissues. Treatments generally last ten to twenty minutes and can be repeated every four hours.

Ultrasound, a technique that uses high-frequency sound vibrations to increase blood supply to a particular area and promote lymphatic drainage from the region, is effective for both rheumatoid and osteoarthritis. Research confirms that ultrasound increases joint mobility, improves blood circulation, and reduces pain.

To keep the joints flexible and mobile, physical therapy may include "passive exercises" in which the therapist gently moves the affected joints to enhance circulation and increase range of motion.

Lifestyle changes: If the patient is overweight, weight reduction techniques can help relieve pressure on the joints.

Proper sleep and rest during periods of severe inflammation are often recommended.

Psychotherapy: Because emotional disturbances are thought to aggravate arthritic conditions, psychotherapy may be suggested.

TRADITIONAL CHINESE INTERPRETATION

Traditional Chinese medicine considers all varieties of arthritis as symptoms of blockage in the flow of energy and/or blood. The Chinese believe that pain and obstruction are intimately linked; if there is an obstruction, there will always be associated pain, and if there is pain, the practitioner immediately seeks out the underlying obstruction.

Arthritis is often referred to as Bi Syndrome; *bi* means obstruction. Although anyone can get arthritis, the Chinese believe Wood and Water types are most vulnerable because of their proclivity to blocked or obstructed energy. Wood energy is prone to obstruction and stagnation (constrained Liver *chi*), while Water energy has a tendency to freeze and solidify; if the underlying imbalance in Wood or Water energy is not corrected, arthritic conditions often develop. Prolonged bouts of Bi Syndrome will also deplete the Liver (Wood) and Kidney (Water) energies, creating a vicious cycle that inevitably weakens the tendons and the bones.

The Chinese believe that four of the Five Devils or pathogenic forces—Wind, Damp, Cold, and Heat—invade the body, causing obstructions and eventually creating arthritic conditions. Each type of blockage involves different symptoms:

• **Wind Bi** involves moving or migrating sensations of pain. Wind is the energy associated with the Liver and Wood energy.

• **Damp Bi** involves a dull, heavy pain that tends to be localized and stationary. Damp weather and/or abrupt barometric changes exacerbate the pain. Dampness is most often associated with imbalances in the Spleen/Stomach orb and Earth energy.

• **Cold Bi** involves severe cramping pains, often described as a "drilling" sort of pain that is fixed in a specific area or areas. Cold is associated with the Kidney and Water energy.

• **Heat Bi** involves pain characterized by an intense burning quality, with redness and swelling around the affected joints. Heat and inflammation are considered disturbances of *yang* energy, and the Large Intestine (the domain of Metal) is the organ most directly associated with this condition.

COMPLEMENTARY TREATMENTS

Diet

Food allergies or sensitivities often play a significant role in both rheumatoid arthritis and osteoarthritis. The typical Western diet, rich in chemical additives, sugars, excess fats, and refined carbohydrates, can weaken the body's defensive energy (the *wei chi*), allowing pathogens to invade the joints. To help prevent and/or reverse arthritis, make sure your diet is rich in complex carbohydrates and fiber, with plenty of fresh vegetables and fruits. Gently steaming your vegetables will help break down the tough cellulose coating and make them easier to digest.

Because acidic buildup in the joints is often connected with arthritis, avoid foods such as red meat, poultry, and animal fats, which can leave acidic residues in the blood and inflame the joints.

The nightshade family of vegetables—tomatoes, eggplants, peppers, and potatoes—may aggravate arthritic conditions. Researchers theorize that the solanum alkaloids in these vegetables inhibit collagen repair in the joints. Consume them sparingly or avoid them completely.

Avoid oranges and orange juice, because the acids in oranges can irritate the delicate joint membranes. Grapefruits and lemons, which are more alkaline in nature, are often well tolerated.

Drink at least eight to ten 8-ounce glasses of fresh, filtered water daily to help the Liver and Kidneys filter food additives and other foreign chemicals from the blood, thus preventing toxins from accumulating in the joints.

Exercise

Exercise is critical for all forms of arthritis. During acute flare-ups, physical therapy (passive exercises, ultrasound, and heat and/or cold applications) will keep the blood circulating. Walking in the fresh air (or on a treadmill, if the weather keeps you inside) and swimming or exercising in a heated pool will help relieve the pain, enhance your circulation, and replenish your vital energy.

Because it relies on gentle stretching movements, *yoga* is a wonderful exercise choice if you suffer from arthritic symptoms. In Chapters 2 through 6 we describe yoga *asanas* corresponding to each of the Five Elements. If you experience any pain or discomfort when trying a particular exercise, seek the guidance of a yoga teacher before continuing. Or take a yoga class and ask your teacher to recommend specific exercises that will help relieve the pain and stiffness in your joints.

Tai chi is an ancient martial art and health-promoting form of exercise that is firmly based in the Taoist philosophy of balance, harmony, and healing from the inside out. The fluid, graceful movements help to invigorate circulation and open up the acupuncture channels to stimulate the flow of *chi*. As with all exercises for arthritis, honor your limits and don't push yourself too hard; with time and repeated practice, you'll find your limits expanding.

In general, we suggest twenty to thirty minutes of exercise daily; adjust the intensity of exercise to your level of pain and degree of inflammation.

Massage is helpful for all types of arthritis because it promotes better circulation and helps the lymph system eliminate toxins from the body. Swedish massage, Rolfing, postural integration, and muscular therapy are particularly effective at breaking up stagnation in the muscles and tendons and promoting lymphatic drainage. The Alexander technique, a unique form of bodywork, teaches ways to change habitual postures or body movements that interfere with the natural flow of energy.

Gentle massage will also ease the pain and reduce the swelling of arthritis. To avoid irritating the skin, lubricate your hands and fingers with massage oil or cream. (Vegetable oil works just as well.) Use long strokes and gentle pressure around (not directly on) the painful or swollen joints.

Sinus Cleanse

In studies conducted in Japan, researchers report that people with autoimmune diseases often have chronic sinus infections (frequently asymptomatic), which can complicate or exacerbate their condition. Periodic sinus cleanses may actually help to calm down a hyperreactive immune system and ease the symptoms.

We recommend a variation of a cleanse suggested by Japanese acupuncturist Kiiko Matsumoto. Put a teaspoon of sea salt and a pinch of baking soda in a cup of lukewarm water, mix well, and pour a small amount of this solution into the cupped palm of your hand. *Gently* inhale through each nostril, moving your head around to circulate the saltwater solution. Let the water drain out of your nose, or spit it out of your mouth; gargle with the remaining solution, and spit it out.

Follow this routine once a day.

Nutritional Supplements

Omega-3 fatty acids (eicosapentaenoic acid or EPA): These anti-inflammatory agents have general supportive effects on the circulatory system and a specific ability to reduce blood cholesterol levels. Omega-3's reduce the joint stiffness and soreness caused by rheumatoid arthritis and improve flexibility.

They are found in cold-water fish such as salmon, mackerel, herring, anchovies, sardines, and tuna. Eat two or three servings of fish weekly, or take a 1,500-mg. supplement daily.

Gamma linoleic acid: GLA has well-documented anti-inflammatory actions and a balancing effect on the immune system. As many researchers and clinicians theorize, arthritis and other autoimmune diseases are caused in part by the body's inability to manufacture GLA and other essential fatty acids. So this is a particularly important supplement for arthritis patients. GLA is available in oil of evening primrose, borage seed oil, and black currant seed oil. Take 1,500 mg. daily.

GLA and omega-3's work well together and are often found in combined formulas. Whether you take them separately or in one formula, make sure you get 1,500 mg. of each daily.

Vitamin C: This vitamin stimulates the immune system, fights free radicals (molecular fragments that attack healthy cells), soothes inflamed tissues, and helps maintain healthy connective tissue. Take 2–4 grams (2,000–4,000 mg.) daily.

Vitamin E: This powerful antioxidant protects the cell walls and joint linings by destroying free radicals, which can attack the joints in arthritic conditions. Take 400 I.U. of d-alpha tocopherol daily; if pain is chronic and persistent, increase to 800 I.U. daily.

Selenium: Selenium stimulates the antioxidant and immune-enhancing effects of vitamin E, as well as antibody formation. Take 200 mcg. daily with vitamin E.

Vitamin B$_6$ and Vitamin B$_5$ (pantothenic acid): These vitamins have anti-inflammatory actions. Take 50–100 mg. of B$_6$ daily and 100–200 mg. of B$_5$ twice daily (200–400 mg. total). Always take any individual B vitamin with a high-potency B-complex vitamin (B-50 or B-100).

Magnesium: Magnesium is considered an antistress mineral, with relaxing effects on both the body and mind. A gentle yet effective muscle relaxant, it relieves muscle cramping and spasms. Magnesium is particularly important for arthritic conditions because it allows calcium to bond into the bone, preventing arthritic deterioration. Take 500–1,000 mg. daily; choose a magnesium supplement that is *chelated with amino acids,* which means it is easier for your body to absorb.

Glucosamine sulfate: This nutritional substance is used as a building block for connective tissue. Studies with osteoarthritis patients indicate that it relieves pain, resolves joint tenderness and swelling, and enhances joint flexibility. Take 500 mg. two to three times daily.

Bromelain: A digestive enzyme derived from pineapple stems, bromelain has strong anti-inflammatory and digestion-supporting properties. In studies with rheumatoid arthritis patients, individuals who took bromelain supplements required significantly lower levels of steroids. Take one tablet approximately half an hour before each meal (three tablets daily).

Chinese Patent Remedies

These famous herbal remedies were formulated for chronic arthritis with gradual onset and/or for arthritis associated with the aging process. As with most Chinese tonic formulas, take the formula until your symptoms subside and your energy returns, then rely on dietary strategies and basic nutritional supplements to maintain good health and ultimate immunity.

Chen Pu Hu Chien Wan ("Walk Vigorously Like Tiger Stealthy Pills"): The Emperor herb in this formula is powdered animal bone—in the old days, herbalists used real tiger bones. Sharing Emperor status is achyranthes root, a well-known blood mover used to break through obstructions and restore normal circulation. Five attending herbs including ginseng, dong quai, gentian, chaenomeles fruit, and honey (as a binder) support the *chi* and the blood and disperse accumulated Damp/Heat in the joints.

This formula comes in bottles of two hundred pills; take twenty pills twice daily.

Du Huo Jisheng Wan ("Angelica Du Huo and Loranthus Pill"): This remedy is used to support the Liver and Kidneys and stimulate the movement of energy and blood through the meridians. The Emperor herb is angelica *du huo,* which helps to break up stagnating energy in the joints and dispel Wind/Damp. Attending herbs include eucommia bark, codonopsis root, rehmannia root, ginger root, poria fungus, cinnamon bark, loranthus, dong quai, and licorice.

This formula comes in bottles of one hundred pills; take nine pills twice daily.

Note: This formula, which contains warming herbs, is *not* recommended for Heat Bi conditions with fever or hot, inflamed joints.

For more acute conditions generally associated with rheumatoid arthritis or acute flare-ups of osteoarthritis, try:

Guan Jie Yan Wan ("Close Down Joint Inflammation Pills"): This gentle but powerful remedy consists of ten herbs that work to initiate vigorous movement of *chi* and blood, helping to eliminate the Damp/Heat from the joints. The Emperor herb is coix seeds, also called Job's tears, a form of barley famous for its ability to dispel Dampness anywhere in the body but particularly in the joints. Attending herbs include eythrina bark, atractylodes, tephania root, achyranthes root, gentiana, cinnamon, ginger, ephedra, and angelica *du huo.*

This formula comes in bottles of three hundred pills; take eight pills three times daily or twelve pills twice daily.

Caution: Because all arthritic formulas are considered "moving" remedies, helping to break through blockages and obstructions and assist the body in eliminating toxic substances, they should not be used in pregnancy.

Herbal Allies

Herbal remedies are aimed at treating the individual rather than the disease itself, so the formulas will vary according to individual needs and symptoms. In herbal medicine, the root causes and underlying constitutional issues are always addressed. If a person suffering from arthritis also experiences difficulty digesting and eliminating foods, the herbal formula should include special digestive and Liver-supporting herbs. If heat and agitation—redness, inflammation, burning pain—are involved, select cooling and/or relaxing herbs.

Dozens of herbs are available to help eliminate toxic wastes, reduce inflammation and swelling, and increase circulation to the affected joints. The following herbs are extremely effective for arthritic conditions:

Celery seed (*Apium graveolens*): This cleansing herb has "blood-moving" qualities that help the body eliminate toxins more effectively. Renowned for its ability to assist the body in eliminating uric acid and other acid accumulations via the Kidneys, celery seed has been used to treat arthritis for hundreds of years.

Devil's claw (*Harpagophytum procumbens*): This traditional African and European remedy is most often used for its gentle but powerful anti-inflammatory actions; in one study, nearly ninety percent of subjects taking devil's claw experienced increased mobility in their joints and a significant reduction in pain and morning stiffness.

Yarrow (*Achillea millefolium*): This herb acts as a powerful circulatory tonic and diuretic, helping the body eliminate toxic wastes through the urine.

Ginger (*Zingiber officinalis*): A warming, nourishing herb, ginger acts as a circulatory tonic, helping the blood move freely through the joints to flush out toxic wastes. Ginger also helps the digestive system work more efficiently, breaking down proteins and other food products that can aggravate arthritis.

Licorice (*Glycyrrhiza glabra*): This all-purpose herb with natural anti-inflammatory actions helps the body put out the "fires" in the joints. When used in any herbal formula, licorice (called "the Great Unifier") helps balance the actions of the other herbs.

You can combine all the herbs listed above or choose any combination of them. One of my favorite formulas for rheumatoid arthritis and gout (a form of rheumatoid arthritis) includes equal parts celery seed, devil's claw, and licorice. For general arthritis or osteoarthritic complaints, I often prescribe licorice, devil's claw, and yarrow (each constituting thirty percent of the formula), with ten percent ginger. The moving, anti-inflammatory quality of the herbs is appropriate for all forms of Bi Syndrome.

Dosage: If you purchase your herbs in a health food store (either in tincture form or, as dried herbs, in capsule or pill form), follow the dosage instructions on the label. Because herbs in dried form tend to lose their potency rather quickly, be sure to check the label for the expiration date.

For information on preparing your own herbs from the root, bark, leaves, flowers, or seeds of a plant, see Appendix II.

In Appendix I, Resources, we offer a list of mail-order sources for high-quality herbs and herbal preparations. For advice on ordering specially made herbal formulas, see pages 394 to 396.

Acupoints

We've selected acupoints on the basis of the individual's presenting symptoms and the diagnosis of Wind, Cold, Damp, or Heat Bi Syndrome. Additional points are determined by the precise location of the pain and other accompanying symptoms. For help locating these and other acupoints, see Appendix III.

Wind Bi Syndrome:

Governing Vessel 12 ("Body's Pillar"): This point supports the *wei chi* (immune) energy, eliminates the Wind Devil, and strengthens the body, mind, and spirit (as its name implies). It is also said to strengthen the back and support the upper body, and it is therefore especially useful for arthritic conditions that affect the upper back, neck, and head, as well as the shoulders and elbows.

Location: Governing Vessel 12 is located on the spine between the third and fourth thoracic vertebrae, approximately at shoulder level.

Gallbladder 34 ("Yang Mound Spring"): Known as "the influential point for the tendons and sinews," this point is used for any problem involving tight, strained, or injured tendons. It supports the tendons and joints and helps to ensure the free movement of energy and blood through the tendinomuscular channels.

Location: Gallbladder 34 is located on the outside border of the calf, in the depression between the two bones (tibia and fibula).

Liver 3 ("Great Rushing"): This point is used to keep the energy and blood moving by eliminating Wind and removing various obstructions.

Location: Liver 3 is located in the webbing between the big toe and the second toe.

Cold Bi Syndrome:

Wet Heating Pads or Moxabustion: This traditional Chinese method, in which an herb or combination of herbs is burned over the affected areas of the body, helps to warm the body/mind/spirit and disperse the Cold. Heat is contraindicated when there is active inflammation of the joints.

Damp Bi Syndrome:

Stomach 36 ("Walks Three Miles"): This point supports the Stomach and Spleen functions, allowing the metabolic fires to disperse the dampness.

Location: Stomach 36 is located three inches below the dimple or depression on the outside (pinky side) of the knee, approximately an inch from the crest of the shinbone, in a groove or natural depression in the muscle.

Spleen 9 ("Fountain of Yin Spring"): This point is used to clear the body's waterways of Damp/Heat conditions and replenish *yin* (fluid) energies.

Location: Spleen 9 is located in the depression on the inside of the lower leg, just below the knee. With your knee bent, slide your fingers along the bone on the inside border of the knee until they stop in a natural depression. This point is often extremely sensitive to the touch.

Heat Bi Syndrome:

Governing Vessel 4 ("Great Hammer"): This point is frequently used to subdue the *yang* energies of the body, mind, and spirit and to remove Heat from the blood.

Location: Governing Vessel 14 is located just below the large protruding vertebra at the base of the neck (the seventh cervical vertebra).

Large Intestine 4 ("Great Eliminator"): This point helps drain and disperse the "stuck" energy in the upper part of the body, particularly in the head and neck areas.

Location: Large Intestine 4 is located in the webbing between the thumb and index finger.

Large Intestine 11 ("Crooked Pond"): This point is used to disperse Heat from the body and remove obstructions.

Location: Large Intestine 11 is located in the lateral (outer) part of the elbow.

Questions to Ask Yourself

The physical symptoms of pain and discomfort associated with all forms of arthritis may express related problems of blockage or obstruction in the mind and the spirit. Use the following questions to talk to your disease, asking your symptoms what they want from you.

- How do I resist change in my life?
- How do I stop myself from achieving my goals?
- Why am I having trouble standing up for myself?
- What is the worst thing that could happen if I let my feelings out?

Many people with arthritis have a strong affinity to Wood and/or Water. If you are a Wood type, your symptoms might be asking you to address these questions:

- How am I constraining or repressing my energy?
- Where am I blocked creatively?
- Am I turning my anger, frustration, and fear against myself? Am I allowing myself to express these emotions?

If you are strongly influenced by Water energy, ask yourself these questions:

- What is my fear preventing me from doing or accomplishing?
- How can I learn to stand up for myself and assert myself with clarity and force?
- Does my physical stiffness have a counterpart in my psyche? Am I too rigid in my beliefs and my behaviors?

A STARTING POINT

Picking and choosing among the many and diverse remedies recommended for arthritis may seem like an overwhelming task. Where should you begin?

The following supplements, herbal remedies, and healing strategies will give you a solid foundation that you can then build upon, using the other remedies suggested in this section when and if you need additional support:

1. *Diet:* Follow the dietary suggestions on pages 287 to 288.
2. *Exercise:* Exercise for twenty to thirty minutes every day.
3. *Nutritional supplements:* Take the general formula for Maximum Immunity.
4. *Essential fatty acids:* Take 1,500 mg. each of omega-3 and GLA oils, or eat at least three deep sea fish meals every week.
5. *Glucosamine sulfate:* Take 500 mg. twice daily.
6. *Du Huo Jisheng Wan:* Take nine pills twice daily.
7. *Western herbal arthritic tonic:* Take a tonic of licorice, devil's claw, and yarrow (each constituting thirty percent of the formula), with ten percent ginger.

Lupus (Systemic Lupus Erythematosis)

Amy was diagnosed with lupus when she was thirty years old. Within two years the disease had attacked her kidneys, causing massive inflammation. Kidney dialysis and massive doses of prednisone, an anti-inflammatory steroid drug, saved her life, but Amy's kidneys were permanently damaged, and she was told that she would have to take steroids for the rest of her life.

"I can't bear the thought of being dependent on drugs," Amy told me. "If there's anything I can do to help my body heal itself, I'm willing to do it." Amy's desire to challenge herself, her grace under pressure, and her unflagging confidence in her body's ability to heal itself pointed to a strong Wood constitution; physical complaints of sudden, sharp pains between her ribs, migraine headaches, and muscle spasms in her neck and shoulders confirmed her affinity to Wood. Because her physical health was fragile and unstable, we used gentle pressure on specific acupoints rather than needles, and we relied on tonic herbs that offered slow but steady support for her immune system.

Progress was gradual, but after a year Amy had weaned herself off the steroids. She started a lupus support group and spent many hours every week helping others learn how to live with their disease. In our work together—which has spanned a period of seventeen years—we both came to appreciate the combined strengths of Eastern and Western medicine. "Western medicine saved my life," Amy explained, "and Eastern medicine gave me back my independence and restored my faith in the future."

WESTERN INTERPRETATION

Lupus is a strange and unique autoimmune disease of unknown origin that affects virtually every part of the body. In autoimmune diseases, the immune system mistakes the self for the enemy and initiates inflammatory reactions in an attempt to expel the invader. In lupus, the body produces antibodies (called antinuclear antibodies) that act indiscriminately to destroy the body's own tissues and organs.

Approximately one million Americans suffer from lupus; ninety percent of the victims are women. The average age of onset is between twenty and forty, with a mean onset of twenty-nine. Although there is a slight genetic risk of inheriting lupus, the risk is much lower than in most diseases—only five percent of people with lupus will have children with the disease. Lupus is not contagious.

With the greatly improved diagnostic and treatment methods available today, more than ninety percent of lupus patients survive the disease, compared to only fifty percent in 1955. The disease begins slowly, and the earliest symptoms are vague and widely varied. People report feeling slightly "off," with fatigue, swollen glands, aching joints, fever, and stomach upset; these general symptoms are associated with many diseases. As time goes by, however, the earlier symptoms intensify, and more debilitating symptoms may appear, including blood abnormalities, kidney disorders, and heart disease.

To help physicians diagnose lupus, the American College of Rheumatology has identified eleven criteria commonly associated with the disease; at least four of them must be present simultaneously to confirm the diagnosis:

1. **Butterfly (malar) rash,** a red rash that covers the nose and cheeks in a distinctive butterfly pattern. Forty to fifty percent of lupus victims have this rare and unusual rash.

2. **Discoid lesions,** scaly, red, disk-shaped rashes or lesions that often erupt on the face, neck, upper torso, or scalp. They affect approximately fifteen percent of people with lupus.

3. **Photosensitivity of the skin** or hypersensitivity to light resulting in a rash following exposure to sunlight. Approximately one third of lupus patients are sun-sensitive.

4. **Mucosal ulcers** or ulcerative sores in the mouth, throat, or nasal linings, experienced by one in eight lupus patients. Similar to cold sores, they are blisterlike in appearance, usually painless, and reflect an immune system imbalance.

5. **Arthritis,** or inflammation of the joints, usually in the peripheral joints such as hands, wrists, feet, ankles, and knees, but often shifting around from one joint to another. Approximately ninety percent of lupus patients suffer from arthritic symptoms at some point in their disease.

6. **Chest and heart problems** caused by inflammation of the mucous linings of the heart or lungs. Twenty-five percent of lupus patients will have pericarditis (inflammation of the membrane surrounding the heart) at some point in their disease, while forty-five percent of lupus patients have pleuritis (inflammation of the membranes lining the lungs and chest cavity). These conditions are painful but not life-threatening.

7. **Kidney problems** related to inflammatory reactions in the kidneys. Approximately fifty percent of lupus victims experience kidney disorders at some point in their illness.

8. **Neurologic disorders** such as seizures or psychotic episodes. They affect about fifteen percent of lupus victims.

9. **Blood abnormalities** such as hemolytic anemia (abnormally rapid destruction of red blood cells); thrombocytopenia (a reduction in platelets); or leukopenia (low white blood cell counts). Virtually all lupus patients have one or more of these blood abnormalities at some point in their illness.

10. **Immune disruptions** confirmed by the following tests:

• **Lupus erythematosus (LE) cell test** determines whether the white blood cells known as phagocytes (which means "cell-eating") are devouring the nuclear core material from other white blood cells. Approximately fifty percent of people with lupus test positive for this test, although people with other autoimmune disorders, especially rheumatoid arthritis, also test positive.

• **Anti-DNA test** determines whether the patient has a heightened level of antibodies to DNA. Abnormal levels of anti-DNA are found in fifty to sixty percent of lupus patients.

11. **High antinuclear antibody levels** (determined by an antinuclear antibody, or ANA test), which indicate that you are producing antibodies to the nu-

clei of your cells. The antibodies tell the phagocytes ("cell-eaters") and macrophages ("big eaters") to consume dead or diseased cells, but in lupus these antibodies are rapidly and continuously produced, causing the immune system to gobble up healthy cells as well. High ANA levels are not exclusive to lupus, although nearly one hundred percent of lupus patients have them.

WESTERN TREATMENT

Western medicine considers lupus a disease of unknown origin that cannot be prevented or cured. Treatment is therefore aimed at controlling and relieving the symptoms while preventing and treating life-threatening complications.

For inflammation and acute flare-ups of the disease, the nonsteroidal anti-inflammatory drugs (NSAIDs)—ibuprofen and aspirin—are often used. Because side effects include gastrointestinal irritation (particularly with aspirin and related drugs known as salicylates), which can lead to ulcers, these drugs are often combined with antacids or anti-ulcer medications like Tagamet or Zantac, to reduce stomach acid and prevent problems. Prescription NSAIDs such as Rufen, Naprosyn, Feldene, and Dolobid can cause headaches, fever, fatigue, allergic reactions, hypertension, blood count abnormalities, and liver disease, especially when used in high dosages over long periods of time.

If NSAIDs are not strong enough to control the inflammation, systemic corticosteroidal drugs (prednisone, Medrol, dexamethasone, cortisone, hydrocortisone) are often prescribed. In the early days of treating lupus, these drugs were often overprescribed, and many patients actually became sick because of their treatment. Today, treatment is much more conservative, and stronger medications are prescribed only when absolutely necessary. Nevertheless, virtually every lupus patient will receive a prescription for a corticosteroid at some point in their disease.

Synthesized to resemble cortisol, a hormone produced by the adrenal cortex, the corticosteroids control symptoms by suppressing the immune system, which in turn reduces the inflammatory response. Side effects include weight gain, increased susceptibility to infection, abnormal bruising or bleeding, unusual hair growth, cataracts, increased risk of developing diabetes, coronary artery disease, elevated blood pressure and cholesterol, facial swelling, sleep problems, and psychological disturbances. Women should be warned that the corticosteroidal drugs can encourage osteoporosis, a weakening of the skeletal bone, increasing the risk of fracture.

For skin lesions and rashes, antimalarial drugs (quinine, Avalen, Plaquenil, Atabrine) are often prescribed and have been found to be extremely helpful for joint problems and fatigue as well.

When the immune system is raging out of control and other methods don't work, powerful immune suppressants like azathioprine (Imuran) or cyclophosphamide (Cytoxan) may be prescribed. Because prolonged use can have severe and even life-threatening side effects, these drugs are reserved for critical interventions, such as severe kidney inflammation.

Many physicians caution against overusing medications, which can create additional problems for the patient. Treatment is geared instead to helping the patient institute various lifestyle changes and stress-reduction techniques. As Dr. Paul Blau states in his book *Living with Lupus:*

> A person who has lupus need not necessarily take any medication. Therapy should be keyed to symptoms—and even so, need not involve drugs. . . . Frequently . . . another "prescription"—a combination of diet modification, rest, and a certain amount of specific exercise—will be wonderfully effective.

TRADITIONAL CHINESE INTERPRETATION

The symptoms of lupus are somewhat paradoxical, from a Chinese point of view. Fatigue, lethargy, and anemia are considered signs of deficient *chi* and blood, while the hot, inflamed joints, butterfly or discoid rashes, mucosal ulcers, heart and lung inflammations (pleuritis and pericarditis), kidney infections, and bladder infections are signs of excess or disturbed *chi* and blood. In traditional Chinese medicine any disorder of the immune system involves the Kidneys, which supply the Lungs with the energy needed to create the *wei chi* (immune energy) and distribute it through the blood vessels and meridians to every cell in the body. Thus, if you have lupus, you might be told that you have a deficient Lung (Metal) *chi* and deficient Kidney (Water) *yin* condition, with brushfires creating heat in the blood.

In other words: Because the body's water (*yin*) supply is deficient, small brushfires (*yang*) are breaking out all over the place. These fires are not true fires, however, because the body doesn't have sufficient fuel (*chi*) to feed them. Blazing heat caused by a deficiency of *yin* rather than a true excess of *yang* creates friction in the system, which contributes to the inflammation in the Kidneys, Lungs, and Heart. The blood heats up, and hot blood rises to the skin (creating the characteristic rashes) or to the head, causing such central nervous system symptoms as seizures and psychotic episodes.

Chinese medicine always focuses on the individual rather than the disease, especially in lupus and other autoimmune diseases whose symptoms are so varied and widespread. Anyone can get lupus, although Water and Metal types seem to be more vulnerable; however, the disease always involves deficient Kidney and Lung energies, and treatment strategies are aimed at building up the Kidney and Lung *chi,* supporting the *yin* energies of the Kidneys and Lungs to cool the blood, and dispersing the raging fires with various acupoints and herbal remedies.

Lupus is definitely a disease that demands respect, but it is no longer a disease to fear. By following the complementary treatment strategies outlined in this section, you will assist your body in its courageous attempts to heal itself. In my experience with hundreds of lupus patients, the great majority go on to live full, healthy, happy lives.

COMPLEMENTARY TREATMENTS

Diet

The vast majority of people with lupus suffer from allergies, including food allergies or sensitivities. To test for food sensitivities, *try the Elimination / Provocation Diet,* or have your blood tested. Blood tests such as the Radio Allergo Sorbent Test (RAST) can detect immune reactions to food by measuring IgG or IgE antibodies to specific food allergens. If you find that you are allergic to a particular food or food group, eliminating that food from your diet may significantly relieve your symptoms.

Cutting down on animal proteins will also help your system return to a state of balance. A number of studies show that reducing the amount of protein you eat and increasing complex carbohydrates will help support kidney function and reduce flare-ups of the disease. If the disease affects your kidneys in any way, you can only benefit by dramatically reducing your protein intake, which automatically eases the burden on your kidneys.

Lupus patients tend to have higher-than-normal cholesterol and triglyceride levels and are therefore at greater risk of coronary artery disease. (As we mentioned earlier, taking steroidal drugs can significantly increase this risk.) For these reasons, it is extremely important to *avoid fatty foods, fried foods, and red meat,* all of which are high in saturated fat.

Partially hydrogenated fats or vegetable oils found in margarines, shortening, and many canned and frozen foods can aggravate inflammatory conditions in the body and contribute to the buildup of arterial plaque, increasing the risk of coronary artery disease. *Use only olive or canola oil for cooking,* and use only cold-pressed polyunsaturated oils (safflower, almond, sesame) or monosaturated oils (olive and canola) for your salads. *Substitute olive oil for butter whenever possible.*

Low levels of stomach acid (hypochorhydria) are common in lupus patients; you might *try eating bitter foods* (endive, escarole, Swiss chard), which stimulate the bitter taste buds on the tongue, increasing stomach acid levels and promoting the production of bile, which is good for both the Liver and the Gallbladder.

Drastically reduce your consumption of sugar, refined carbohydrates, coffee, and all caffeine products, including soft drinks and chocolate. These antinutrients, which take more from the body than they give back, can aggravate inflammatory conditions.

Exercise

Follow the exercise regimens suggested for your particular constitutional type in Chapters 2 to 6, but avoid strenuous, jarring exercises like running, racquetball, tennis, or long-distance bicycling, which can further inflame the joints and tissues. Gentle walks, swimming, and yoga exercises will increase circulation, build endurance, and lift your spirits.

We recommend twenty to thirty minutes of exercise daily.

Avoid Overexposure to the Sun

One third of people with lupus are sensitive to ultraviolet light (sunlight and fluorescent light), which can trigger skin reactions and acute flare-ups of the disease. Avoid overexposure to the sun, wear a hat and long sleeves when outside (even on cloudy days), and use a strong sunscreen, preferably one without PABA, which causes allergic reactions in many lupus patients.

Certain plants containing chemicals called psoralens—limes, lemons, figs, celery, parsley, and parsnips—enhance photosensitivity. Certain drugs also heighten photosensitivity, including the antibiotic tetracycline, the anti-inflammatory drug Feldene, and various antihypertensive, sulfa, antiseizure, and antidepressant drugs.

Skin Treatments

Hypersensitive, dry, and flaky skin is a common problem for lupus sufferers. While numerous commercial brands of moisturizing creams are available, natural creams and ointments may offer you better results in the long run. For dry, itchy skin, try chickweed (*Stellaria media*) cream or ointment. Other gentle yet effective herbal creams include calendula ointment, Self-Heal Salve (a combination of prunella, burdock, St. John's wort oil, and calendula), vitamin E and aloe ointment, and Purple Gold Ointment, a Chinese herbal preparation. These products are available in many health food stores, or they can be ordered (see Appendix I).

Sinus Cleanse

For an excellent sinus cleanse, see page 289.

Nutritional Supplements

Vitamin C: Vitamin C helps create and maintain collagen, the body's connective tissue, which is found in the skin, joint linings, ligaments, vertebral disks, and capillary walls—all vulnerable areas for people with lupus. A powerful antioxidant and immune system stimulant, vitamin C helps your cells resist damage from free radicals, reducing the chance of injury and inflammation. Vitamin C will also help to lower blood cholesterol levels by assisting the body in its efforts to metabolize and eliminate cholesterol, thus protecting you against coronary artery disease.

Take 2,000–4,000 mg. (2–4 grams) daily; during acute flare-ups, take up to 10,000 mg. daily in 1,000-mg. doses every hour or two. If you experience diarrhea or loose bowels, cut back until the symptoms disappear.

Beta-carotene: Beta-carotene promotes healing of the skin and mucous linings of the body, including the lungs, urinary system, stomach, and intestines, making it an excellent supplement for lupus patients. A powerful antioxidant with specific supportive effects on vision and eyesight, beta-carotene may also reduce the risk of developing cancer. Beta-carotene is converted into vitamin A in the intestines, but it has none of the toxicity associated with large doses of vitamin A. Take 25,000 I.U. daily.

Vitamin E: This powerful antioxidant has protective effects on cell membranes and tissues. Whenever there is inflammation in the body (and in lupus inflammations rage in many areas of the body), the destructive molecular fragments known as free radicals proliferate; like vitamin C and other antioxidants, vitamin E protects the cell membranes and tissues of the body against free radical damage. Vitamin E also supports the immune system against viral invaders and relieves many arthritic symptoms. Take 400 I.U. daily; increase to 800 I.U. daily during acute flare-ups.

Selenium: Selenium enhances the antioxidant actions of vitamin E and helps reduce inflammation in many acute, degenerative diseases. Take 200 mcg. daily with vitamin E.

B-complex vitamins: These vitamins help maintain the proper functioning of the nervous system, alleviating fatigue, calming shattered nerves, easing anxiety, and generally supporting and balancing all body systems. Take a B-50 or B-100 complex.

Zinc: Zinc is essential in the formation of collagen and supports the skin and tissues; it also promotes immune function and seems to have an anti-inflammatory action, especially for the joints and blood vessels. Take 20–30 mg. daily and up to 60 mg. during acute flare-ups.

Pycnogenol (Proanthocyanidan): This nutrient is considered fifty times more powerful than vitamin E in its antioxidant actions, working hard to protect the body's cells from destruction by the highly unstable and reactive free radicals. Pycnogenol stabilizes collagen structures within the body, protecting the skin, joints, tissues, and organs. Its anti-inflammatory and immune-enhancing effects and its ability to cross the blood/brain barrier to prevent oxidative damage to nervous tissues while simultaneously strengthening blood vessels make pycnogenol a particularly appropriate supplement for lupus and other autoimmune diseases. To reach tissue saturation, take 10 mg. per 10 pounds of body weight; after ten days cut the dosage to 50 mg. daily.

Omega-3 fatty acids (eicosapentaenoic acid or EPA): These fatty acids act as natural anti-inflammatory agents, with general supportive effects on the circulatory system and a specific ability to reduce blood cholesterol levels. The best food source of omega-3 fatty acids is certain oily fish—salmon, sardines, herring, mackerel, anchovies, and albacore tuna. Other rich sources of omega-3's are flaxseed, flax meal, flax oil, hemp oil, and walnuts. Eat fish rich in omega-3's three times a week, or supplement your diet with 1,500 mg. daily.

Gamma linoleic acid: GLA is a valuable ally in protecting the cells from degenerative changes and reducing inflammation throughout the body. Numerous research studies support claims that GLA reduces the symptoms of arthritis, inflammatory skin conditions, premenstrual syndrome, and inflammations in general. GLA is found in oil of evening primrose, borage seed oil, and black currant seed oil. Take 1,500 mg. daily.

Betaine hydrochloric acid: HCl is particularly useful for those lupus patients who have low levels of stomach acid (a relatively common problem); supplementing with HCl supports the digestive process, helping to reduce the "renegade" proteins that can cause autoimmune responses. Take one 5–10 grain (64-mg.) pill with each meal.

Caution: For some individuals with high stomach acid levels, HCl can irritate the stomach, causing heartburn or acid reflux and increasing the risk of gastric ulcers. If you have ulcers, or if you experience any negative reactions to HCl, discontinue use.

Chinese Patent Remedies
Restorative Pills or He Che Da Zao Wan ("Placenta Great Creation Pills"): While there are many Chinese patent herbal remedies that will relieve the indi-

vidual symptoms associated with lupus, we recommend this formula to address the underlying Kidney (Water) and Lung (Metal) deficiencies. Specifically formulated to nurture and support Kidney, Liver, and Heart *yin* functions, this famous remedy also builds and nourishes the blood, gently subduing the rising fire (inflammatory) signs so common in lupus. The Emperor herb is human placenta extract; attending herbs include rehmannia root, asparagus root, codonopsis root (an herb similar to ginseng but slightly cooler and less expensive), poria fungus, and tortoise shell.

This patent remedy is available in bottles of two hundred small pellets or pills; take eight pills three times daily or twelve pills twice daily.

Liu Wei Di Huang Wan ("Six Flavor Rehmannia Pills"): If you object to the use of animal parts (tortoise shell) or human placenta extract in the above formula, you could try this gentle substitute. It is the classic formula to support the *yin,* especially Kidney *yin,* with six herbs including rehmannia root as the Emperor herb, cornus fruit, dioscorea root, moutan bark, poria fungus, and alisma root.

Take eight pills three times daily or twelve pills twice daily.

These Chinese patent remedies are gentle and can be safely combined with any of the following Western herbs. If you need help choosing the most effective formula or combination of herbs for your symptoms, consult an experienced herbalist.

Herbal Allies

The following herbs can be used alone or combined in a single formula. Popular formulas available at health food stores offer different combinations of these herbs, or you can contact a qualified herbalist, who will mix up a formula tailored to your specific needs.

Marshmallow root (*Althea officinalis*): This wonderful healing herb has mucuslike qualities that help restore the integrity of all the mucous membranes of the body, including the mouth, nose, urinary, respiratory, and digestive systems. Healthy mucous linings naturally prevent inflammations from flaring up; if the mucous membranes are hot and inflamed, marshmallow root will coat the tissues and cool them down.

Dandelion root (*Taraxacum officinalis*): This superlative Liver tonic is traditionally used for what herbalists call "toxic conditions" such as arthritis, skin inflammations, and red or inflamed rashes. Dandelion helps the Liver filter the blood and eliminate toxins; when the blood is flowing smoothly and efficiently, the cells and tissues are well lubricated and less likely to become hot and inflamed.

Nettles (*Urtica dioica*): Nettles is so rich in nutrients, particularly iron and vitamin C, that it could be considered a complete food. Used for hundreds of years in numerous countries and cultures for skin diseases (including rashes, eczema, and psoriasis) allergic reactions, and as a general support for the immune system, nettles is also a gentle but powerful Kidney tonic. For lupus victims, the healing qualities of this herb are unsurpassed.

Vervain (*Verbena officinalis*): Vervain helps to ease the nerves and support the nervous system in general, and it has been used with great success to relieve many symptoms of depression, anxiety, and nervous exhaustion. Its antispasmodic qualities contribute to its usefulness in treating allergies, particularly allergic asthma, and its bitter qualities make it a good Liver tonic and cooling remedy to extinguish the raging fires of lupus.

Licorice (*Glycyrrhiza glabra*): A wonderful balancing herb for lupus, licorice has soothing and restorative effects on the body's delicate mucous membranes. Its anti-inflammatory properties help to soothe the fires of lupus, while its supportive and balancing effects on the adrenal gland will help you cope with physical and emotional stress. *Caution:* If lupus has affected your Kidneys or if you have high blood pressure, use licorice only under professional supervision.

Echinacea (*Echinacea angustifolia* or *Echinacea purpura*): A powerful immune stimulant, echinacea has antimicrobial, antibacterial, antiviral, and antifungal qualities. Also known as one of the best alterative (blood-cleansing) herbs, it actively supports and cleans the blood, working to prevent and treat skin diseases and disorders ranging from rashes (as in lupus) and hives to eczema and psoriasis.

Because echinacea stimulates the immune system, some herbalists believe it should not be used for autoimmune problems, in which the immune system is already overstimulated. Research and clinical experience show, however, that echinacea is an adaptogenic herb, working to balance and modulate the immune response, whether it is sluggish or overexcited.

Dosage: If you purchase your herbs in a health food store (either in tincture form or, as dried herbs, in capsule or pill form), follow the dosage instructions on the label. Because herbs in dried form tend to lose their potency rather quickly, be sure to check the label for the expiration date.

For information on preparing your own herbs from the root, bark, leaves, flowers, or seeds of a plant, see Appendix II.

In Appendix I, Resources, we offer a list of mail-order sources for high-quality herbs and herbal preparations. For advice on ordering specially made herbal formulas, see pages 394 to 396.

Acupoints

Lung 9 ("Great Abyss"): This point helps to balance the immune system by supporting the Lung in its production of *wei chi,* helping the Lung circulate blood and *chi* throughout the body, and circulating and distributing the *wei chi* to the various organs and tissues. For autoimmune diseases, Lung 9 seems to balance the *wei chi,* while in immunodeficient diseases, it helps to strengthen and support the immune system. By helping to move the blood, this point enables the body to eliminate excess Heat in the blood, the cause of such symptoms as rashes and inflamed joints or organs.

Location: Lung 9 is located on the wrist crease, approximately half an inch in from the thumb. Press with your thumbs or forefinger, then massage gently in small circular movements.

Conception Vessel 3 ("Central Pole"): This is the point where three *yin* meridians—the Liver, Spleen, and Kidney—intersect with the Conception Vessel, the central *yin* meridian. Stimulating this point taps into a deep reservoir of cooling, healing *yin* energy and distributes the fluid energy to every organ in the body.

Location: Conception Vessel 3 is located on the midline of the lower abdomen, about three inches above the pubic bone. Massage gently in small circles, moving in a clockwise direction.

Kidney 3 ("Great Mountain Stream"): This point recharges the battery pack of the Kidneys, nourishing every aspect of Kidney function, including the *yin, yang, chi,* and *jing* (inherited essence). Since lupus puts a significant drain on the Kidneys, stimulating this point will help replenish and invigorate the depleted Kidney energy.

Location: Kidney 3 is located in the depression between the inside ankle bone and the Achilles tendon. Find the tender spot, and massage in a circular, clockwise pattern with your thumb or fingers.

Questions to Ask Yourself

The symptoms of disease can be imagined as the body's way of asking us to pay attention. Something is wrong; yet in lupus and other autoimmune diseases, no one is quite sure what went wrong, why or how it went wrong, or what to do about it. The disease itself eludes our understanding and our powers to make it go away.

Use the following questions, which pertain to all autoimmune diseases, to talk to your body, asking your symptoms what they want from you. Be sure to pay attention to the individual symptoms associated with your disease. If you have a butterfly rash, for example, ask yourself what might be getting under your skin or why you seem to be thin-skinned at this point in time.

- How am I turning against my self?
- How do I prevent myself from getting what I want from life?
- If my disease signifies a lack of distinction between self and nonself, is something preventing me from knowing who I really am?
- What am I getting from my symptoms? What do my symptoms prevent me from accomplishing?

Lupus always involves deficient Lung (Metal) and Kidney (Water) energies. In Chinese thought, Metal energy relates to aesthetics, high ethical standards, and a basic need for quality rather than quantity. Grief is the emotion associated with

Metal. If you are strongly influenced by Metal, consider these observations and questions:

- I hold myself to incredibly high standards—what can I do to create more reasonable expectations for myself?
- I tend to be hypercritical of my own behavior: How can this disease help me let go of my perfectionist tendencies and allow me to accept who I am?
- I often feel overwhelmed by a sense of sadness and loss—how can I express my grief and let go of it?

Water energy tends to be reflective and introspective. Although inherently adaptable, Water can freeze up and harden, contributing to physical and emotional inflexibility. Fear is Water's primary emotion. If you have a strong affinity to Water, think about these questions:

- I tend to isolate myself from others—why don't I allow myself to be supported? What am I afraid of?
- How can I ask for support and not feel like a failure?
- I fear being out of control, and I fear death: How does my disease help me deal with these fears? Why am I holding on to my fear?

A STARTING POINT

Picking and choosing among the many and diverse remedies recommended for lupus may seem like an overwhelming task. Where should you begin?

The following supplements, herbal remedies, and healing strategies will give you a solid foundation that you can then build upon, using the other remedies suggested in this section when and if you need additional support:

1. *Diet:* Follow the dietary suggestions on pages 302 to 303.
2. *Exercise:* Exercise for twenty to thirty minutes every day.
3. *Nutritional supplements:* Take the general formula for Maximum Immunity.
4. *Essential fatty acids:* Take 1,500 mg. of GLA and 1,500 mg. of omega-3 (EPA) oils daily.
5. *Restorative pills:* Take twelve pills twice daily.

6. *Western herbal tonic:* Take a tonic consisting of equal amounts of dandelion root, nettles, licorice, and vervain.

Chronic Fatigue Syndrome

Jennifer was twenty-one years old when she left her childhood home in rural Tennessee for the glamorous and exciting life she had always dreamed about in New York. With her three roommates she partied almost every night, attending plays, gallery openings, and nightclub acts. Jennifer's professional life was equally demanding, and after working for just two years at a Wall Street investment firm, she was promoted to an executive position.

A year later she married another executive at the firm. Every day Jennifer and her husband would work ten or twelve hours, and every night they would go out to dinner and a show or join friends for drinks. Five hours of sleep was the norm. Exercise and relaxation were reserved for the weekends, when they drove to their country home, where they busied themselves with golf, hiking, or skiing and entertained an endless stream of friends and relatives.

Jennifer's natural exuberance, outgoing personality, and passion for socializing indicated excessive Fire energy. Over time her frenetic lifestyle depleted her Fire, and she began to experience physical and emotional problems. Vigorously healthy all her life, she began to suffer from recurrent colds and flus, which she just couldn't shake. One winter she caught a flu that simply wouldn't go away; her body ached all over, and with every passing day she became more fatigued and dispirited. When the exhaustion became incapacitating—she literally couldn't force herself out of bed in the morning—Jennifer asked for an extended leave of absence from her job. In the next three months she consulted six doctors, none of whom could diagnose her disease; instead, each doctor offered her pain medications, antidepressants, sleeping pills, or anti-inflammatory drugs to relieve her symptoms.

Eventually one of her doctors conducted a series of blood tests, which confirmed the diagnosis of Epstein-Barr virus, otherwise known as chronic fatigue syndrome.

"What's my prognosis?" Jennifer asked.

"There's no cure yet," the doctor explained, "although drugs are available to relieve your symptoms. According to the most current medical literature, the disease simply has to run its course, which can last from two to ten years."

Jennifer broke down and cried. After a week of tears and anger, she decided "enough is enough," and began to make plans for her recovery. She asked for an extended medical leave from her job, moved permanently to the country home, where her husband joined her on weekends, and called me to schedule weekly acupuncture sessions. Together we worked out a series of dietary changes, which included eliminating dairy products, red meat, and most refined and processed foods, while increasing the amounts of fresh fruits and vegetables she consumed. Every day Jennifer took vitamins A, C, and E and other nutritional supplements she had never heard of before: omega-3 and gamma linoleic acid (GLA) supplements, coenzyme Q-10, and pycnogenol.

To build up Jennifer's deficient Fire energy, strengthen her Liver, and support her immune system, I prescribed an herbal tonic consisting of echinacea, isatis, dandelion, milk thistle, astragalus, and licorice. During the acupuncture sessions she reflected on her former frenetic lifestyle and the changes she could make to support her body, mind, and spirit.

Over the next four months Jennifer's energy began to return. Six months after she began acupuncture treatments, she claimed that she was "eighty-five percent my old self"; after a year she pronounced herself "one hundred percent cured." The cure did not come without some sacrifice and many dramatic changes in her lifestyle. She quit her Wall Street job and moved permanently to the country, where she enrolled in graduate school to earn her master's degree in social work. Every day without fail she swims laps at the local YMCA, where she also attends evening yoga classes. She stopped smoking and limits herself to one glass of wine a day. Four times a year she has an acupuncture "tune-up" session.

Jennifer now works as a private psychotherapist. She has had no recurrence of her disease.

WESTERN INTERPRETATION

Chronic fatigue syndrome (CFS) has been called by many names: "Yuppie flu," chronic mononucleosis, neuromyasthenia, chronic Epstein-Barr, or chronic fatigue immune deficiency syndrome (CFIDS). Approximately two thirds of people diagnosed with chronic fatigue syndrome are women, with the average age of onset in the late thirties or early forties.

The Centers for Disease Control have compiled a list of criteria used to define chronic fatigue syndrome by its symptoms. The major criteria include:

- **Fatigue:** "Persistent or relapsing, debilitating fatigue" in a person with no previous history of fatigue is the most common symptom associated with chronic fatigue syndrome. Fatigue is considered debilitating when it cuts your activity level in half for at least six months.
- **Chronic sore throat and / or swollen glands.**
- **Myalgias,** chronic muscle aches or pains (the kind you get when you have the flu).
- **Arthralgias,** chronic aches or pains in the joints.
- **Sleep disturbances:** difficulties falling asleep, disturbed sleep.
- **Cognitive disturbances,** including the inability to focus, poor memory, distractability, light-headedness, difficulty solving problems (especially math problems).
- **Emotional disturbances,** especially depression.
- **Gastrointestinal problems,** including constipation, diarrhea, irritable bowel, persistent nausea, and sensitivities to foods formerly tolerated.

Chronic fatigue syndrome is considered a multicausal illness—a disease caused by many different factors. The Epstein-Barr virus is considered a factor in the disease, but ninety percent of us carry this virus with no ill effects. Why do some people with the Epstein-Barr virus develop CFS while the rest of us don't? The answer clearly resides in the affected individual—a weakened immune system can no longer control the virus, which proliferates and further drains the body's defensive energy.

What impairs the immune system? Long-term, unrelieved stress, dietary influences, toxins in the environment and in the home, excess use of alcohol, tobacco, prescription or recreational drugs, a chronic illness such as repeated colds and flus, or major surgeries can overburden the immune system, which is then unable to protect the body against invasion by other pathogens. Paul Cheney,

M.D., one of the first investigators into chronic fatigue syndrome, theorizes that the disease is related to an intracellular dysfunction, in which the mitochondrion—the intricate energy factory located within each individual cell—is somehow disrupted and unable to produce energy sufficient to combat and destroy the free radicals circulating within the system. As a result, free radicals proliferate, destroying healthy cells and causing many of the symptoms of chronic fatigue syndrome.

Sudden onset of the disease is typical; approximately seventy-five percent of people with CFS claim they can pinpoint the exact moment when the crushing fatigue and chronic aches and pains began. No one is immune from this disease, which crosses all boundaries, races, cultures, and socioeconomic groups. The illness is not contagious.

Laboratory tests cannot diagnose chronic fatigue syndrome, although blood levels of certain viruses, especially Epstein-Barr, may be elevated. Laboratory tests used to rule out other chronic illnesses with similar symptoms include a complete blood count and profile, thyroid profile, tests for Lyme disease, stool test for parasites, and viral antibody tests. Although these tests often yield important information about the patient's general state of health, the symptoms outlined by the Centers for Disease Control remain the major diagnostic criteria for CFS.

Recovery is gradual; three of four patients report eighty to ninety percent improvement within two to five years. The disease takes its toll on the patient's emotional life, however: The divorce rate among CFS patients is seventy-five percent, and the suicide rate is six times the national average.

WESTERN TREATMENT

Chronic fatigue syndrome, like so many chronic immune disorders, is a disease of unknown origin that defies medical science's efforts to find a cure. Treatment generally consists of symptom relief. Drugs such as pain-killers, tranquilizers, antidepressants, and sleeping pills are commonly prescribed. Ritalin, a mild nervous system stimulant and antidepressant, may be prescribed to increase energy and elevate mood. While these drugs provide short-term relief from symptoms, they can also stress the liver and kidneys, providing an additional strain on an already overstressed system.

The antiviral drug acyclovir has been used to control the Epstein-Barr virus and other viruses that might contribute to the disease, but clinical trials with this drug have been disappointing.

Antacid drugs like Tagamet, Zantac, and Axid, which are traditionally used to block the production of stomach acid in the treatment of heartburn, hiatal hernias, or ulcers, also block the histamine receptors on the T-cells and act as immune system stimulants. Preliminary research with CFS patients appears promising, as these drugs seem to increase energy and stamina.

Doxepin, a standard antidepressant drug with antihistamine effects, has been used successfully to relieve insomnia and induce relaxation.

Kutapressin, a liver extract, seems to possess immune-supporting effects and may have antiviral properties as well; preliminary evidence indicates that it may relieve fatigue and promote endurance in CFS patients.

TRADITIONAL CHINESE INTERPRETATION

The Chinese consider chronic fatigue syndrome a deficiency disease—specifically, a deficiency of Spleen *chi* and Kidney *chi*. The Spleen is unable to derive the necessary energy from food, and the Kidneys are unable to generate the "fire" necessary to spark the life-force, which feeds our ambition, drive, and will power.

A long-term deficiency in *chi* and *wei chi* energy seems to be at the root of the problem. People with chronic fatigue syndrome are literally "burned out"—after years of running on the fast track, they suddenly run out of energy. The Chinese would explain it this way: When an individual is in the "Wood" mode, living under chronic stress, staying up late and not getting enough sleep, eating on the run, forgetting to exercise, and generally neglecting to take care of herself, the *chi* is gradually depleted, which in turn drains the *wei chi* and increases susceptibility to disease.

Such a diagnosis would never be considered an indictment of specific individuals, for most people who have this disease are blessed with abundant reserves of energy and previously handled the stress for years without ever getting sick. If the stress continues, however, the Liver will begin to feel the strain. The Liver supports digestive functioning by filtering impurities and waste products from the blood, and when the Liver is stressed, toxins build up and overwhelm the digestive system. Since Wood (Liver) energy is said to control Earth, symptoms such as poor digestion, bloating, and gas often appear, along with ulcers and irritable bowel syndrome. These gastric disorders eventually deplete Kidney and Spleen energies, leading to the symptoms of chronic fatigue syndrome.

Treatment is geared to supporting the Liver, Spleen, and Kidneys. Every patient is treated individually, depending on their constitutional type and the symptoms that create the most distress.

COMPLEMENTARY TREATMENTS

Diet

Food allergies and sensitivities are common in people with chronic fatigue syndrome. As with all chronic immune disorders, the first step should be to test for possible allergies, using blood tests or the Elimination Provocation Diet (see pages 105 to 107).

Whether or not you have food allergies, you will need to make changes in your diet in order to support the activities of your immune system. Choose foods that are loaded with nutrients. Unprocessed fruits and vegetables, whole grains, beans, nuts, and seeds should be the foundation of your new diet.

Avoid red meat and dairy products, which are extremely difficult to digest and use up vital energy that you need for healing. If you eat meat, eat only *organic* fish and chicken. Although it's common knowledge that chicken and beef are fed large quantities of antibiotics and steroids, few people realize that farm-reared fish, spawned in plastic trays and kept in pens or cages for their entire existence, receive antibiotics and other drugs in their food, a widespread practice that has already led to the spread of antibiotic-resistant fish diseases.

Choose "wild" fish over farm-reared fish whenever possible. For information on ordering "wild" fish, see the Resources section in Appendix I.

Limit or eliminate sugar, honey, corn syrup, and sugar substitutes—antinutrients that give the body nothing in return for the energy they require for digestion and processing. Sugar-rich foods and refined carbohydrate products (white breads, white pastas, flour products) burden the immune system and encourage the buildup of bacteria, which can lead to yeast infections and candidiasis. You should avoid fermented foods like soy sauce and vinegar because they contain yeast and can encourage yeast infections.

Avoid caffeine, another antinutrient that can stress the already overstimulated Liver and adrenal glands. Although it may seem that caffeine gives you energy, it actually drains precious energy from your already depleted system.

Avoid all trans-fatty acids and partially hydrogenated oils found in fried, greasy, and highly processed foods; these products release free radicals, unstable, highly reactive molecules that can attack cell membranes and tissue linings, causing irritation, inflammation, damage, and disease.

Be sure to *drink at least eight to ten 8-ounce glasses of fresh, filtered water each day,* to replenish essential body fluids and help the Liver and Kidneys to remove toxins from the blood.

Exercise

People with chronic fatigue syndrome tend to feel more debilitated and exhausted when they exercise; in fact, one of the criteria for diagnosing this disease is a crushing sense of fatigue that forces you to cut back on your activity. If you are experiencing severe fatigue, it would be best to avoid all forms of strenuous exercise; remember, *strenuous* is a relative term that for some might mean walking up and down the stairs twice a day or pushing a cart around the grocery store.

No matter how tired you feel, however, it is important to move around in order to keep the blood and *chi* from stagnating and worsening your condition. In the active stages of chronic fatigue syndrome, walking is your best bet. Begin by walking for five minutes twice a day. As you begin to feel better, gradually work up to twenty to thirty minutes daily. You might also enjoy yoga and tai chi exercises, which will open up the meridians to stimulate the flow of energy and blood and speed up the healing process.

Nutritional Supplements

Vitamin C: This powerful antioxidant and immune-supporter has antihistamine actions in higher doses. Antihistamine actions are extremely important in chronic fatigue syndrome, since seventy-five percent of CFS patients have elevated histamine levels with related symptoms of nasal congestion, itching, and digestive problems. Take 5,000–10,000 mg. (5–10 grams) daily. The best way to take vitamin C is in 1,000-mg. doses every two or three hours so that the body can use what it needs and excrete the rest. If you experience loose bowels or diarrhea, reduce the dosage until the symptoms disappear.

Beta-carotene: Beta-carotene, which is converted in the intestines into vitamin A, protects the body tissues from infections and free radical damage. Take 25,000 I.U. daily.

B-complex: The B vitamins function as coenzymes, assisting in numerous biochemical interactions and providing energy for every cell in the body. In addition to their energizing metabolic functions, the B-complex vitamins also improve nervous system functioning and help relieve fatigue, stress, anxiety, depression, and irritability. Take a B-100 complex vitamin daily.

Magnesium: Magnesium is an extremely important supplement for people with chronic fatigue syndrome. An intracellular nutrient, magnesium assists the mitochondria in their job of releasing energy for the cell, helping to restore normal energy levels. Used with great success to combat stress, anxiety, fatigue, muscle cramps and pains, nerve pains, and insomnia, magnesium also has a protective effect on the heart, stabilizing heart rhythms, regulating blood pressure, and preventing the formation of blood clots. Take 500–1,000 mg. daily.

Omega-3 fatty acids and gamma linoleic acid (GLA): These nutrients work to protect the cells and tissues of the body by reducing inflammation and supporting the immune system. You can purchase them separately (take 1,500 mg. GLA and 1,500 mg. omega-3) or combined in one formula (take 1,500 mg. *twice* daily).

Coenzyme Q-10 (ubiquinone): This supplement supports the digestion and stimulates the immune system; it is particularly important for CFS patients because it appears to work at the cellular level, helping the mitochondria manufacture energy; in fact, some researchers theorize that CFS is related to faulty mechanisms at the mitochondrial level of the cell. Take 20–30 mg. twice daily.

Pycnogenol (proanthocyanidan): This extremely powerful antioxidant (reputedly fifty times more powerful than vitamin E and twenty times more powerful than vitamin C) also functions as a natural antihistamine, relieving allergic reactions. To reach tissue saturation, take 10 mg. for each 10 pounds of body weight for the first ten days, then reduce the dosage to 50 mg. daily.

Chinese Patent Remedy
Bu Zhong Yi Qi Wan ("Support the Center, Benefit Energy Pills"): This gentle formula strengthens and supports the Spleen and Kidneys and specifically aids digestion and boosts energy levels. The Emperor herbs are ginseng and astragalus, both excellent immune- and energy-supporting herbs; attending herbs include dong quai to support the blood and improve circulation; atractylodes, citrus peel, ginger root, cimicifuga root, and jujube fruit, all of which support the digestive system to eliminate dampness in the system and ease feelings of fatigue and lethargy; bupleurum, a Liver tonic that breaks through obstructions and boosts energy; and licorice, "the Great Unifier," which helps all the other herbs work harmoniously together.

Take twelve pills twice daily.

This Chinese patent remedy can be safely combined with any of the following Western herbs. If you need help choosing the most effective formula or combination of herbs for your symptoms, consult an experienced herbalist.

Herbal Allies
For chronic fatigue syndrome three different categories of herbs help to relieve the symptoms and strengthen both the *wei chi* and the *chi*:

- herbs to boost energy and support immune function
- herbs to fight infection and viruses
- herbs to help the Liver and Kidneys cleanse the blood and eliminate toxins

Siberian ginseng (*Eleutherococcus senticosus*): This powerful energy tonic works wonders when your strength and stamina are faltering. Ginseng balances adrenal function, relieving many of the harmful effects of stress and tension. As the physical and emotional stress caused by chronic fatigue syndrome is intense, Siberian ginseng will build up your energy reserves and help you channel the stress so that it doesn't become overwhelming. Although we don't usually recommend ginseng for women because of its slight testosteronal qualities, when your energy level is low and convalescence is expected to take months or even years, ginseng is a wonderful restorative herb for both men and women.

Astragalus (*Astragalus membranaceous*): This Chinese herb is used primarily to support the immune system and promote energy. Recent studies confirm its ability to increase the production of interferon, a substance produced by the immune system's lymphocytes, macrophages, and T-cells in response to viruses and other intracellular microorganisms. Interferon protects your cells from invasion by viruses and bacteria by preventing these microorganisms from replicating. Particularly effective for what the Chinese call "wasting/exhausting" diseases (chronic immune disorders), astragalus has been shown to increase significantly the life expectancy of AIDS patients.

Licorice root (*Glycyrrhiza glabra*): A soothing and restorative herb, licorice has anti-inflammatory properties and supportive effects on the adrenal glands that help mitigate stress.

Goldenseal (*Hydrastis canadensis*): Goldenseal has powerful antimicrobial and antiviral actions and supports both the Liver and the immune system. Proven to be effective in the treatment of Epstein-Barr virus, goldenseal is a valuable ally in the treatment of chronic fatigue syndrome.

Echinacea (*Echinacea angustifolia* and *Echinacea purpura*): This powerful antibiotic, antiviral, antimicrobial, and antifungal agent has impressive immune-supporting actions. It is often combined with goldenseal for increased effectiveness.

Milk thistle (*Carduus marianus* or *Silybum marianum*): A superb Liver tonic, milk thistle contains a constituent called silymarin, which increases the flow of bile, helping the Liver metabolize and eliminate numerous toxins.

Wild indigo (*Baptisia tinctoria*): Another powerful antimicrobial herb, wild indigo is extremely valuable when fighting viral and bacterial infections. Especially effective in treating infections of the ear, nose, throat, and lymph glands, wild indigo reduces the inflammation often associated with infections and acts as a "lymphatic cleanser," assisting the lymph system in its job of removing debris.

Dosage: If you purchase your herbs in a health food store (either in tincture form or, as dried herbs, in capsule or pill form), follow the dosage instructions on the label. Because herbs in dried form tend to lose their potency rather quickly, be sure to check the label for the expiration date.

For information on preparing your own herbs from the root, bark, leaves, flowers, or seeds of a plant, see Appendix II.

In Appendix I, Resources, we offer a list of mail-order sources for high-quality herbs and herbal preparations. For advice on ordering specially made herbal formulas, see pages 394 to 396.

Acupoints

Kidney 7 ("Recover Flow"): This point is used to fortify and intensify the energy flowing in and through the Kidneys. Particularly useful for deficient *chi* and *yang* conditions, it helps to spark the energy systems within the body; its most important target is the immune system.

Location: Kidney 7 is located between the Achilles tendon and the leg bone, approximately two inches above Kidney 3, in a natural depression that is often tender to the touch.

Conception Vessel 6 ("Sea of Energy"): This point is often used to strengthen the Kidneys and ignite Kidney *chi* energy. Whenever the body's "spark" is low or flickering, this point will add "fire" to the system, boosting sexual energy, supporting digestion, promoting healthy bowel movements, and warming the body from the inside out. *Note:* When fires are flaring up and inflammation is widespread, it's best to avoid using this point.

Location: Conception Vessel 6 is located on the midline of the lower belly, about two inches below the belly button. Massage it with the thumb or fingers in small circular movements.

Lung 9 ("Great Abyss"): This is a powerful immune-enhancing acupoint that helps to build and support the *wei chi,* circulate *chi* and blood, and break through blockages. Stimulating this point will give you the energy you need to break through the stagnation that characterizes chronic fatigue syndrome.

Location: Lung 9 is located on the transverse crease of the wrist, approximately half an inch in from the thumb side. Massage it with your thumb or fingers in slow, circular, clockwise motions.

Questions to Ask Yourself

Chronic fatigue syndrome often involves imbalances in Wood (Liver) and Water (Kidney) energy. When you work too hard, exercise too strenuously or not enough, get insufficient sleep, eat greasy or fatty foods, and rely on artificial stimulants like coffee, alcohol, or nicotine, you stress your Liver and deplete your vital energy. Over time the Liver *yin* (fluid) energy is drained, and friction begins to build up in the system, further draining the body's Water reserves and putting the entire system in danger of overheating.

Questions relating to Wood and Water imbalances may help you understand the nature and scope of your disease:

- I've been living in the fast lane for years, but now my energy is scattered and diffuse: How does my disease allow me to slow down and pay attention to myself?
- Was I trapped by my former lifestyle? Is my illness a way of breaking out of my imprisonment and searching for an entirely new way of life?
- What can I do to keep myself more focused and in touch with my basic needs?
- How has my disease served me? How has it injured me?
- I feel too tired to control anything in my life—how can I use this sense of disease and learn to let go and lose control?
- If I can't take care of myself, how can I let others take care of me? How do I learn to ask for help, friendship, love?

Perhaps the most common symptom associated with CFS is the sense of being "sick and tired." Use the following questions to understand the nature of your distress and what your disease is trying to communicate to you.

- What makes me feel sick and tired? What do I want to change in my life?
- How can I bring more joy and enthusiasm into my life? At what point in my life was I filled with joy? How can I re-create those feelings now?
- How do my symptoms help me pay attention to myself and my needs?
- What do my symptoms prevent me from doing, accomplishing, or being?

As you meditate on these questions, make a list of the steps you can take to overcome your feelings of being trapped and out of touch. Ask yourself: "What can I do to get what I really want—and deserve—from life?"

A STARTING POINT

Picking and choosing among the many and diverse remedies recommended for CFS may seem like an overwhelming task. Where should you begin?

The following supplements, herbal remedies, and healing strategies will give you a solid foundation that you can then build upon. Use the other remedies suggested in this section when and if you need additional support.

1. *Diet:* Follow the dietary suggestions on pages 317 to 318.
2. *Exercise:* Exercise for twenty to thirty minutes every day.
3. *Nutritional supplements:* Take the general formula for Maximum Immunity; increase the vitamin C dosage to at least 5,000 mg. daily.
4. *Coenzyme Q-10:* Take 20–30 mg. twice daily.
5. *Pycnogenol:* Take 50 mg. daily.
6. *Bu Zhong Yi Qi Wan:* Take twelve pills twice daily.
7. *Western herbal formula:* Take equal amounts of astragalus, Siberian ginseng, echinacea, licorice, and goldenseal.

Type II Diabetes (Adult Onset Diabetes Mellitus)

"I hate needles," fifty-six-year-old Evan told me, "but if your acupuncture needles can help me avoid insulin shots, I'm willing to give them a try." Recently diagnosed with adult-onset diabetes, Evan was under a great deal of stress. His job, to which he had devoted himself for more than twenty years, was in jeopardy; the company was undergoing a major reorganization, and every month new layoffs were announced. Hoping to prove that he was indispensable, Evan arrived at work at six A.M. and left every evening at eight or nine. He wasn't getting enough sleep or exercise, he was always eating on the run or snacking on M&M's and coffee ("my favorite foods"), and his relationship with his wife and three children was deteriorating as his stress level continued to rise.

A classic Earth type, Evan loved sweets and found it extremely difficult to control his cravings. Chronic headaches, a yellow-green tinge around his mouth, a subtle sweet smell to his perspiration, and a tendency to worry and fret over minor setbacks confirmed an imbalance in Earth energies.

The first and most important treatment strategy involved Evan's diet. He agreed to go through his kitchen cabinets and remove all processed and refined foods, switching to whole-grain pastas, breads, and cereals, and increasing his intake of fresh vegetables and fruits. He also agreed that it was counterproductive to spend so much time worrying about his job. Reassuring himself that he was experienced, intelligent, and highly capable, he realized that even if he lost his job, he could find another one; and if he couldn't find another job, early retirement was a distinct possibility. "I have a great pension plan, and I'd love to spend more time with my wife and children," he said. "I've definitely got options."

Dietary changes, weekly acupuncture sessions, nutritional supplements, and an herbal formula of goat's rue, devil's club, and dandelion root helped to stabilize Evan's blood sugar. Two years later, with his job still intact, he claims that he's a changed man. "I've got a disease that I can control," he said. "I consider myself a lucky man."

WESTERN INTERPRETATION

Diabetes is a disease of carbohydrate metabolism in which the normal insulin mechanisms malfunction and the cells are unable to oxidize and utilize carbohydrates. Carbohydrates are an important and immediate source of energy for the body; as unused carbohydrates accumulate, the diabetic begins to feel weak and drained of energy. No matter how much food diabetics consume, they are improperly nourished because their bodies are unable to use the energy circulating in the blood.

The reasons for the malfunction are extremely complex, but an automobile metaphor may help you understand the basic problem. Insulin is the "spark" delivered by the distributor (the pancreas) that ignites a series of chemical and electrical reactions, which allow the gas (blood sugar or glucose) to be utilized by the cylinders (the cells) so that the car can run smoothly and efficiently. If the spark (insulin) is too weak or too strong, the car sputters and eventually stalls out.

Diabetes is sometimes described as a disease of three excesses: excess thirst, excess appetite, and excess urination. In addition to the three excesses, the symptoms include elevated blood sugar, sugar in the urine, and general weakness and fatigue. Because bacteria and other microorganisms thrive on sugar, the excess sugar in the blood provides a fertile breeding ground for infection. Deprived of their essential carbohydrate energy, the body's macrophages and white blood cells have a harder time fighting infection, and relatively minor infections can rage out of control, leading to dangerous complications such as ulcers and gangrene.

Without the energy available from carbohydrates to aid in metabolism, proteins and fats accumulate in the blood and can eventually damage the blood vessels by slowing down circulation, which can cause heart and kidney problems and lead to vision dysfunctions, nervous system problems, and permanent organ damage. Circulatory problems also increase the risk of infection.

When the liver works overtime to create its own sugar for the body to use as energy, fats and proteins are broken down from the body's muscles and nerves, leading to muscle wasting and additional nervous system dysfunctions. The sugars released by the body as it breaks down its own tissues are called ketones, and they are a poor substitute for the energy-rich carbohydrate sugars. General metabolic problems lead to improper fat metabolism, which can cause atherosclerosis, or hardening of the arteries—which, in turn, contributes to poor circulation in the lower extremities.

There are two distinct forms of diabetes mellitus: juvenile-onset (Type I) diabetes and adult-onset (Type II) diabetes. In Type I diabetes the insulin-producing cells in the pancreas aren't working to produce insulin, while in Type II diabetes the body's cells become insensitive to insulin. Five percent of diabetics have juvenile onset diabetes, which is treated by insulin injections and continual monitoring of blood sugar levels. Type II diabetes, which affects ninety-five percent of diabetics, is responsive to dietary changes and various drug therapies.

The seventh leading cause of death in the United States, adult-onset diabetes can develop in anyone, although the following groups are most susceptible: people who are obese (over forty percent of diabetics have a history of obesity); people over forty years of age; women; and individuals with a family history of diabetes.

Diagnostic tests for diabetes include urinalysis for sugar in the urine and blood tests such as the fasting blood sugar test or the glucose tolerance test, which show the body's ability to utilize carbohydrates.

WESTERN TREATMENT

When you are diagnosed with Type II (adult-onset) diabetes, your doctor will suggest that you make a drastic reduction in your sugar intake. If you are overweight, you will be asked to go on a strict weight-loss diet. For most people these two strategies—restricting sugar and losing weight—are sufficient to stabilize the blood sugar.

If the blood sugar cannot be controlled with diet, the next treatment strategy is oral hypoglycemic agents, or drugs that lower blood sugar levels. For the most part these are sulfa drugs (Diabinese, Glucotrol, Micronase, Orinase) that stimulate the pancreas to produce more insulin and assist the cells in utilizing the sugar available to them. Unfortunately, these drugs work to control blood sugar levels in only sixty percent of patients; furthermore, they lose their effectiveness over time, and they can cause hypoglycemic reactions. Other relatively rare side effects include allergic skin reactions, headaches, indigestion, and fatigue.

If sulfa drugs are unable to control your blood sugar levels, your physician may suggest insulin injections and a home monitoring device to help you regulate and control your insulin levels. While insulin therapy often works to stabilize blood sugar levels, the diabetic eventually becomes dependent on taking synthetic insulin because the pancreas, which is no longer required to produce insulin, stops working and may begin to atrophy. Blood sugar fluctuations are common in insulin-dependent diabetics and create additional stress on cells, tissues, and organs.

Diabetes causes many serious, even life-threatening complications, including increased susceptibility to infection, nerve disorders (tingling sensations, numbness or pain, loss of nerve function, muscle weakness), diabetic foot ulcers, retinal problems (diabetes is the leading cause of blindness in the United States), kidney problems, and atherosclerosis (buildup of plaque on the artery walls).

TRADITIONAL CHINESE INTERPRETATION

The Chinese call diabetes "the great wasting and thirsting disease," a name that vividly portrays the excessive thirst, hunger, and urination associated with this illness, as well as the wasting away of the cells and tissues because the body cannot effectively utilize carbohydrate energy.

According to traditional Chinese medicine, diabetes is caused by eating too many sweet and/or fatty foods, which deplete the Earth energies (Spleen/ Pancreas) and interfere with digestive processes. As more sweets and fats are consumed, Earth is forced to work even harder, which generates heat in the system. As heat accumulates, the body draws on its water (*yin*) reserves to extinguish the smoke and fire; over time, the *yin* is seriously depleted. Because *yin* originates in the Kidneys, diabetes is considered a Kidney *yin* deficiency disease as well as a deficient Earth disease.

Deficient Kidney *yin* affects the ability of the Triple Heater—the only organ within the Chinese classification system that is solely functional and has no structural counterpart—to "mist" the body with life-giving water and to provide the power needed to circulate the blood and *chi*. When the Triple Heater malfunctions, circulation falters, digestion breaks down, and both the bladder and bowels are affected. In the upper heater (called the Misting), deficient *yin* creates the first wasting—great thirst—because the depletion of the body's Water supply triggers the desire for replacement fluids, which is experienced as thirst. As the body's fluid supplies continue to decrease, the *chi* (vital energy) diminishes, for *chi* depends on a sufficient *yin* supply in order to function properly. In the middle heater (called the Factory), deficient *chi* levels create a craving for food (excessive hunger) to replenish the dwindling energy supply. The third wasting occurs in the lower heater (the Swamp), where the deficient *chi* is unable to hold the urine in its place, causing excessive urination.

Treatment strategies vary depending on the individual's constitutional type (Wood, Fire, Earth, Metal, or Water), general state of health, lifestyle choices, emotional balance, and spiritual yearnings. In all cases, however, the Spleen/ Pancreas *chi,* Kidney *chi,* and Kidney *yin* will need support and nourishment. As the *yin* begins to build up, it will naturally resolve many of the false Fire signs and symptoms associated with diabetes; herbs and acupuncture treatments will also help to drain the excess heat from the Misting, the Factory, or the Swamp.

COMPLEMENTARY TREATMENTS

Although the following complementary treatments are specifically recommended for adult-onset (Type II) diabetes, Type I diabetics can also benefit enormously from them. With dietary changes, daily exercise, nutritional supplements, herbal remedies, and acupuncture, many Type I diabetics can significantly lower the amount of insulin they use on a daily basis and at the same time protect themselves against many of the complications associated with the disease.

Diet

Blood sugar disorders like diabetes (hyperglycemia) and hypoglycemia (low blood sugar) are increasing at an alarming rate, and many researchers believe the Western diet—high in refined carbohydrates, sugar, fat, and animal products, and low in fiber, fresh fruits and vegetables, and whole grains—is responsible. People whose diets include hefty amounts of fat and sugar (the typical "Western-style diet") are five to ten times more likely to be diabetic than those who restrict fats and refined sugars and consume sufficient complex carbohydrates in the form of vegetables, fruits, and whole grains.

The average American consumes 32 teaspoons of sugar every day, or 125 pounds of sugar in one year. "Mainlined" sugar sets off an alarm system in the pancreas, which releases insulin in an attempt to remove the excess sugar from the blood and make it available to the cells. When insulin is pumped into the bloodstream, it distributes blood sugar to the cells and eliminates any surpluses, leading to a precipitous drop in blood sugar levels, which in turn creates a hypoglycemic or low blood sugar reaction. Hypoglycemia leads to a craving for sweets (the body's way of asking you to put more sugar in the blood), irritability, and fatigue. Because sugar is critical to normal brain function, low blood sugar can also lead to cognitive and emotional problems ranging from headaches to blurred vision, foggy thinking, memory deficits, depression, irritability, and mood swings.

When your body cries out for more sugar to alleviate these distressing symptoms, you will probably reach for sugar-saturated foods like cookies, candies, or pastries. After eating these foods, your blood sugar will rise steeply, and for an hour or so you'll feel better. Soon enough, however, the pancreas releases extra insulin, the blood sugar drops like a rock, and you're back where you started.

This could go on forever (with your emotions fluctuating along with your blood sugar), except at some point you may develop insulin resistance, a condition in which your cells close their doors to insulin, which leads to rising blood levels of both glucose and insulin. The overworked pancreas releases more insulin in response to the elevated blood sugar levels, which can trigger diabetes.

Diet is the major cause of adult-onset (Type II) diabetes; it can also be the primary healing agent. To prevent and/or cure diabetes, follow these dietary strategies:

STEP 1: The first and most important rule in the prevention and treatment of Type II diabetes is: *Stop eating sugar and refined carbohydrate products.* To satisfy your body's need for carbohydrate fuel, eat plenty of fresh fruits and vegetables and increase your intake of complex carbohydrates (rice, whole wheat, oatmeal, whole-grain breads and pastas, and potatoes). If you have a weight problem, try to get most of your carbohydrates from fruits and vegetables.

Refined Carbohydrate Products
- White bread and rolls
- Doughnuts
- Cakes
- Pastries
- Candy
- Soft drinks
- Pasta (except whole grain)
- Italian and French breads
- Bagels (except whole grain)
- Most breakfast cereals

STEP 2: *Reduce harmful fats in your diet.* Here's a quick rundown on ways to reduce the "bad" fats and increase the "good" fats in your daily diet.

Reduce the "Bad" Fats
- Eliminate red meat from your diet.
- Remove the skin from chicken and turkey (and buy organic—nonchemically treated—varieties whenever possible).

- Drastically reduce or eliminate dairy products (milk, cream, cheese, butter, ice cream, yogurt); when you use dairy products, use nonfat varieties.
- Avoid all "partially hydrogenated" products, which include margarine, solid vegetable shortening, fried fast foods, cookies, cakes, frostings, pies, pastries, crackers, frozen french fries, and packaged microwave popcorn.
- Avoid polyunsaturated oils (safflower, walnut, sunflower, sesame, corn, soybean, and cottonseed) in cooking; these oils become chemically unstable when heated.

Increase the "Good" Fats

- Use monounsaturated oils (olive, canola, peanut, avocado, flaxseed) in salads and for all cooking needs; extra-virgin, cold-pressed olive oil is the best choice.
- Eat fatty fish (salmon, sardines, herring, mackerel, bluefish, and albacore tuna) three times a week.
- If you are allergic to fish or simply don't like the taste, take omega-3 and/or gamma linoleic acid (GLA) supplements, available in most health food stores; follow the directions on the product label.

STEP 3: *Increase the fiber in your diet.* Fiber tends to bulk up in the intestine, making the elimination of waste products more efficient. Glucose molecules also latch on to the fibrous material, allowing a gradual release of sugar into the bloodstream and reducing the risk of a sugar overload, which can trigger a diabetic attack.

STEP 4: *Avoid overeating.* Overeating stimulates excess insulin production, which initiates the series of actions and reactions that can lead to adult-onset diabetes. If you need help in your efforts to lose weight and avoid sugar-rich foods, ask your health care practitioner for advice on sensible diet and exercise regimens.

STEP 5: *Drink eight to ten 8-ounce glasses of fresh, filtered water every day.* Diabetes is considered a serious *yin* deficiency condition, characterized by excessive dryness and thirst. Sufficient water in the system helps the Liver and Kidneys work more efficiently and assists the bowels in their efforts to eliminate waste products. Water is also a natural appetite suppressant.

Some Final Suggestions

+ Onions and garlic contain sulfur compounds and can help reduce your blood sugar levels; add them to anything and everything.
+ Avoid alcohol, caffeine, and all recreational drugs, which drain the energy from your Liver, Kidneys, and Spleen/Pancreas at a time when they desperately need support.

Exercise

Diabetics tend to be overweight, and overweight people are less likely to exercise regularly. If you incorporate exercise into your weight-loss program, you'll lose weight faster and feel better doing it.

Most diabetics have an affinity to Earth or Water. Earth types tend to enjoy slow, easy, nonjarring exercises like swimming, yoga, light aerobics, and tai chi. Exercises that feature a rhythmic flow and graceful, supple movements are important to Water types: Water sports, cross-country or downhill skiing, brisk walks, bicycle rides, and workouts on home fitness machines typically appeal to Water. The gentle stretching nature of yoga and tai chi exercises are also supportive to Water energy.

As a general rule, Water types enjoy exercising alone, while Earth types like to have company when they exercise.

Exercise for twenty or thirty minutes every day.

Nutritional Supplements

Guar gum: This plant fiber is extremely useful in the prevention and/or treatment of diabetes and hypoglycemia. Glucose molecules latch on to the fibers, causing sugar to be released slowly into the bloodstream, which reduces stress on the pancreas. The dietary fiber in fruits and vegetables helps stabilize glucose levels, but few of us eat enough fresh produce to affect significantly the blood sugar. Guar gum supplements are therefore an important addition to our daily fiber intake.

Take one or two capsules before each meal, or follow the directions on the product label. Be sure to drink lots of fresh, filtered water to help the fiber bulk move swiftly and efficiently through the digestive tract.

Chromium: Chromium stabilizes blood sugar levels, improves glucose tolerance, lowers insulin levels, decreases low-density lipoproteins ("bad" cholesterol) and increases high-density lipoproteins ("good" cholesterol). Chromium increases the efficiency of insulin so you need less insulin to deliver the blood sugar to the cells; if you are deficient in chromium, your pancreas may compensate by producing more insulin.

Chromium is available in the following forms: chromium chloride, chromium polynicotinate, chromium picolinate, or chromium-enriched brewer's yeast (which is also chock full of B vitamins). Take 200 mcg. daily if you are prone to diabetes and want to prevent the disease; take 200–400 mcg. *twice* daily (400–800 mcg. total) if you have been diagnosed with diabetes.

Vanadium: Vanadium, like chromium, works to regulate the blood sugar and lower elevated blood sugar levels; it also helps to lower cholesterol levels and may be helpful in treating atherosclerosis and heart disease. Take 7.5–15 mg. *with* chromium.

Vitamin C: This is an essential supplement in diabetes, because insulin is needed to help the cells absorb the vitamin; when insulin levels are low, there is a greater likelihood of a vitamin C deficiency. Vitamin C's strong immune-stimulating and antioxidant actions also help strengthen the body's resistance to disease. Take 2,000–4,000 mg. (2–4 grams) daily.

Vitamin E: Vitamin E protects the cell linings from free radical damage (common in diabetes) and reduces nerve cell damage, which diabetes often causes. Vitamin E is also a wonderful preventive supplement for hypoglycemia and diabetes. Take 400–800 I.U. daily.

Selenium: Selenium works synergistically with vitamin E to enhance its immune-supporting, antioxidant effects. Take 200 mcg. daily with vitamin E.

B-complex vitamins: These vitamins help to prevent and treat diseases and disorders of the nerves (neuropathies) and retina (retinopathies), both very common in diabetes. The B vitamins also reduce the negative impact of stress on all body systems. Many of the individual B vitamins such as niacin, niacinamide, biotin, B_6, and folic acid are used to prevent and treat various diabetic symptoms. Take a B-100 complex daily.

Zinc: Zinc plays a role in preventing diabetes, as it improves glucose tolerance and supports immune function; people with a zinc deficiency are more likely to have diabetes. Take 30–50 mg. daily.

Chinese Patent Remedies

Yeuchung Pills ("Jade Spring Pills"): This extremely effective formula is designed to treat Type II diabetes, or what the Chinese used to call "sugar urine disease." Formulated to nurture and support the *yin* essence, especially the *yin* of the Kidney, Spleen/Pancreas, and Lung, the five herbs in this formula (rehmannia root, pueraria root, trichosanthes root, licorice, and schisandra fruit) work to subdue the Heat and reduce dampness and phlegm. It is available in either powder or pill form. In powder form, take one capful four times daily; in pill form, take one vial four times daily.

Liu Wei Di Huang Wan ("Six Flavor Rehmannia Pills"): This formula contains six gentle, supportive herbs to strengthen the *yin* and support Kidney and Spleen energies. Rehmannia, the archetypal herb to support the body's *yin* essence, reigns as Emperor; attending herbs include cornus fruit, dioscorea root, moutan bark, poria fungus, and alisma root. Used for diabetes and other *yin*-deficient conditions that involve dry skin, dry mucous membranes, excess urination, and muscle wasting, this formula can be taken for long periods of time to treat such symptoms as restlessness, chronic low back pain, dizziness, and ringing in the ears. Take eight pellets three times daily or twelve pellets twice daily.

These Chinese patent remedies are gentle and can be safely combined with any of the following Western herbs. If you need help choosing the most effective formula or combination of herbs for your symptoms, consult an experienced herbalist.

Herbal Allies

The following herbs can be used alone or combined in a single formula. Popular formulas available at health food stores offer different combinations of these herbs, or you can contact a qualified herbalist, who will mix up a formula tailored to your specific needs.

Goat's rue (*Galega officinalis*): Goat's rue has been used in Europe to treat diabetes for centuries. One of the herb's main constituents, galegine, acts as a hypoglycemic agent, helping to balance blood sugar levels and assisting the cells in metabolizing and assimilating fats and proteins.

Devil's club (*Oplopanax horridum*): Devil's club is the premier herb for balancing blood sugar levels. Considered part of the ginseng family, it grows abundantly in the Pacific Northwest and is sometimes called armored ginseng or northwest ginseng. A soothing digestive tonic and metabolic stimulant, devil's club also seems to help people lose weight, an added bonus for diabetics.

Dandelion root (*Taraxacum officinalis*): This gentle but powerful liver tonic helps the body eliminate toxic overloads. An excellent digestive bitter tonic, dandelion also supports the digestion and assimilation of food and drink, and it strengthens the pancreas as well.

Ginkgo (*Ginkgo biloba*): Ginkgo is one of the oldest recorded plant medicines. It has been used successfully for centuries to treat a wide range of diseases and symptoms, including memory loss, dizziness, ringing in the ears, headaches, visual problems, and cold hands and feet, as well as many emotional and psychological problems, particularly depression. Modern scientific research now offers convincing support for ancient claims about this herb.

An extremely effective circulatory stimulant, ginkgo specifically targets the peripheral areas of the head, eyes, brain, hands, and feet—the areas most directly affected by circulatory problems in diabetes. Recent studies suggest that ginkgo may help protect against diabetic retinopathy—deterioration of the retina that can lead to blindness.

Dosage: If you purchase your herbs in a health food store (either in tincture form or, as dried herbs, in capsule or pill form), follow the dosage instructions on the label. Because herbs in dried form tend to lose their potency rather quickly, be sure to check the label for the expiration date.

For information on preparing your own herbs from the root, bark, leaves, flowers, or seeds of a plant, see Appendix II.

In Appendix I, Resources, we offer a list of mail-order sources for high-quality herbs and herbal preparations. For advice on ordering specially made herbal formulas, see pages 394 to 396.

Acupoints

Spleen 3 ("Great Brightness"): This is the "master point" of the Spleen meridian, meaning that it provides strong support for Earth energies and the organs associated with Earth (Spleen/Pancreas and Stomach). Since Earth is considered the mother of Metal (Lung energies), this strong supportive point benefits the Lungs and generally supports immune *(wei chi)* functions; in diabetes, however, its most important function is to help the digestive system operate efficiently and effectively.

Location: Spleen 3 is located on the inner part of the foot, along the arch in the depression on the side of the big toe. Gently massage with your fingers in a circular, clockwise motion.

Spleen 6 ("Three Yin Meeting"): This is one of the most important acupoints for supporting the *yin* energy of the body, mind, and spirit. In diabetes, it is said, for every glass of water you drink, you urinate two glasses' worth; by stimulating this point, you will help to replace this vital, life-giving water. Spleen 6 also supports the Spleen and Stomach energies, promoting healthy digestion and the proper assimilation of nutrients.

Location: Spleen 6 is located approximately three inches above the interior ankle bone, in a depression next to the tibia. Gently massage with your fingers in a circular, clockwise motion.

Conception Vessel 12 ("Sea of Nutritive Energy"): This point helps to balance Earth energies, specifically the energy of the Spleen/Pancreas and Stomach. Assisting the digestive system in its metabolism of *chi* and blood, it makes sure to route properly the leftover "sludge" to the intestines for elimination. If you suffer from chronic sugar cravings, fatigue, or general feelings of sluggishness, stimulating this point will help support the pancreas and digestive system to resolve these problems, which are common in diabetics.

Location: Conception Vessel 12 is located on the midline of the stomach, approximately two inches below the lower end of the breastbone or about four inches above the belly button. Gently massage it with your fingers in a clockwise, circular motion.

Questions to Ask Yourself

Because diabetes is fairly common among Earth types and is considered an Earth-deficient disease, the following questions may help you understand the widespread impact of an Earth imbalance:

- How do I take nourishment away from myself in order to nourish those around me?
- What can I do to take care of myself?
- Why do I have difficulty asking for what I need or want?
- What would happen if my wishes were fulfilled?
- How do I use food to fulfill my emotional needs?
- What does food insulate and protect me from? What do I need to be protected from?
- What's eating me up inside?

While Earth imbalances are often connected with diabetes, many of the physical symptoms of this disease relate to a deficiency in Water—achy or weak lower back, cold hands and feet, tendency to edema (water retention), fear, phobias, fatigue, lack of will, and loss of motivation. The Chinese believe that Water's tendency to get caught up in excessive brooding or reflection weakens the functions of the Spleen, which in turn increases the body's vulnerability to diabetic or hypoglycemic reactions.

To help you understand better the underlying Water (Kidney) imbalances, ask yourself these questions:

- How do my fears—of rejection, humiliation, pain, and death—prevent me from making myself heard?
- How can I learn to stand up for myself and my beliefs?
- What can I do to restore my motivation and will to live?
- How can I accept my mortality without living in fear of it?

A STARTING POINT

Picking and choosing among the many and diverse remedies recommended for adult-onset (Type II) diabetes may seem like an overwhelming task. Where should you begin?

The following supplements, herbal remedies, and healing strategies will give you a solid foundation that you can then build upon. Use the other remedies suggested in this section when and if you need additional support.

1. *Diet:* Follow the dietary suggestions on pages 329 to 332.
2. *Exercise:* Exercise for twenty to thirty minutes every day.
3. *Nutritional supplements:* Take the general formula for Maximum Immunity.
4. *Chromium:* Take 200–400 mcg. twice daily.
5. *Vanadium:* Take 7.5–15 mg. daily.
6. *Guar gum:* Take one or two capsules before each meal, followed by a full glass of water.
7. *Western herbal remedy:* Take equal amounts of goat's rue, devil's club, dandelion root, and ginkgo.

11. LEVEL FOUR: THE ORGANS

Darkness within darkness.
The gateway to all understanding.

—*Tao Te Ching*

At the *wei chi* and *chi* levels, the symptoms of chronic illness tend to be *yang* in nature, with acute flare-ups, high fevers, and severe, throbbing pain. As disease penetrates deeper into the body's kingdom, infiltrating the blood and threatening the organs themselves, the symptoms become more *yin*—long-lasting, deep-rooted, ever-present. Over time, energy drains from the system, gradually depleting the body's vital reserves, and deeply affecting the mind and spirit.

"When the pathogen travels from the yang [exterior] level to the yin [interior], the symptoms will quiet down and the patient will become more withdrawn," observed Huang Di, the Yellow Emperor. Anyone who has lived for months or years with a serious debilitating illness knows the truth of this statement. As the disease penetrates deeper into the tissues and organs, it seems to burrow into the soul itself, and you find that all your attention is drawn inward, toward the sickness at the center.

To understand the depth and breadth of disease at this level, we need to spend a moment discussing the Chinese concept of *zang* and *fu* organs. Traditional Chinese medicine views organs as centers or zones of activity rather than strict anatomical structures, and it separates them into *yin (zang)* and *yang (fu)* orbs. The Heart, Liver, Spleen, Lungs, and Kidneys are the five solid *zang* organs that store and preserve the precious *chi* and blood and oversee the innermost work-ings of the body. In *The Yellow Emperor's Classic* the *zang* organs are said to be "full but never filled" because the *chi* and blood are constantly circulating as each or-gan nourishes and supports the other organs with vital energy.

The Stomach, Small Intestine, Large Intestine, Bladder, Gallbladder, and Triple Heater are the six hollow *fu* organs responsible for processing foods and fluids, eliminating the "impure" particles, and transporting the "pure" ele-ments to the vital organs, where they are refined into *chi* and blood. Because the *fu* organs are constantly eliminating and transporting materials, taking them in and then letting them pass through, they are said to be "filled but never full."

The *zang* organs are most immediately and powerfully affected by chronic im-mune disorders because they are responsible for creating and transforming blood, *chi,* and *wei chi,* which are essential to all life processes. When disease pen-etrates deep into the body's kingdom, it settles in the *zang* organs and disrupts their vital functions, threatening life itself.

Each of the *zang* organs is also associated with a spiritual (nonmaterial) qual-ity or essence, which is considered critical to the patient's health and well-being. The Yellow Emperor described the spiritual manifestations of the *zang* organs as follows:

> The spirit of the heart is known as the shen, which rules mental and creative functions. The spirit of the liver, the hun, rules the nervous system and gives rise to extrasensory perception [intuition]. The spirit of the spleen, of yi, rules logic or reasoning power. The spirit of the lungs, or po, rules the animalistic instincts, physical strength and stamina. The spirit of the kidneys, the zhi, rules the will, drive, ambition, and survival instinct.

The disturbance of a *zang* organ by illness will have a powerful impact on the patient's spirits. Thinking processes may become jumbled and confused, creative energies drain away, ambition falters, perceptions are distorted, and the will to live gradually dissipates. When it becomes clear that the disease is chronic and perhaps even incurable, the patient may feel overwhelmed by anger, grief, fear, and panic. These emotions contribute to the wear and tear on the body, mind, and spirit, further overburdening the immune system and obstructing the healing process.

If your spirit and will to live are strong, you will significantly increase your chances of halting and even reversing the disease process. Only when hope dies and the will to live weakens is the condition considered life-threatening. "When there is spirit, the prognosis is positive," counseled Qi Bo. "When the spirit is gone, the condition is very grave."

In this final chapter we focus on the two most dreaded diseases of modern times: cancer and AIDS. Both diseases represent a massive assault on the immune system, in which a pathogen overpowers the *wei chi,* disrupts the smooth flow of *chi,* and disturbs the blood. In both cancer and AIDS the disease penetrates deep into the system, eventually threatening the vital organs—the elite royal guards at the center of our very being. Although the situation is serious, it is not irreversible, for the organs have astonishing powers of regeneration and renewal.

In traditional Chinese medicine, cancer and AIDS are viewed as external manifestations of a progressive breakdown in the body's defenses. Either the pathogen is so virulent that even a vigorous immune system cannot repel it, or the immune system is so weakened by neglect and improper lifestyle choices that the pathogen meets with little resistance. While the Chinese always emphasize the patient's responsibility in preventing serious illness through diet, exercise, meditative techniques, and harmonious relationships, harsh words are leveled at "inept and careless" physicians who allow illness to progress to the point where it threatens the vital organs. "A physician who is incompetent in medical skills fails to stem the patient's disease from deteriorating," admonished Qi Bo. "Consequently, when the condition becomes grave, the physician gives a prognosis of death or incurable when the disease actually could have been reversed earlier. This behavior is completely intolerable."

No matter how lethal the pathogen or how diminished the forces of the immune system, as long as the mind is focused and the spirit is strong, there is reason for hope. At this stage of illness, the physician's major responsibility is clear: to "guide the patient's mind and moods in a positive way," as Huang Di phrased it, by giving the patient the confidence he or she needs to conquer illness and remain focused on the task at hand. So many people afflicted with a chronic, "incurable" illness feel betrayed by their body's inadequacies and imprisoned by its defects, perceiving their disease as an external manifestation of internal weakness and failure. When the mind labels the body "invalid," the body hears the message, and responds accordingly. In both human and animal studies, feelings of helplessness and loss of control have a profoundly negative impact on the body's ability to resist and recover from disease. If you believe that your illness somehow invalidates your existence, you give it the opportunity to do just that, for what you cannot challenge in your mind, you cannot hope to defeat in your body.

Finding reason for hope may be your greatest challenge, for Western medicine tends to take a somewhat fatalistic attitude toward disease at this level. While physicians aggressively treat the symptoms and while patients struggle valiantly to maintain their strength and composure, an overall sense of futility accompanies the diagnosis of AIDS and many types of cancer. In fact, many Western doctors believe that offering hope to patients with serious, potentially terminal illnesses is a cruel subterfuge and elect instead to give their patients an honest assessment of the odds against them. In his book *Healing Words,* Dr. Larry Dossey tells about a letter he received from a woman with AIDS whose doctor told her the disease was "uniformly fatal." These words seemed to cut through her, slashing deep into her heart and soul. "Why do I feel like my own physician is *killing* me?" she asked.

This woman's anguish is mirrored in another patient's experiences, witnessed by Dr. Bernard Lown in his introduction to Norman Cousins's book *The Healing Heart.* As Dr. Lown recounts, a middle-aged woman with congestive heart failure had survived for more than a decade with her disease, continuing her work as a librarian, raising her children, and staying active in her community. Every week she visited the cardiac outpatient clinic where she received her weekly medications and talked to her doctor, a professor of cardiology at Harvard Medical School, who had followed her through the course of her illness. On this particular occasion, her doctor arrived with a group of attending physicians, greeted her warmly, and then announced to the other doctors, "This woman has T.S." Minutes later she was hyperventilating, drenched with sweat, her pulse racing.

Dr. Lown, one of the attending physicians, was astonished at the patient's rapid descent from apparent health to serious illness and asked her if she could explain what had caused her so much anxiety. "I know what T.S. means," she said. "It means I'm a Terminal Situation." Dr. Lown reassured her that T.S. is simply an acronym for tricuspid stenosis, the medical term for her heart condition, but his words came too late to save her. She died later that same day of intractable heart failure.

I find it amazing that two simple, seemingly innocuous letters—T.S.—had the power to destroy this woman's belief in her ability to recover from her disease. Her mind communicated the message of imminent collapse, and her body, perceiving that all was lost, gave up the struggle. Her faith in her body's ability to keep fighting was destroyed, her hope drained away, and she died.

Another story, originally told by Dr. Lown, affirms the power of a kind or reassuring word to reduce panic, inspire confidence, and, in miraculous ways, stimulate the life-force. It involves the case of Mr. B., a patient who had suffered a massive heart attack and whose prognosis was grim. When Dr. Lown visited during morning rounds, the patient was breathing through an oxygen mask and seemed unaware of the doctor's presence. As he reviewed Mr. B.'s medical history, Dr. Lown explained to the attending staff that his patient had a wholesome, very loud third-sound gallop, actually a poor sign indicating imminent heart failure. Over the next few days, to everyone's amazement, Mr. B.'s condition improved, and eventually he was discharged from the hospital.

Several months later during a routine checkup, Dr. Lown expressed amazement at Mr. B.'s miraculous recovery and asked him if he could explain what happened to change the course of events. "Doctor, I not only know what got me better," said Mr. B., "but even the exact moment when it happened.

"I was sure the end was near and that you and your staff had given up hope. However, Thursday morning, when you entered with your troops, something happened that changed everything. You listened to my heart; you seemed pleased by the findings and announced to all those standing about my bed that I had a 'wholesome gallop.' I knew that the doctors, in talking to each other, might try to soften things. But I knew they wouldn't kid each other. So when I overheard you tell your colleagues I had a wholesome gallop, I figured I still had a lot of kick to my heart and could not be dying. My spirits were for the first time lifted, and I knew I would live and recover."

Mr. B. believed he had a chance to recover (a belief actually based on a misinterpretation of his diagnosis), and with just that little bit of faith and renewed hope, his body responded. The cure didn't come from without—it emanated from within.

In modern times, with all the dazzling brilliance of high technology, we have come to imagine a cure as something instantaneous, even magical, with the primary healing energy supplied by some outside agent—a doctor's wisdom, a powerful drug, a drastic surgical intervention. "Cure me!" we say when we are sick with a cold or flu. "Cure me!" we pray when we are diagnosed with a chronic, incurable disease. With that urgent request for a cure, we hope for an end to pain and fear, a reason to believe, to have faith, to live again with passion and grace.

As a healer who has witnessed time and time again the miraculous healing capabilities of the human body, I feel honored with a powerful responsibility: to restore the hope and the will to live of my patients by caring for them even—and especially—when their disease has been labeled incurable. When I hear the anguished words "Cure me!" I translate the request as "Care for me!" and I immediately respond with the words, "I will take care of you." When I speak these words, my patients' fear and distrust begin to subside, for what they really want is for someone to care for them and to care what happens to them.

I believe that we must redefine what we mean by "cure." We must focus our energies on creating a positive healing environment in which curing is possible even when the disease itself is "incurable." To have another human being care for you and care what happens to you, always treating you as a person with a body *and* a mind *and* a spirit, is the real meaning of *cure.*

In a deeper metaphorical sense, chronic illness can actually become the cure for what ails you, the paradoxical "god that comes through the wound." When you are broken apart by illness—whether it is an affliction of the body, mind, or spirit—you become more fully conscious of life itself. When you are sick and in despair, you begin to discover the depth of your need for others—the need to be cared for and to be taken care of—and at the same time you are forced to journey deep inside yourself to discover your own healing potential.

At the moment when the breakthrough occurs, people afflicted with chronic disease sometimes speak of an epiphany—a sudden insight, an intense appreciation for the simple, once-overlooked pleasures of life, an overwhelming sense of peace that comes even in the midst of pain and confusion. The disease, which reminds you of your immediate vulnerability and inevitable mortality, releases you into a new awareness of the gift of life.

If we rethink curing as synonymous with caring, we find many examples of "the god coming through the wound":

• Afflicted by rheumatoid arthritis and chronic emphysema, ninety-year-old Pablo Casals spent several hours every day playing the piano and cello. When he placed his twisted fingers on the piano keys and began to play a piece by Bach, a small miracle unfolded. His back straightened and his body uncoiled as his fingers moved in graceful waves over the keys. After playing several selections, Casals stood up and, with no trace of a stoop, walked to the kitchen table, where he ate a hearty breakfast. An hour-long walk and several hours of work were followed by lunch and a nap. Temporary inactivity stiffened his joints, but in the afternoon when he played the cello, his frozen limbs unthawed once again, and the miracle of rejuvenation repeated itself.

Every day, several times during the day, Casals's disease was "cured," not by powerful medicines or technological interventions but by the creative energies released by his love of music and the melodies that flowed through his veins, as essential to his well-being as blood and oxygen.

• Diagnosed with a terminal illness while still in his internship at the University of Oklahoma, Dr. Lauran Eugene Trombley was "cured" by his illness, which pointed the way not to death but to "a new way of life." In the act of compressing his life, his illness stripped away all the extraneous details and focused his energies into a fierce, undying hunger for experience:

> I found that all of my senses seemed more acute, though I believe that I simply paid more attention to what was going on around me and, in a way, I found myself hungering for every sensory experience that I could absorb. In many ways the world seemed to offer more beauty, and there was a heightened awareness of sounds and sights which in the past I may have only casually observed or simply not have paid much attention to at all. . . . Aside from the sensory and affective sensitivity that I had seemed to acquire, there appeared to me to be a culmination of all the learning experiences that I had in my professional career, which, in a compressed space of time, became the foundation for practically a new way of life.

♦ Susan was thirty years old when she discovered a black mole on her breast. Biopsies confirmed a malignant melanoma, and surgeons performed a radical mastectomy. For five years Susan visited her doctor on a regular basis for tests and checkups to make sure that the cancer was still in remission. Twice a year the reminder cards came, and every time they arrived, she experienced a renewed fear that the disease had returned.

One day she walked into her doctor's office and asked to be taken off the mailing list. "Every time I get a reminder card in the mail, I'm flooded with feelings of fear and panic," she explained. "It's been five years now, and the cancer hasn't returned. I'd like to live my life as a healthy person who defeated a disease rather than a sick person waiting for the disease to take control again."

The doctor complied with her wishes, trusting Susan to call him when and if she needed help; ten years later she remains cancer-free.

Each of these patients had a chronic, "incurable" disease. Each patient decided to go his or her own way, seeking a long-term "cure," a word whose meaning goes beyond the idea of freedom from pain and discomfort to convey the image of a journey and the message that life goes on even in the shadow of chronic illness. As their experiences attest, such a life can be more richly imagined and deeply felt than the experience of life before illness struck.

In each case, part of the "cure" was the realization that illness is not a place that we are forced to inhabit but rather a perspective on life that can expand rather than diminish our passion for life. When Pablo Casals's swollen fingers moved with delicate precision over the piano keys, he was no longer an old man with crippling arthritis but a healthy, vibrant human being whose love for music transcended the pain and disfigurement of his disease. When Dr. Trombley regarded the world with a dying man's eyes, his senses sharpened and a whole new world opened up before him. And when Susan asked her doctor to stop sending reminder cards, she threw her weight on the side of life rather than death.

These men and women learned how to live with chronic illness and remain healthy in mind and spirit. Once they accepted the long-term nature of their illness, they stopped trying to push the unwelcome guest out the door and instead politely suggested that the visitor take a seat, saying, in effect, "Since you're here, you might as well pull up a chair, but don't expect to monopolize the conversation."

The words *incurable* and *invalid* were not part of their vocabulary. "Cancer literally cured my life," said Susan. "I was selfish, driven, and stressed out before the illness, and I rarely took the time to pause or reflect. Now I've got cancer, and even though it's in remission, I'm no longer so utterly self-absorbed. It's as if there were only room for this one cloud, all my other clouds became absorbed by it, and suddenly the sun broke through."

In the process of learning how to live with chronic disease, these people created a healing environment in which life was affirmed rather than denied. They remained positive and optimistic, refusing to give up hope—refusing even to entertain the idea that hope might not be available to them. Working hard to become active participants in their own recovery, they gained a sense of control over their lives. A renewed passion for life and a sense of connection to others and to the world itself filled the space broken open by illness.

Cancer

When Caryn was thirty-five years old, she was diagnosed with lung cancer. After surgeons removed her middle right lung lobe, she was told that she had a ninety-percent chance of complete recovery. Seven months later a CT (computerized tomography) scan revealed that the cancer had spread to the lower lobe of her right lung. The surgeon scheduled another operation to remove the remainder of Caryn's right lung, and she began an intensive cycle of chemotherapy.

Caryn's doctors were not optimistic about her future. "I suggest a 'wait and see' approach," her pulmonologist said. "If the cancer returns, I'm afraid there isn't anything else medical science can do for you except to make you comfortable and relieve your pain."

To prevent the nausea that often occurs with chemotherapy, Caryn took five different antinausea drugs, experiencing such side effects as weakness, fatigue, and general irritability. Sick and filled with despair, she called me, hoping to learn about herbs that might alleviate her discomfort and strengthen her immune system. Although she was extremely thin and appeared fragile, her posture told a great deal about her spirit: Head high, chin up, back straight, and shoulders squared, she had a strong inner structure and an unshakable faith in her body's healing capabilities. A proclivity to dry hair and dry skin, hay fever, and chronic sinus problems confirmed a strong affinity to Metal. As we worked together and her energy gradually returned, a secondary affinity to Water became evident in her strong will to live and in her ability to persevere despite all the odds against her.

Two months after Caryn began complementary treatments, a CT scan revealed that the cancer had spread to her left lung, and her oncologist pronounced the dreaded verdict: "You have stage IV terminal cancer." When Caryn called her pulmonologist, hoping for a different opinion, he agreed that her condition was hopeless. A social worker suggested that she accept the incurable nature of her disease and try to live each day to the fullest.

Despite the grim prognosis, Caryn refused to give up. She spent dozens of hours in the library, researching both conventional and experimental treatments, and dozens more hours on the phone, talking to clinicians, researchers, and pharmacists actively involved in cancer research and treatment. After countless meetings and phone calls, she was accepted into Boston's New England Medical Center cancer program, where she was treated with Taxotere, a drug extracted from the yew tree and recently approved by the FDA for cancer treatment.

To complement the Taxotere treatments, Caryn created her own recovery program, which included daily exercise, dietary changes, vitamin and mineral supplements, herbal tonics, acupuncture, meditation, and psychotherapy. These complementary therapies, Caryn believes, invigorated her immune system, giving her body the strength it needed to combat the cancer cells, increased her energy level, and reduced the overall side effects of the chemotherapy treatments. Most important, by taking an active part in treatment, Caryn gained a sense of control over her life, which, in turn, reduced her fears and gave her reason to hope.

After four Taxotere treatments, Caryn felt that her immune system needed a rest, and she informed her doctors that she had decided to discontinue chemotherapy. Two years later she claims that she feels stronger and more energetic than she has at any time in her illness.

Caryn firmly believes that hope and faith in her body's innate healing capabilities were more powerful than anything her doctors could offer her. Even more important than hope or faith, however, was her willingness to become an active participant in her own recovery. In a recent letter to one of her doctors, Caryn described the benefits of the hard work she has invested in her recovery:

I face my cancer every day and work very hard fighting it. In doing so, I have become a fully functional person, living a fulfilling life, thriving, not just surviving—despite having cancer. This has been an extremely difficult task, and I suspect that most cancer patients would not choose to do what I am doing, but I am not by any means the average cancer patient. It is now two and a half years since I was diagnosed with terminal cancer. At this point my focus is on obtaining the best health possible in order to strengthen my own self-healing abilities. I believe that this is why I am very much alive and doing very well.

WESTERN INTERPRETATION

Cancer is our most dreaded disease. When you consider the statistics, it's not hard to understand why:

- One million people in the United States will be diagnosed with cancer this year; more than half will die from their disease.
- Since 1950, the incidence of cancer has increased by 44 percent.
- Between 1973 and 1987, lung cancer increased by 32 percent, melanoma by 83 percent, and non-Hodgkin's lymphoma by 52 percent; breast, prostate, and kidney cancers have also increased significantly.
- Cancer is the leading cause of death in people between the ages of 35 and 64.
- Cancer kills more women in the United States than any other disease; every year more than 40,000 women die from breast cancer alone.
- By the year 2000, researchers believe, cancer will surpass heart disease as the number-one cause of death in this country.
- Fifty-nine percent of Americans believe that they are likely to get cancer; only three percent expect to contract AIDS.

Cancer has plagued human beings since ancient times—the bones and skulls of Egyptian and Peruvian mummies embalmed five thousand years ago show signs of the disease—and yet it continues to elude a medical cure. Why does cancer continue to escalate despite billions of dollars spent on research into various treatments and cures?

Cancer is, to put it simply, the growth of abnormal cells. When functioning normally, the body regulates cell growth, manufacturing new cells to replace dead and dying ones and then sending a clear signal to stop when enough cells have been produced. In cancerous cells, the stoplight malfunctions, and the green light is always on. In a big city, the inevitable result of a malfunctioning stoplight is a massive traffic jam with fender benders, pileups, and frustrated drivers creating all kinds of chaos. In the body, with its one trillion cells, the results are similar, with masses of cells piling up and blocking normal traffic lanes.

As the cancer cells multiply, they form masses of cells called tumors, which press against surrounding cells, causing damage and destruction to healthy tissues. Benign tumors are distinct and well-defined; for the most part, they are polite and keep to themselves. Cancerous tumors, on the other hand, are rude and disorderly, directly invading their neighbor's space and breaking off from the mother tumor like undisciplined children to travel through the bloodstream or lymph system to distant neighborhoods, where they create havoc and mayhem.

Kinds of cancer: Cancer cells come in three basic families:

1. **Carcinomas,** the most common form, begin in the cells lining the various organs—the mucous lining of the skin and the respiratory, gastrointestinal, and urinary tracts, as well as the breasts, prostate gland, and thyroid gland.
2. **Sarcomas** arise from other body tissues, including the muscles, bones, and connective tissues.
3. **Leukemias and lymphomas:** Leukemia is a disease of the tissues in the bone marrow, spleen, and lymph nodes, while lymphomas arise from lymphatic or immune system cells.

Diagnosis: The American Cancer Society lists seven warning signs of cancer:

1. Any unusual bleeding or discharge
2. A lump that doesn't go away or grows rapidly
3. A sore that doesn't heal within two weeks
4. An obvious change in bowel or bladder patterns

5. Persistent cough or hoarseness in the voice
6. Persistent indigestion or difficulty swallowing
7. Changes in a wart or mole

Note: Pain is not usually considered a warning sign of early cancer.

If you or your doctor notice any of these early warning signs, a series of diagnostic tests will be conducted, including a complete physical examination, blood tests, chest X-ray, stool tests, and urinalysis. Tumors often can be felt as a lump or nodule below the surface of the skin or mucous membrane; if a tumor is discovered, a biopsy is performed, in which a piece of tissue is removed from the tumor and then examined to determine if the cells are benign (normal cells) or malignant (cancerous).

Your doctor may also order high-tech diagnostic tests, including CT (computerized tomography) scans, which give detailed pictures of your body that are analyzed by computer; MRI (magnetic resonance imaging) scans, which use radio waves to deliver the information to the computer to be analyzed; ultrasound, which uses sound waves to create computerized pictures of the interior of the body; and endoscopy, in which the doctor uses a special instrument to examine the hollow organs or body cavities.

If abnormal growths or tumors are discovered in any of these procedures, a biopsy is typically scheduled to determine if the growth is benign or malignant.

CAUSES: Numerous theories have been offered to explain why cancerous cells start to reproduce in the body, though many of them are hotly debated. The most commonly accepted theories include:

The Viral Theory: According to this theory, a virus is hidden within the genes in the cells. At some point, and for some unknown reason, the virus is released, causing the normal cellular mechanisms to malfunction.

The Oncogene Theory: A newer version of the viral theory, the oncogene theory holds that approximately twenty genes called "proto-oncogenes" mutate into oncogenes, which cause cancer within the cell.

The Tumor Suppressor Gene Theory: This theory was proposed as an extension of the oncogene theory to help explain why cancer often occurs in the absence of photo-oncogene mutations. According to this theory, anti-oncogenes, or tumor suppressor genes, roam the body to inhibit the actions of the oncogenes and prevent cancer. If the tumor suppressor genes mutate or malfunction, oncogenes gain the advantage and cancerous cells multiply.

The Epigenetic Theory: One of the oldest theories about cancer causation, the epigenetic theory is being reconsidered by many cancer researchers. According to this theory, the cytoplasm—the part of the cell that surrounds the nucleus—is frozen at an early stage of the cell, resulting in a breakdown of the signaling mechanisms that control genetic activity. Consequently, the developing cells lose their "voice" and cannot communicate essential information to the chromosomes or the genes themselves, leading to alterations in genetic activity that in turn cause mutations and malignancies.

The Immune Deficiency Theory: According to this theory cancer cells exist in everyone but are controlled by a vigorous immune system; when the immune system is weakened by radiation, environmental pollution, stress, toxic chemicals in food or water, or unhealthy lifestyle habits, normal cells mutate and cancerous cells replicate. Few people contest this theory, which has been validated by recent environmental disasters like the nuclear meltdown at Chernobyl in 1986 and the Love Canal tragedy, where toxic wastes dumped into an old canal caused unusually high incidences of assorted cancers and nerve, respiratory, and kidney disorders. One year before the meltdown at Chernobyl, two cases of thyroid cancer were diagnosed in children who lived in the area; between 1987 and 1994, 236 cases were diagnosed.

WESTERN TREATMENTS

Present methods of treating cancer include surgery, radiation therapy, chemotherapy, and immunotherapy. Increasing numbers of physicians are incorporating various alternative or complementary therapies into their treatment regimens, possibly in response to the fact that many of their patients will use these therapies whether the doctor sanctions them or not. Nearly half of all cancer patients consider or try alternative therapies, spending more than $10 billion on un-orthodox treatments each year. The average cancer patient spends more than $100,000 on various treatments to combat the disease.

In this section we'll concentrate on those treatments generally accepted and widely used by the medical community.

Surgery: When performed at an early stage in the development of cancer, before the cancer has metastasized and spread to other organs, surgery can literally "cure" cancer. When detected early enough, cancers of the skin, breast, stomach, bowel, and uterus can be cured completely by surgery. The surgeon removes the tumor and some of the adjacent normal-appearing tissue to make sure that all cancerous tissues are removed; the surrounding tissue is examined by a patholo-gist, who determines if it is free of malignancy. The lymph nodes may also be biopsied to make sure the cancer hasn't spread to the lymphatic system.

Radiation therapy: More than half of all cancer patients in the United States re-ceive radiation therapy (X-rays or gamma rays), which destroys cancerous tu-mors. Although radiation is often successful with such cancers as early Hodgkin's disease, lymphosarcoma, inoperable local prostate cancer, localized tumors of the head, neck, larynx and cervix, testicular cancer, and childhood leukemia, nu-merous studies show that radiation does not cure most cancers and rarely ex-tends life expectancy.

Many researchers and clinicians are concerned about the fact that radiation, particularly when used for cancers against which it is not effective, may actually promote the development of cancer. Research shows that people who have radi-ation are more likely to have their cancer metastasize; studies published in the prestigious medical journal *Lancet* suggest that radiation following breast surgery may increase death rates.

Radiation therapy can reduce pain and suffering and, when used against cer-tain cancers, save lives. However, because radiation also harms healthy tissues, even to the point of encouraging the development of cancer, it should always be used with care and deliberation. Patients are well advised to ask their doctors whether radiation promotes a cure or increases life expectancy for their partic-ular type of cancer. If you are still uncertain, ask for the available scientific liter-ature supporting radiation's effectiveness.

Chemotherapy: Chemotherapy, which uses toxic chemicals to combat cancer, is the most popular form of cancer treatment in the United States, with $1.5 billion spent annually on various cancer drugs. The toxicity of these drugs is undisputed—one popular class of chemotherapy drugs known as nitrogen mustards is closely related to the poisonous mustard gases used in World War I. More than sixty varieties of the nitrogen mustards are on the market today, and they are taken by half a million Americans. One frequently prescribed derivative of mustard gas, Cytoxan, causes such side effects as nausea, vomiting, loss of appetite, hair loss, blood abnormalities, heart damage, and lung damage. Cytoxan is also carcinogenic—that is, it can actually cause cancer. Platinol, another best-selling cancer drug, can cause seizures, hearing loss, nerve damage, and kidney damage.

Although hundreds of billions of dollars have been spent on developing research and chemotherapy treatments for cancer, the results have been extremely disappointing except for a few relatively rare cancers—acute lymphocytic leukemia, Hodgkin's disease, Burkitt's lymphoma, choriocarcinoma, lymphosarcoma, Wilms's tumor, and Ewing's sarcoma. The most common forms of cancer don't respond at all to chemotherapy, or they react with only a temporary shrinkage in tumor size. Even when the tumor shrinks in response to chemotherapy agents, life expectancy remains the same in two out of three cases.

Chemotherapy saves the lives of only two to three percent of cancer patients, raising serious questions about the indiscriminate practice of giving toxic chemicals to cancer patients. In *The Immortal Cell* cancer researcher Gerald B. Deremer writes:

> Chemotherapy does kill the cells of the research models used to test drugs. It will also kill patients. But it does not effectively kill human tumors *before* it kills patients.
>
> In the nineteenth century, bloodletting was considered good medicine by physicians the world over. Chemotherapy is the bloodletting of our day, with the added horrors of toxic side effects and the added price tag of billions of wasted research dollars.

Immune supportive therapy (cell transfer therapy or biological therapy): These innovative cancer treatments, developed within the last twenty years, are designed to activate the immune system by injecting immune system cells directly into the patient's bloodstream. Animal studies were initially promising, but many researchers believe the statistics on human mortality and the steady rise in cancer rates in the last twenty years raise doubts about the effectiveness of these costly, often painful treatments.

New variations of biological therapy using substances like monoclonal antibodies and interleukin appear more promising, and cancer researchers remain hopeful that biological therapy will eventually prove helpful in the treatment of cancer.

TRADITIONAL CHINESE INTERPRETATION

In Chinese medicine all cancers are considered different manifestations of constrained Liver *chi*. Because the *chi* commands the blood and keeps it moving in its proper pathways, any disorder in *chi* will lead to disorders in the blood. As the circulation slows down, the blood congeals and becomes stagnant, marking the first stage in the potential development of cancerous tumors.

Why does the Liver *chi* become constrained and obstructed? The Chinese are most suspicious of stress—particularly excessive or prolonged stress—and long-term exposure to toxic chemicals in the form of pollutants in the air or water, toxins in food, and various drugs including alcohol and cigarettes.

All toxic substances are first processed in the digestive system. If toxins begin to build up and accumulate in the intestines, they preoccupy the *chi,* which gets tired and sluggish. "Stagnant *chi*" weakens the Liver, interfering with the Liver's role of maintaining the free and easy flow of blood, energy, and emotions, which in turn contributes to obstructions that can lead to cancer. Treatment strategies are designed to invigorate the *chi* and restore the free flow of energy in the digestive system and the Liver to eliminate the obstructions.

When constrained Liver *chi* is the main cause of cancer, symptoms include general irritability, sudden emotional outbursts, tightness in the throat, pains on the sides of the body (particularly near the rib cage), headaches (typically near the temples), and red, itchy, or inflamed eyes.

The Chinese also view deficient Spleen/Pancreas, Lung, and Kidney *chi* as contributing to the development of cancer because these organ systems are directly involved in stimulating and nourishing *chi* and *wei chi* energy. Deficient *chi* in these vital organs saps the body's natural defenses, making it easier for diseases of all types, including cancer, to take root and thrive. If the Kidney *chi* is deficient, the Kidneys are unable to provide adequate support for the Liver, which eventually leads to constrained Liver *chi,* congealed blood, and cancer. The Lungs are responsible for creating and distributing *wei chi* to all the vital organs; a deficiency of Lung *chi* will cause a breakdown in this vital function, weakening the body's defensive energy and resistance to disease. A deficiency in Spleen *chi* results in inefficient digestive processes, which can lead to an excessively moist, mucus-filled environment that encourages the growth of cancerous cells.

COMPLEMENTARY TREATMENTS

In Asia and Europe, and increasingly in the United States, complementary treatment methods including herbs, nutritional supplements, and acupuncture are often combined with or substituted for orthodox Western treatment strategies. Approximately fifty percent of cancer patients either consider using or have used alternative treatments, spending more than $10 billion on these therapies. In Europe, herbal therapy for cancer is considered mainstream; Europeans spend significantly less money on their health care than U.S. cancer patients, yet the statistics clearly show that they enjoy longer life expectancies.

Although cancers behave differently depending on the type of cell that is growing and multiplying, the complementary treatments discussed in this section apply equally to all types of cancer.

Diet

Step 1: Eliminate animal protein. Red meat, white meat, and dairy products are difficult to digest and contain numerous toxins that stress an already overburdened system.

Step 2: Avoid harmful fats. Harmful fats include saturated fats (beef, pork, lamb, chicken, duck, and whole-milk products, including cheese, butter, milk, cream, and ice cream) and trans-fatty acids found in margarine, vegetable shortening, fast food french fries, and hundreds of products that come bottled, canned, or frozen, containing the words "partially hydrogenated vegetable oils" on the label. Research conclusively proves that these chemically altered fats promote cancer.

Step 3: Eat organic (nonchemically treated) foods whenever possible. If you eat meat, eat only organic beef and poultry. Buy or grow your own organic fruits and vegetables, freezing or canning the produce for use in winter months.

Step 4: Avoid refined and processed foods. Chemicals are carcinogenic, and most of us eat them every day. More than three thousand chemicals are added to our foods to give them longer shelf lives, enhance their flavor, create color, and impart texture; on the average we consume nine *pounds* of chemicals along with our food and beverages every year. To protect yourself against cancer, take every step possible to cut down on the chemicals contained in fast, processed, and refined foods.

Step 5: Increase your intake of whole grains. Whole grains include, among others, whole wheat, brown rice, millet, oats, barley, corn, and rye. If you have cancer, we recommend a diet consisting of fifty to sixty percent whole grains.

Step 6: Increase your intake of fruits and vegetables. If your digestion is strong and vigorous, raw fruits and vegetables are fine; if you are prone to digestive disturbances, eliminate raw foods and gently steam the vegetables or sauté them in olive oil to loosen up the cellulose coating and ease the strain on your digestive system.

Step 7: Increase your intake of fiber. Vegetables, fruits, and whole grains provide significant amounts of dietary fiber, which is essential for a healthy digestive system. Without fiber to bulk the food and move it quickly and efficiently through the stomach and intestines, the digestive system gets sluggish. When digestion falters, undigested food particles escape through the walls of the colon and into the body fluids. The immune system comes to the rescue, gobbling up the "renegade" proteins; however, because those same cells are needed elsewhere to maintain health and fight infections, the immune system is slowly but surely drained of vital energy.

To sum up the problem: A malfunctioning digestive system can lead to immune dysfunction. The solution: Consume sufficient dietary fiber in the form of whole vegetables, whole fruits, whole grains, and supplemental fiber (see "Nutritional Supplements," pages 360 to 363) to restore balance and harmony.

Step 8: Drink eight to ten 8-ounce glasses of fresh, filtered water every day.
Avoid city water, which is treated with chlorine and other disinfecting agents. If you drink well water, have it periodically tested for contaminants.

For information on water-filtering systems, see Appendix I, Resources, page 399.

Step 9: Avoid nitrites and nitrates. Hot dogs, sausage, salami, pepperoni, bologna, bacon, and smoked meats contain nitrates and nitrites, salts of nitric and nitrous acid, which have been shown to cause cancer in laboratory animals and are linked with stomach, colon, and esophageal cancers in humans. A recent study conducted at the University of North Carolina at Chapel Hill showed that children who ate hot dogs had twice the risk of brain tumors when compared with children who didn't eat hot dogs. Research at the University of Southern California School of Medicine in Los Angeles showed that children who ate more than twelve hot dogs a month had nearly ten times the risk of leukemia when compared with children who didn't eat hot dogs.

Step 10: Reduce or eliminate your alcohol intake. A recent study conducted at the Harvard School of Public Health showed that even modest amounts of alcohol (approximately two drinks a day) can increase the risk of breast cancer; convincing evidence exists to suggest that alcohol is implicated in stomach, throat, and colon cancers as well.

Step 11: Sit down and eat slowly. Stress is a major factor in the development of cancer. Don't add to your stress by wolfing down your food or eating on the run. Eat slowly, savoring each and every bite. Food is medicine; as the Chinese philosopher Lin Yutang put it, "The Chinese do not draw any distinction between food and medicine." Offer your food a relaxed and stress-free environment in which it can work its healing wonders.

Step 12: Stop smoking. We include cigarette smoking under "diet" because nicotine has a direct effect on the appetite. The right food can do wonders for your health, but nicotine destroys many essential nutrients before your body can use them. Researchers estimate that each cigarette you smoke shortens your life by 5.5 minutes. At that rate, it doesn't matter how many organic fruits or vegetables you eat or how much fresh, filtered water you drink.

The link between smoking and cancer, lung disease, and heart disease is undisputed. You've undoubtedly heard the many statistics confirming the connection between smoking and cancer; here's a frightening statistic linking heart disease and nicotine: Men below the age of forty-five who smoked fifteen cigarettes or more a day were *nine times more likely to die of coronary heart disease* than men of the same age who did not smoke.

Secondhand smoke is also bad for your health. Stop smoking, make sure your environment is smoke-free, and give your new, healthy diet a chance to work.

Exercise

Regular movement and exercise promote the circulation of blood and *chi* throughout the body. Since all forms of cancer involve blockages or stagnation of *chi* and blood, exercise is an extremely important part of any cancer-prevention or cancer-treatment program. Both yoga and tai chi exercises stimulate the flow of energy and blood; these ancient healing methods will also help you develop what Zen Buddhists call "the right mind"—the ability to eliminate distracting thoughts and focus on what is happening right here, right now. If you feel strong enough to try more vigorous exercises, by all means do so.

In general, *Wood types* enjoy aggressive, competitive sports like running, mountain biking, backpacking, racquetball, and solitary workouts on fitness machines; if you are a Wood type, make sure your strength and endurance are sufficient to engage in these or other demanding exercises. Water and winter sports like swimming, boating, fishing, skiing, and skating are ideal for *Fire types,* as are gentle, nonjarring exercises like walking and bike riding. Slow, easy, noncompetitive exercises like walking, swimming, yoga, and tai chi appeal to *Earth types.* Exercises that encourage rhythmic, regular breathing like running, backpacking, mountain climbing, and aerobic workouts are particularly beneficial for *Metal types*: The deep breathing, stretching, and meditation involved in yoga and tai chi are also perfectly suited to Metal. *Water types* enjoy any exercise that emphasizes flow and fluidity, including swimming, jogging, brisk walking, cross-country skiing, yoga, and tai chi.

If your energy is sufficient, exercise twenty to thirty minutes every day.

Nutritional Supplements

Vitamin C: As an antioxidant and free radical scavenger, vitamin C works to prevent cancer-causing substances from gaining a foothold in the body, and it stimulates macrophages and T-cells, which play a critical role in fighting cancer. An important agent in the synthesis of collagen fibers, vitamin C also supports your body's ability to isolate cancerous growths, preventing them from invading healthy tissues.

In a major treatment study conducted in Scotland and published in 1976 by Dr. Linus Pauling (two-time winner of the Nobel Prize for chemistry) and Dr. Ewan Cameron, a Scottish surgeon who had treated cancer patients for thirty years, one hundred terminal cancer patients were treated with an average of 10,000 grams of vitamin C. They lived over four times as long (and experienced dramatic improvements in the quality of life) as a control group receiving the same basic treatment but without the addition of vitamin C.

Numerous studies conducted around the world confirm vitamin C's immune-enhancing activities, although mainstream medicine for the most part remains unconvinced. In this one area, we must be strong in our criticism of Western medicine and its refusal to acknowledge the many benefits of vitamin C therapy. If your doctor does not approve of taking megadoses of vitamin C, we counsel you to ignore his or her advice in this regard. Vitamin C can't hurt you, and the chances are good that daily doses will improve your physical health and emotional well-being and possibly prolong your life.

Take 1,000 mg. every one or two hours, up to 10,000–15,000 mg. (10–15 grams) daily; if you experience loose bowels or diarrhea, cut back on your dosage until the symptoms disappear.

Vitamin E: A powerful antioxidant, vitamin E protects the cells against cancer-causing free radicals. In combination with other antioxidants, particularly selenium and beta-carotene, vitamin E is effective in preventing cancer. Studies show that vitamin E can prevent the transformation of nitrate-containing foods into nitrosamines, which cause cancer; other studies show that higher blood levels of vitamin E reduce the incidence of chemically induced breast cancer in laboratory animals. Women who have higher levels of vitamin E in their blood are significantly less likely to get breast cancer than those who have low blood levels of the vitamin.

To help prevent cancer, reduce the negative effects of chemotherapy or radiation therapy, and provide general support to the immune system, take 800 I.U. daily.

Selenium: Selenium is a powerful immune stimulant, antioxidant, and anticarcinogen. Laboratory animals given selenium in their diets were protected against a wide range of carcinogens. Another study analyzing blood-bank data from seventeen countries around the world showed that areas with low levels of selenium in the diet experienced higher levels of leukemia and cancers of the breast, colon, rectum, prostate, ovary, and lung.

In a 1996 study reported in the *Journal of the American Medical Association,* 1,312 patients with a history of basal cell or squamous cell carcinoma of the skin were treated with 200 mcg. daily of selenium for approximately four and a half years; the incidence of lung, colorectal, and prostate cancers was significantly reduced, and total cancer mortality decreased by fifty percent.

Selenium works synergistically with vitamin E; for optimal anticancer, antioxidant, and general immune-supporting actions, take 200 mcg. daily with 800 I.U. vitamin E.

Vitamin A: Vitamin A helps to maintain the structural integrity of the cells and promotes healthy functioning of the mucous linings, particularly the linings of the respiratory, gastrointestinal, and genito-urinary tracts, protecting these areas from cancer. In numerous studies conducted around the world, vitamin A has been shown to prevent cancer and halt the progression of the disease.

For cancer we recommend vitamin A instead of beta-carotene or mixed carotenes. Recent studies indicate that vitamin A is an extremely effective anticancer agent; the effects of beta-carotene on cancer are still being evaluated. Take 50,000 I.U. daily—25,000 I.U. in the morning and 25,000 I.U. in the evening. If you are undergoing chemotherapy or if your cancer is aggressive and actively spreading, larger doses of vitamin A may be appropriate: however, because of the possible toxicity of large doses, be sure to seek professional advice.

B-complex vitamins: These vitamins support the immune system and help the body deal more efficiently with stress. Because stress is clearly implicated in immune dysfunction and susceptibility to cancer, the B vitamins are essential to prevent cancer. Chemotherapy significantly reduces the level of B vitamins in the tissues, so be sure to take a B-vitamin complex during chemotherapy treatments. Take a B-100 complex daily.

Omega-3 fatty acids: These nutrients are essential to promoting optimal cell integrity by helping to establish and maintain healthy cell membranes. Natural anti-inflammatory agents, omega-3's reduce the irritation and inflammation of the cells, which, in turn, lowers the risk of cancer. The best food source of omega-3 fatty acids is certain oily fish—salmon, sardines, herring, mackerel, anchovies, and albacore tuna. Other rich sources of omega-3's are flaxseed, flax meal, flax oil, hemp oil, and walnuts.

Eat fish rich in omega-3's three times a week, or supplement your diet with 1,500 mg. daily.

Gamma linoleic acid: GLA is a valuable ally in protecting your cells from degenerative changes and reducing inflammation throughout the body; recent studies show that it may inhibit cancer development. GLA is available in oil of evening primrose, borage seed oil, and black currant seed oil. Take 1,500 mg. daily.

Acidophilus (*Lactobacillus acidophilus* and/or *Lactobacillus bifidus*): This valuable adjunct to cancer prevention and treatment supports the health and integrity of the stomach and bowels by breaking down potential irritants and carcinogens (including the cancer-causing nitrates and nitrosamines) into harmless substances. By supporting bowel integrity, acidophilus also supports immune function, thereby reducing the risk of cancer.

We recommend enteric-coated capsules, which are coated to survive the acid bath in the stomach and release in the intestines, where they are needed. In general we prefer a combination of *Lactobacillus acidophilus* and *Lactobacillus bifidus*; take one capsule with each meal.

Shark cartilage: Shark cartilage may inhibit the process of angiogenesis, in which blood vessels are created to feed tumors, allowing the cancer to grow and spread. As a result, it may control the metastasis of the cancer. Research is promising but still in its infancy, and the cost of treatment can be high; however, for those who can afford it, shark cartilage may confer substantial benefits in the prevention and treatment of cancer.

Chinese Patent Remedies

To prevent cancer or to support the immune system during cancer treatment, we highly recommend the following Chinese patent remedies. The first one supports and nourishes the Liver, which because of its detoxification functions is always involved in cancer, while the second acts as a gentle immune tonic. You can take these remedies separately or combine them into an effective yet completely safe herbal tonic.

Hsiao Yao Wan ("Relaxed Wanderer Pills"): This formula supports and nourishes the Liver, encouraging the free and easy movement of *chi* and blood through the meridians and blood vessels. When the *chi* and blood flow vigorously and smoothly, they are able to remove obstructions (tumors) in their pathway. Bupleurum is the Emperor herb in the formula, working to restore the flow of Liver *chi*; seven attending herbs (peony root, dong quai, poria fungus, atractylodes, ginger, licorice, and mint) offer additional support to the *chi* and blood and aid the digestive system.

Take eight pills (actually tiny pellets) three times daily, or twelve pills twice daily.

Shen Qi Da Bu Wan ("Ginseng and Astragalus Great Tonifying Pills"): This formula is specifically designed to boost energy and enhance immune functions. The formula consists of two energy-boosting, immune-enhancing herbs—astragalus and ginseng. Codonopsis root is often substituted for ginseng in the patent remedy, for it mimics ginseng in its actions but is less costly and more appropriate for long-term use.

Take eight pills (pellets) three times daily, or twelve pills twice daily.

These Chinese patent remedies can safely be combined with any of the following Western herbs. If you need help choosing the most effective formula or combination of herbs for your symptoms, consult an experienced herbalist.

Herbal Allies

Three different kinds of herbs are important for cancer:

1. Herbs that support immune function (echinacea, astragalus, the healing mushrooms, and oats)
2. Herbs that promote the health of the Liver (dandelion and milk thistle)
3. Herbs that help the lymph system eliminate toxins from the body efficiently and effectively (red clover, yellow dock, and licorice)

Echinacea (*Echinacea angustifolia* or *Echinacea purpura*): This Native American herb was used by natives and white settlers to treat a myriad of afflictions, including snakebites, burns, wounds, fevers, infections, toothaches, and sore throats. Today, herbalists use echinacea as a general immune system stimulant. It gears up the immune system in two basic ways: by increasing the production of T-cells and by protecting haluronic acid, the cement that holds the cells together and strengthens their resistance to encroaching cancer cells or pathogenic invaders (viruses, bacteria, fungi, and parasites).

Astragalus (*Astragalus membranaceous*): This herb has been used for thousands of years in China as a general energy and digestive tonic to combat fatigue and speed recovery from wounds or disease. Extensively researched for its immune-enhancing effects in the treatment of HIV/AIDS, astragalus significantly increases the production of interferon, a powerful immune enhancer produced by the body, and it is particularly useful for the serious depletion of energy commonly experienced by cancer patients undergoing invasive therapies such as chemotherapy or radiation therapy.

Healing mushrooms: Certain mushrooms have been used in China and Japan for thousands of years for their immune-enhancing and energy-supporting effects. In the past twenty years researchers in the East and West have confirmed the antiviral, antimicrobial, and anticancer properties of Shiitake (*Lentinus edodes*), Maitake (*Grifola frondosa*), *Coriolus versicolor* (also known as *Trametes versicolor*), and Reishi (*Ganoderma lucidium*) mushrooms. Recent research indicates that *Coriolus versicolor* increases T-cell immunity and shrinks tumors, increases the survival rate of many types of cancer, and reduces recurrence of the disease. The British medical journal *Lancet* recently reported the results of a five-year study showing significant improvement and an increase in long-term survival for gastric cancer patients who used *Coriolus* extract. The well-studied Reishi mushroom contains polysaccharides that have been shown to enhance immune function by suppressing the growth of implanted tumor cells and increasing T-cell and macrophage counts.

All these healing mushrooms also enhance interferon production, an essential cancer-fighting element of the immune system.

Oats (*Avena sativa*): This gentle, healing herb relaxes the nervous system, relieves stress, and promotes a sense of well-being. Traditionally used in restorative tonics to combat the effects of stress and disease on an embattled system, oats support the body on a very deep level by providing life-giving energy and nourishment in easy-to-digest form.

Dandelion root (*Taraxacum officinalis*): This premier herb for liver support helps the liver in its job of eliminating toxins. Dandelion also has inhibitory (antitumor) effects on cancer cells. Dandelion root has been used in China for centuries in the treatment of breast cancer.

Milk thistle (*Silybum marianum*): This gentle but powerful liver tonic and cleanser has been used extensively and successfully in severe liver diseases such as cirrhosis and chronic hepatitis. A powerful aid in the detoxification process, milk thistle has proven to be a valuable ally in the treatment and prevention of cancer.

Red clover (*Trifolium pratense*): Famous for its blood-cleansing abilities, red clover has been used for many years to prevent and treat cancer. Researchers at the National Cancer Institute have recently confirmed red clover's antitumor properties. Because of its blood-cleansing actions, red clover has traditionally been used for numerous "toxic" conditions, particularly skin problems such as eczema, psoriasis, boils, and cysts. This same quality makes red clover helpful for cancer, for it supports the lymphatic drainage of toxins from the tissues. We consider red clover one of the most important herbs for treating all kinds of cancer; it is also extremely effective in reducing the side effects of chemotherapy.

Yellow dock (*Rumex crispus*) is a lymphatic cleanser and Liver tonic with stimulating effects on the flow of bile. By supporting the Liver, helping the body clean up debris, and stimulating the bile and lymph in their detoxification duties, yellow dock is an extremely important ally in the prevention and treatment of cancer.

When combined with burdock, another blood cleanser that works to dislodge toxins, yellow dock promotes the elimination of toxic substances. Yellow dock's gentle, stimulating effect on the bowels encourages elimination of toxins and contributes to the relief of numerous skin problems.

Full of nutrients, especially iron, yellow dock is a valuable remedy for anemia as well as for the depletion of red blood cells and platelets that occurs during chemotherapy and radiation therapy. Any condition involving accumulated toxins—skin problems, digestive sluggishness, arthritis, HIV/AIDS, and cancer—will benefit from treatment with yellow dock.

Licorice (*Glycyrrhiza glabra*): This nourishing herb has specific immune-supporting, anti-inflammatory, and antiviral actions. The Chinese call licorice "the Great Unifier," for it pulls together all the herbal components in a formula and helps them work together as a team.

Caution: Avoid licorice if you have high blood pressure, for in large doses it can cause water retention; slippery elm (see page 249) is a good substitute.

A well-rounded, supportive formula that I often use for cancer patients includes red clover as a lymphatic cleanser; echinacea as an immune booster and general support for the lymph system; yellow dock as a liver tonic and lymphatic agent; dandelion as a liver tonic; astragalus as a pure immune tonic; and licorice as a stabilizing herb to support the immune system and balance the adrenal glands. Or you could try the following prepared herbal formula:

Essiac: This herbal prescription was allegedly handed down by a Native American medicine man to a Canadian nurse named Renée Caisse to use for treating cancer. (Essiac is the nurse's name spelled backward.) The four herbs in the formula include burdock root, a blood and lymphatic cleanser; sheep sorrel, an herb with a sour, lemony taste; turkey rhubarb root, which has strong laxative properties to help eliminate toxins; and slippery elm bark, a soothing healing agent that specifically affects the mucous membranes and tissues of the body. Modern research confirms this herbal formula's beneficial effects for cancer prevention and treatment.

Essiac can be purchased ready-made in a product called Flor-Essence, available at most health food stores, or you can prepare the formula yourself. *The Essence of Essiac* by Sheila Snow gives step-by-step instructions on purchasing dried herbs and making the herbal brew.

Dosage: If you purchase your herbs in a health food store (either in tincture form or, as dried herbs, in capsule or pill form), follow the dosage instructions on the label. Because herbs in dried form tend to lose their potency rather quickly, be sure to check the label for the expiration date.

For information on preparing your own herbs from the root, bark, leaves, flowers, or seeds of a plant, see Appendix II.

In Appendix I, Resources, we offer a list of mail-order sources for high-quality herbs and herbal preparations. For advice on ordering specially made herbal formulas, see pages 394 to 396.

Acupoints

Conception Vessel 17 ("Sea of Tranquillity"): This powerful immune-stimulating point provides strong support for the Lung energies, which produce the *wei chi* (immune energy). It also nourishes the Heart, which houses the *shen* (spirit), thus relieving the anxiety and depression that so often accompany serious chronic illness.

Location: Conception Vessel 17 is located on the center of the breastbone, directly above the thymus gland (the originating source of the T-cells). Gently massage this point with your fingers, using circular, clockwise motions.

Liver 3 ("Great Rushing"): This point helps to relieve stagnation and restore the flow of *chi* and blood, breaking up obstructions that can contribute to cancer.

Location: Liver 3 is located on the upper part of the foot, in the depression in the webbing between the big toe and the second toe. Gently massage it in circular, clockwise motions.

Kidney 3 ("Great Mountain Stream"): This point replenishes the reservoirs of *chi* and *yin* (water), strengthening immune function and relieving fatigue and depletion.

Location: Kidney 3 is located in the depression between the inside ankle bone and the Achilles tendon. It is often sore to the touch. Gently massage it in circular, clockwise motions.

Lung 9 ("Great Abyss"): This point assists the Lungs in their job of producing *wei chi* (immune energy), then circulating it through the body, mind, and spirit. A pivotal point for supporting the blood vessels, it enhances overall circulation, which is essential in the treatment and prevention of cancer.

Location: Lung 9 is located on the crease on the palm side of your wrist, in a natural hollow at the base of the thumb (about half an inch in from the side of the wrist). Gently massage it in circular, clockwise motions.

Questions to Ask Yourself

Before we discuss the positive metaphors and images you can use to better understand your disease and its meaning in your life, we want to warn you about the negative metaphors that have captured the public's attention in recent years. Some people contend that cancer is the physical manifestation of unexpressed anger or fear; others argue that the disease represents the inability to stand up for oneself. The implication is that cancer patients are somehow responsible for their illness; if they were more "together" emotionally, they wouldn't be sick.

Emotions obviously play a part in illness, but the interplay of body, mind, and spirit is too complex to reduce to a standard formula or pat response. The following questions will help you to accept your disease as part—but not all—of you. According to Chinese philosophy, health and sickness ebb and flow just as night fades into day and day into night. When darkness reigns, keep your eyes open for the light breaking forth on the distant horizon.

Questions relating to Liver (Wood) imbalances may help you understand the nature and scope of your disease:

- What can I do to break through the obstacles confronting me?
- How can I keep myself from being overwhelmed?
- If cancer represents some form of being stuck or blocked, in what ways do I feel trapped and unable to move forward?
- Am I somehow holding back my creative energies? How do I prevent myself from expressing my creativity to others?
- Have I lost hope in the future? Can I envision a goal that would bring joy—and hope—back into my life?

Spleen/Pancreas (Earth) deficiencies are considered a precursor to cancer. If you are strongly influenced by Earth energy, you might ask yourself:

- When I feel lonely or undernourished, how can I nurture myself in positive, constructive ways? What steps can I take to avoid overindulging in sweets or junk food when I feel anxious or depressed?
- What concerns me most about this disease? What am I most worried about?
- This disease demands a lot of my time and energy: How can I set aside space and time to take care of myself?
- How can I allow others to care for me and take care of me?

Lung (Metal) deficiencies can lower your resistance to all forms of disease. Metal types appreciate quality and refinement, and they tend to hold themselves (and others) to impossibly high standards. If you are a Metal type, ask yourself:

- What is missing in my life? What essential qualities am I lacking?
- At some level cancer represents disorder and loss of control: How can I maintain order and harmony in my life?
- How can I nurture my passion for life?
- What is my disease teaching me about my life? What do the symptoms want from me?

In Chinese thought Kidney (Water) deficiencies are often related to physical and emotional inflexibility; fear is Water's primary emotion. If you have an affinity to Water, ask yourself:

- Is there something I am afraid to face?
- How can I allow myself to be supported by others and still maintain my independence?
- I have difficulty with trust and confidence: What can I do to restore my faith in my body's self-healing capabilities and have confidence in my future?
- If I had only one more day to live, would I feel that my work was completed? Could I move on with gratitude for all that I have been privileged to experience?

Imbalances in Fire can drain the immune system's energy and vitality. If you are a Fire type, the following questions might be relevant:

- In what ways do I inhibit my natural enthusiasm and passion for life?
- Why am I having difficulty communicating my thoughts and feelings to others?
- What can I do to define and protect my emotional boundaries so that I don't become overwhelmed by other people's problems?
- How can I balance my need for excitement and activity with time to rest and renew my energy?

A STARTING POINT

Picking and choosing among the many and diverse remedies recommended for cancer may seem like an overwhelming task. Where should you begin?

The following supplements, herbal remedies, and healing strategies will give you a solid foundation that you can build upon. Use the other remedies suggested in this section when and if you need additional support.

1. *Diet:* Follow the dietary suggestions on pages 356 to 359.
2. *Exercise:* Exercise for twenty to thirty minutes every day.
3. *Nutritional supplements:* Take the general formula for Maximum Immunity, but increase the dosage of vitamin C to 1,000 mg. taken every few hours, up to 5,000–10,000 mg. (5-10 grams) daily.
4. *Omega-3 and GLA oils:* Take 1,500–3000 mg. of each daily.

5. *Shen Qi Da Bu Wan:* Take eight pills three times daily or twelve pills twice daily.
6. *Western herbal formula:* Take a tonic of equal parts red clover, echinacea, yellow dock, dandelion, astragalus, and licorice.

HIV/AIDS (Human Immunodeficiency Virus, Acquired Immune Deficiency Syndrome)

Kevin, thirty-six years old, had been HIV positive for more than ten years when he called me. "I feel healthy and strong," he explained over the phone, "but I know my immune system is working overtime, and I want to do what I can to help my body heal itself."

When Kevin walked into my office, the entire room seemed to light up with his radiant energy. Thin and athletic, with delicate features and clear, smooth skin, his enthusiasm for life was contagious. His rosy cheeks, affectionate nature, and vibrant personality confirmed the influence of Fire, although an affinity to Metal was also obvious in his need for order and discipline and his embrace of the simplicity and purity of spiritual disciplines.

While the acupuncture sessions and herbal formula (consisting of astragalus, eleutherococcus ginseng, licorice, and isatis) seemed to give Kevin more energy, we agreed that the most valuable part of the sessions was the time we spent talking, sharing ideas about AIDS, telling stories about friends who had the disease, and trying to find, as Kevin put it, "the light in the darkness." An eternal optimist, Kevin refused to bow down before his disease, but he also insisted that AIDS was not his enemy. "AIDS has transformed my life," he told me. "For ten years I've lived with death. I can't avoid it or pretend it's not there, right in the room with me. But I'm still alive—isn't that amazing? And every moment of these ten years has been precious, with not one wasted moment. I may not live to be seventy-five—although I haven't ruled that out—but if you put together all the individual moments when I've been completely captured by the beauty and wonder of my existence, they add up to a full, complete life."

After we had been working together for two years, Kevin moved back to the West Coast to be with his family. We talked on the phone periodically, and Kevin continued to share his insights about the light in the darkness. In our last conversation Kevin told me that he had been reading the *Tao Te Ching* by Lao-tzu and had a favorite new quotation:

> *Darkness within darkness.*
> *The gateway to all understanding.*

Fourteen years after he was diagnosed with HIV, Kevin developed Kaposi's sarcoma; he died a few weeks later from histoplasmosis, an opportunistic infection often associated with AIDS. He had just celebrated his fortieth birthday.

WESTERN INTERPRETATION

The first AIDS cases were reported in 1981, when a researcher at the University of California at Los Angeles asked the Centers for Disease Control to investigate an outbreak of five cases of a rare and unusual pneumonia. The CDC concluded that the infection overwhelmed its victims (all homosexual men) because their immune systems were severely compromised. More cases of these rare opportunistic infections were reported in New York and San Francisco, and the AIDS epidemic had officially begun.

Today nearly 22 million people worldwide are infected with the HIV/AIDS virus. Most of the victims live in Africa and Asia. In the United States, over three hundred thousand AIDS cases have been diagnosed, and more than one million Americans are HIV positive, meaning that the virus is discovered in their body fluids even though they have no signs of AIDS. AIDS is the leading cause of death among males in the twenty-to-fifty-year range, and it is spreading rapidly. Experts estimate that by the year 2000 one in every hundred people worldwide will have AIDS.

When researchers discovered the HIV retrovirus in 1984, they were hopeful that a vaccine would be created to prevent and cure the disease. But the virus proved too clever, rapidly mutating and wrapping itself in a cloak of protein that differed in subtle but significant ways from the protein coats worn by other HIV viruses. The immune system works diligently to unbutton and defrock one virus, only to be confronted with dozens of others wrapped in cloaks with different configurations of buttons and snaps. One researcher reported that eighteen of nineteen strains of HIV taken from AIDS patients were structurally different, indicating an astonishing mutation rate.

While the immune cells are preoccupied with undressing the viral invaders one by one, the virus turns on them, killing or wounding millions of healthy cells. More immune cells come running to rid the body of the virally infected cells. Now the immune system itself has become the target as healthy immune cells attack HIV-infected immune cells, leading to what one researcher called "immunological suicide."

Cause: What caused the HIV virus to be unleashed in the first place? Nobody knows for sure, although many researchers believe the virus has been around for decades, even centuries, just waiting for the right opportunity to expand its reach. In her provocative and disturbing book *The Coming Plague,* Laurie Garrett describes the complex of events occurring in the early 1970s that gave the obscure HIV virus its long-awaited opportunity to spread throughout the world:

> Between 1970 and 1975 the world offered HIV an awesome list of amplification opportunities: multiple partner sexual activity increased dramatically among gay North American and European men and among African urban heterosexuals; needles were introduced to the African continent on a massive scale for medical purposes, and then resupplied so poorly that their constant reuse on hundreds, even thousands, of people was necessary; heroin use, coupled with amphetamines and cocaine, soared in the industrialized world; waves of other sexually transmitted diseases swept across the same regions, lowering affected individuals' resistance to disease and creating genital and anal portals of entry for the virus; the global blood market exploded into a multibillion-dollar industry; primate research expanded; and governments all over the world turned their backs, convinced, as they were, that the age of plagues and pestilence had passed.

Transmission: The HIV virus is transmitted from one person to another through body fluids. The *only* way to get AIDS is to intermix your body fluids (blood, urine, saliva, or semen) with the body fluids of an HIV/AIDS infected individual. Common means of transmission include sexual contact, IV-drug use, and transfusions containing HIV-contaminated blood. A mother can also pass the virus to her unborn child through the placenta, where blood and fluids are interchanged.

Progression of the Disease: HIV/AIDS progresses in four stages:

1. *The acute onset phase,* which represents the immune system's initial response to the newly acquired virus. The symptoms are similar to those associated with any other viral syndromes and include fever, aching muscles and joints, swollen glands, and sore throat. These symptoms may appear a few days or many months after initial exposure.
2. *The asymptomatic phase,* in which the individual with HIV appears normal and feels healthy. While there are no overt symptoms, beneath the surface devastating changes are taking place as the HIV virus penetrates and mutilates the body's cells. This stage lasts from a few months to ten or more years.
3. *The stage of lymph gland abnormalities,* in which lymph glands in the neck, groin, under the arms, and other areas become swollen and tender; nonspecific flu-like symptoms such as fevers, chills, aching muscles, nausea, digestive disturbances, diarrhea, and fatigue become chronic and intensify as time goes by.
4. *The stage of opportunistic infections,* in which there is a startling decrease in the ratio of T-helper cells to T-suppressor cells, indicating a severely compromised immune system. A myriad of rare "opportunistic" infections occur and reoccur, draining the patient's physical and emotional resources.

Most of the opportunistic infections associated with the fourth and final stage of AIDS are caused by microbes to which we are all exposed regularly or that we carry within us at all times. In AIDS the severely weakened immune system can no longer control these microbes, and they proliferate, causing such life-threatening infections as:

• **Pneumocystic pneumonia,** a rare pneumonia seen in sixty percent of patients with AIDS.
• **Candida albicans,** a common yeast infection that runs amok in AIDS patients, causing "thrush" and systemic yeast infections. Oral thrush (candida of

the mouth, tongue, and throat) and systemic candida (when the yeast proliferates internally and multiplies in the digestive or respiratory tract) are extremely common in AIDS patients.

- **Kaposi's sarcoma,** a rare form of skin cancer that affects approximately
eighty percent of AIDS patients.
- **Histoplasmosis,** a fungus that attacks virtually any part of the body. In individuals with vigorous immune systems, this condition is usually responsive
to treatment, but in AIDS patients the beleaguered immune system is often
unable to combat the fungus. Histoplasmosis is the leading cause of death in
AIDS patients.
- **Toxoplasmosis, herpes simplex, tuberculosis, and CMV (cy-
tomegalovirus)** take a major toll in AIDS victims, causing serious, life-
threatening symptoms and often proving fatal.

WESTERN TREATMENT

The cure for AIDS remains elusive, and in all likelihood it will remain so for
at least the near future because of the rapid mutation levels of the HIV virus.
Although numerous drugs have been developed over the years to treat AIDS and
its related diseases, only one drug significantly prolongs the AIDS patient's life—
AZT (azidothymidine, also known by its trade name Zidovudine). AZT was originally created as a cancer-fighting drug and works by targeting reverse
transcriptase, the enzyme used by the HIV virus to inject its genetic material into
the cells of the host. Preliminary research indicates that in HIV-positive individuals, AZT postpones stages 3 and 4 for one to two years.

The first drug approved for treatment of AIDS, AZT remains the drug of
choice, even though its long-term use can cause side effects ranging from unpleasant (headaches, nausea) to life-threatening (severe anemia and bone marrow suppression). Furthermore, while AZT seems to be highly effective when
first used, after a year or so of treatments the symptoms emerge again, often
with renewed vigor.

A new class of drugs called protease inhibitors work to inhibit the virus's protease, the enzyme produced by HIV and needed for replication. If the HIV replication process can be slowed down, the progression of the disease should also
slow down. While the protease inhibitors show great promise in reducing the

symptoms of AIDS and increasing life expectancy for AIDS victims, many researchers are concerned about the development of tolerance and resistance to these new drugs. To temporarily avoid the problem of resistance and tolerance, a patient can take a combination of AZT and the protease inhibitors, but the average annual cost of such treatments can be prohibitively expensive, exceeding $10,000.

TRADITIONAL CHINESE INTERPRETATION

The Chinese would agree with Western medicine that AIDS is a multistage phenomenon. In the first stage, which is marked by an invasion of Wind/Cold or Wind/Heat, the physician notes the typical cold/flu symptoms with fever, swollen glands, aching muscles, and fatigue. In most cases the patient's pulses appear superficial and tight to the touch, indicating that the body is attempting to fight off invading pathogens. Acupuncture and herbal treatments are carefully selected to support the *wei chi* (immune energy) in order to help the body, mind, and spirit resist the attack. Various lifestyle changes are suggested as an important part of the treatment regimen.

If the immune system is strong and the patient complies with treatment, the Chinese believe there is a good chance to defeat the HIV virus in this first stage. Research conducted in China in the 1980s, which showed significant increases in survival rates of cancer patients who received a combination of Chinese herbs and acupuncture along with conventional therapies as compared with patients who received only conventional treatment, prompted similar research in the United States. In one study, titled the Immune Enhancement Project, AIDS patients who were given a combination of Chinese herbs reported a significant reduction in their symptoms. In a 1988 paper published in the *Journal of Clinical Laboratory Immunology*, University of Texas researcher Dr. D. Chu discussed his studies showing that the herb astragalus helped restore failing immune systems and brought T-cell functioning back to normal levels.

If the patient ignores the early symptoms and neglects to take proper care of himself, or if the doctor fails to detect the developing disease, the virus goes into hiding for several years—the asymptomatic stage—only to reemerge in the third and fourth stages of lymph gland abnormalities and opportunistic infections. In the latter stages of the disease, the doctor notes the depletion of *chi* and blood and the accompanying symptoms of fatigue, swollen glands, low-grade fever, weight loss, and chronic coughing. Careful examination of the patient reveals Lung, Spleen/Pancreas, and Kidney deficiencies. Since these are the organs responsible for creating and maintaining sufficient levels of *chi,* a deficiency in any one of them will have a serious impact on the immune system's ability to resist disease or recover from an existing disease. A depletion of *chi* in these vital organs will further weaken the *wei chi,* leaving the individual vulnerable to infection and disease.

More aggressive measures, including stronger herbal formulas, more frequent acupuncture sessions, strict dietary changes, and various lifestyle changes, are prescribed to prevent the *chi* and blood deficiencies from progressing. If these strategies are not successful, the disease will eventually deplete the body's reserves of *yin* and *yang,* leading to such symptoms as fever, night sweats, and a dry, irritating cough. The Wind, Heat, and Cold Devils can further complicate matters; if Wind/Cold or Wind/Heat conditions persist, they can cause yeast infections, thrush, digestive upsets, diarrhea, chronic nausea, lethargy, and thought disturbances.

When the *chi* is no longer able to keep the blood moving properly, the blood begins to stagnate, leading to "heat in the blood" or "blood stasis" with signs and symptoms such as tuberculosis, Kaposi's sarcoma, pneumocystic pneumonia, and the other opportunistic infections that characterize the fourth and final stage of AIDS.

COMPLEMENTARY TREATMENTS

Diet

What you eat—or don't eat—directly affects your immune system's ability to resist disease. A healthy diet is critical in all chronic immune disorders, but for HIV/AIDS patients, eating well can literally mean the difference between life and death. Most AIDS patients die from the opportunistic infections that take advantage of their severely weakened immune systems. By adding certain foods to your diet and eliminating others, you will give your immune system the energy it so desperately needs to mount an effective counterattack.

Step 1: Increase your protein intake. Because your metabolic needs escalate with this disease, you will need to include generous amounts of high-quality protein in your diet. High-cholesterol foods are generally not a problem for HIV-positive individuals, because cholesterol levels tend to decrease as the disease progresses. If at all possible, buy organic (nonchemically treated) meat, fish, and poultry. Dairy products are not the best protein choice, because yeast infections and thrush, common problems for HIV/AIDS patients, thrive on these foods.

Step 2: Avoid harmful fats. Research conclusively proves that chemically altered fats, especially saturated fats and trans-fatty acids, can promote cancer and heart disease, both major risks for immune-compromised individuals.

Step 3: Avoid refined and processed foods. Such foods contain few nutrients and numerous chemicals that burden the Liver and preoccupy the immune system. We *strongly* suggest that HIV/AIDS patients avoid alcohol and cigarettes, which contain toxic chemicals that can drain vital immune energy.

Step 4: Increase your intake of whole grains. These include whole wheat (unless you are allergic or sensitive to wheat), brown rice, millet, oats, barley, corn, rye, and potatoes.

Step 5: Increase your intake of fruits and vegetables. They should make up approximately thirty percent of your diet. Use organic fruits and vegetables whenever possible. If your digestion is strong and vigorous, raw fruits and vegetables are fine, but if you are prone to diarrhea (a common symptom in HIV/AIDS), eliminate raw foods and gently steam the vegetables or sauté them in olive oil to loosen up the cellulose coating and ease the strain on your digestive system. If you are prone to yeast infections (thrush, candida), eliminate fruit juices, because the sugars encourage the growth of yeast in the digestive system.

Step 6: Increase your intake of fiber. Vegetables, fruits, and whole grains provide significant amounts of dietary fiber, which is essential for a healthy digestive system; a properly functioning digestive system significantly eases the burden on the immune system.

Step 7: Drink eight to ten 8-ounce glasses of fresh, filtered water every day. Fresh, pure water is essential to the integrity of every cell in your body. Water dilutes the blood, making it easier for the Liver to filter toxins and foreign substances from the blood, and it dilutes the urine, easing the Kidneys' job of filtering and separating toxins.

For information on water-filtering devices, see Appendix I, Resources, page 399.

Step 8: Avoid nitrates. Hot dogs, sausages, salami, bologna, and smoked meats contain nitrites and nitrates, substances that have been proven to cause cancer in laboratory animals and humans. Because their immune systems are severely compromised, HIV/AIDS patients are vulnerable to cancer and should avoid all products containing nitrates.

Step 9: Sit down and eat slowly. Stress is a major factor in the development of chronic immune disorders and can speed up the progression of HIV/AIDS. Avoid additional stress by not rushing your meal and savoring your food.

Exercise

Eating the right foods can build up vital energy reserves, but regular exercise is necessary to circulate the energy to the cells and tissues of the body. If you are HIV positive with no active symptoms, we strongly recommend a full exercise regime. Refer back to Chapters 2 through 6 for specific exercise advice to match your affinity to Wood, Fire, Earth, Metal, or Water.

Many AIDS patients rely on yoga and tai chi exercises to gently build their energy and lift their spirits. These ancient healing methods will help restore a sense of balance and harmony in your life, even in the midst of serious illness.

Nutritional Supplements

A high potency multivitamin and mineral supplement: Such a supplement will ensure that you are getting all the essential micronutrients. Ask your health care practitioner or health food store owner to suggest a good formula from a reputable company.

Vitamin C: This powerful antioxidant and immune supporter works to preserve the integrity of the cells and tissues of the body and to speed up the recovery process when injury occurs. Numerous research studies indicate that vitamin C helps the body combat bacterial, viral, and fungal diseases, which are common in HIV/AIDS.

Take 6,000–10,000 mg. daily in 1,000-mg. doses every few hours.

Beta-carotene (or mixed carotenes): This nutrient increases the number of T-helper cells—the cells that are targeted and destroyed by the HIV virus. Beta-carotene is converted to vitamin A in the intestines, but unlike vitamin A, it has no toxic side effects. If you take large doses for long periods of time, you may experience a slight orange-yellow discoloration of the skin (which also occurs if you eat too many carotene-rich foods like carrots); if this bothers you, reduce the dosage, and your skin color will return to normal. Take 100,000 I.U. *twice* daily, for a total of 200,000 I.U.

Vitamin E: This powerful antioxidant prevents oxidative stress to the cells, tissues, and organs, protects cell membranes, and assists the cells in their attempts to repel invasion by the HIV virus. Take 800 I.U. daily.

Selenium: Selenium works synergistically with vitamin E to enhance its positive effects. Selenium's anti-inflammatory and antioxidant qualities help protect cell membranes and tissues, reducing the risk of various cancers. In recent studies with HIV/AIDS patients, researchers report that selenium prevents the HIV virus from reproducing by injecting an HIV replication "birth control" into the system. Because selenium levels tend to be reduced in HIV positive and AIDS patients, take up to 600 mcg. daily.

B vitamins: These vitamins are considered the "spark plugs" for the body's biochemical machinery, helping the cells metabolize energy from food and drink, ensuring proper nervous system functioning, mitigating stress on all bodily systems, and providing essential support to the immune system. Take a B-100 complex daily.

Acidophilus (*Lactobacillus acidophilus* and/or *Lactobacillus bifidus*): These friendly bacteria work to nourish and heal the entire digestive system, helping to keep yeast and fungal infections under control and protecting against opportunistic infections in the digestive tract. *Always* take acidophilus if you have a yeast infection or if you are taking antibiotics, for it reintroduces friendly bacteria into the colon and helps restore normal bodily functions. We recommend enteric-coated capsules, which are coated to survive the acid bath in the stomach and release in the intestines where they are needed. In general we prefer a combination of *Lactobacillus acidophilus* and *Lactobacillus bifidus.*

Essential fatty acids (EFAs): Omega-3 fatty acids help to establish and maintain healthy cell membranes. They act as natural anti-inflammatory agents, reducing the irritation and inflammation to the cells, which, in turn, reduces the risk of cancer. The best food source of omega-3 fatty acids is certain oily fish—salmon, sardines, herring, mackerel, bluefish, and albacore tuna. Other rich sources of omega-3's are flaxseed, flax meal, flax oil, hemp oil, and walnuts. Eat fish rich in omega-3's three times a week, or supplement your diet with 1,500–3,000 mg. daily.

Gamma linoleic acid: GLA protects the cells against degenerative changes and reduces inflammation throughout the body. GLA is available in oil of evening primrose, borage seed oil, and black currant seed oil; take three to six 500-mg. capsules daily.

Note: Each 500-mg. capsule contains 35–40 mg. GLA, for a total of 100–250 mg. GLA daily.

Thymus gland extract: This extract stimulates immune function and can reduce both the number and the severity of recurrent infections in HIV/AIDS patients. The immune system's T-cells are manufactured in the thymus gland, which is larger than the heart at birth but weakens and atrophies as we age to the point where it may not be detected on X-rays. To help regenerate thymus function, take two to three 250-mg. tablets daily.

In his book *The Body Doesn't Lie,* John Diamond, M.D., suggests another way of stimulating the thymus: the Thymus Thump. With the fingertips of one hand, tap hard ten or twelve times on the bony area between your breasts (the breastbone). You can repeat this invigorating exercise as often as you want throughout the day.

Zinc: Zinc can rejuvenate immune function by stimulating the thymus gland to release hormones that in turn increase the production of T-cells. In one study, subjects ranging in age from 50 to 80 took 30 mg. of zinc for six months and experienced a forty percent increase in the hormone thymulin and nearly doubled the thymus gland's production of interleukin-1, a T-cell stimulator. Nutritional supplements often combine zinc, thymus extract, and other antioxidants. Take 30–50 mg. daily.

Chinese Patent Remedies

The patent remedies recommended below gently support the immune system and can be used without fear of any ill effects.

Bu Zhong Yi Qi Wan ("Support the Center, Benefit Energy Pills"): This general tonic was designed to support the immune and digestive systems. The Emperor and Empress herbs in this formula are ginseng and astragalus, which work to "support upright *chi*," giving you strength and stamina. Attending herbs include licorice root, which has immune-supporting and anti-inflammatory actions; dong quai, which supports the blood and nourishes the *yin* essence (so often depleted in AIDS); atractylodes, citrus peel, and ginger, all of which support the digestion and assimilation of nutrients; bupleurum to assist the Liver; cimicifuga to prevent the blood from collecting and stagnating; and jujube berries to calm the spirit.

Take eight pills three times daily, or twelve pills twice daily.

If you experience more *yin*- and *chi*-deficiency signs—night fevers and "rising heat" signs such as dry, irritated cough, hot itchy eyes, headaches, irritability, insomnia, and night sweats—try the following formula:

Ren Shen Yang Ying Wan ("Ginseng Supportive and Nourishing Pills"): This formula is often used to restore energy, relieve fatigue, and combat deficient *yin* or "rising heat" signs (fevers, night sweats, headaches, irritability). Extremely safe, it can be used for prolonged periods of time. It strengthens the *chi* of the Kidneys, Spleen, and Lungs, nurtures the heart, calms the spirit to relieve restlessness, anxiety, and insomnia, supports immune function, and slows aging. The herbs used in the formula fall into four categories: herbs to support *chi* and immune function (ginseng and astragalus root); herbs to support the *yin* and blood (dong quai, peony root, and rehmannia root); herbs to promote digestion (atractylodes, poria fungus, and orange peel); and herbs to harmonize the Heart and calm the spirit (ziziphus berries, schisandra fruit, and polygala root).

Take twelve pills twice daily.

These Chinese patent remedies can be safely combined with any of the following Western herbs. If you need help choosing the most effective formula or combination of herbs for your symptoms, consult an experienced herbalist.

Herbal Allies

The list of herbs to relieve symptoms of HIV/AIDS is endless, because the complications and infections associated with the disease are so diverse and involve so many body organs. Many of the opportunistic infections associated with HIV/AIDS can be life-threatening, so be sure to consult with your doctor and/or complementary health care provider for advice on combining standard medical treatments with complementary healing approaches.

In this section we list six gentle but effective herbs that have been used with great success to support the immune system of HIV/AIDS patients and combat infections caused by viral, bacterial, and fungal invaders.

Astragalus (*Astagalus membranaceous*): The fame of this ancient Chinese herb has spread to the West due to its impressive immune-enhancing actions. Experiments with mice and human subjects show that astragalus stimulates the production of interferon, a protein that inhibits viral multiplication. Astragalus is one of the most frequently used herbs in the treatment of HIV/AIDS.

Echinacea (*Echinacea angustifola* and *Echinacea purpura*): Echinacea was originally used as a Native American wonder herb to promote the healing of wounds and speed recovery from disease. Recent research in Germany substantiates echinacea's antimicrobial, immune-enhancing actions. Echinacea also protects haluronic acid, the cement that gives the cells their strength and integrity, allowing them to repel viral and bacterial invaders. Used successfully for immune-deficiency and autoimmune diseases, echinacea's protective actions make it a key player in the treatment of HIV/AIDS.

Licorice (*Glycyrrhiza glabra*): This is an extremely effective anti-inflammatory, antiviral, adrenal-supportive, and immune-enhancing herb. Japanese research confirms that licorice inhibits the growth of viruses by inactivating the active particles within the virus. In a recent study, HIV-positive patients received a daily dose of 200–800 mg. of glycyrrhizin (licorice) intravenously; after eight weeks, their T-cell counts increased and liver functioning improved.

Osha root (*Ligusticum porteri*): This traditional Native American herb has potent antiviral, immune-enhancing, and allergy-alleviating actions. In Chinese medicine the herb isatis is often used in HIV/AIDS treatment; if you have difficulty finding osha root, you can substitute isatis.

Shiitake mushrooms (*Lentinus edodes*): These mushrooms stimulate the immune system, increasing the production and the effectiveness of interleukin-1 and -2, crucial immune-stimulating substances produced by the T-helper cells that assist in many aspects of immune function.

Dandelion (*Taraxacum officinalis*): As the premier liver tonic, dandelion assists the liver in its vital role of detoxification. If the liver is working efficiently, it prevents fewer toxins from escaping into the bloodstream, where they can preoccupy the immune system.

Dosage: If you purchase your herbs in a health food store (either in tincture form or, as dried herbs, in capsule or pill form), follow the dosage instructions on the label. Because herbs in dried form tend to lose their potency rather quickly, be sure to check the label for the expiration date.

For information on preparing your own herbs from the root, bark, leaves, flowers, or seeds of a plant, see Appendix II.

In Appendix I, Resources, we offer a list of mail-order sources for high-quality herbs and herbal preparations. For advice on ordering specially made herbal formulas, see pages 394 to 396.

Acupoints

The following five acupoints can be used together to support the immune system by stimulating and invigorating Kidney (Water) and Spleen/Pancreas (Earth) energies:

Conception Vessel 4 ("Gate at the Source"): Known as the *tantien* or "center" point, this point is said to connect directly to the Kidney *chi* reserves, which are used to ignite and sustain all the vital functions. Some acupuncturists call this point "Life Gate Fire" because of its ability to rebuild *chi,* relieve fatigue and exhaustion, enhance immune function, rekindle sexual energies, and promote general well-being.

Location: Conception Vessel 4 is located on the midline of the lower belly, halfway between the umbilicus (belly button) and the pelvic bone.

Kidney 3 ("Great Mountain Stream"): This point invigorates and supports all aspects of Kidney functioning, including the *chi, yin,* and *yang.* As generators of both *yin* and *yang* energies, the Kidneys provide support for fatigue, depressed immune (*wei chi*) function, lower back pain, general debility, and depression.

Location: Kidney 3 is located in the depression between the inside ankle bone and the Achilles tendon. Use your fingers to poke around in the valley until you feel the tender spot.

Lung 9 ("Great Abyss"): Traditionally used to strengthen Lung functions and support the production of *wei chi* to boost immune function, Lung 9 helps the body to fight off foreign invaders. It also improves the circulation of *chi* and blood, which in turn supports the body's immune functions.

Location: Lung 9 is located on the palm side of the wrist, on the crease of the wrist, in the depression at the base of the thumb.

The following two points—Spleen 6 and Stomach 36—are often used together to help the digestive system function efficiently and to support the Lungs' ability to produce *wei chi* (defensive energy). When these points are simultaneously needled or massaged, their positive actions are said to be multiplied.

Spleen 6 ("Three Yin Meeting"): This point is used to support the *yin* energies, which HIV/AIDS often depletes, and to invigorate the digestive system, which is also depleted and sluggish in HIV-positive individuals. Nourishing the *yin* and the blood, Spleen 6 helps with insomnia, irritability, restlessness, night fevers or sweats, and dryness anywhere in the body. Because Spleen 6 helps to build Spleen and Stomach energy, it is often used for digestive problems including bloating, gas, heavy or aching limbs, lack of enthusiasm, feelings of being weighed down, fatigue, and lethargy.

Location: Spleen 6 is located approximately three inches above the interior ankle bone, in a depression just to the side of the tibia (shin) bone.

Stomach 36 ("Walks Three Miles"): This point is a powerful stimulator and supporter of energy formation in general and digestion in particular. In the old days, when traveling monks journeyed long distances from one monastery to another, they would needle or press this point to enable themselves to walk another three miles.

Location: Stomach 36 is located approximately three inches below the dimple or depression on the outside (pinky) side of the knee and one inch from the crest of the shinbone, in a groove or natural depression in the muscle.

Questions to Ask Yourself

Several years ago hundreds of people became seriously ill after eating ice cream infected with salmonella bacteria. The fascinating part of this story centers not on the people who got sick but on those who didn't—for only ten percent of those people who ate the tainted ice cream actually became ill. The bug was the same; the people were different.

When exposed to the same virus, some people get sick and others don't; among those who get sick, some progress rapidly in their disease while others stay relatively healthy. This truth holds in every disease, no matter how virulent, and HIV/AIDS is no exception. If you are HIV positive or if you have AIDS, you must keep this thought foremost in your mind: *You are not powerless.* The HIV virus is as virulent as any virus on this earth and more deceptive than most, yet thousands of infected individuals have been able to live healthy, productive lives as their immune systems work steadily and consistently to contain the virus and slow its progress.

The gardeners within have powerful muscles. Provide them with a healthy environment, let them know that you believe in their power to heal, and they will respond by working diligently to restore balance and harmony. To regain a sense of your innate powers of healing, ask yourself these questions:

- In what ways do I allow myself to feel defenseless?
- What can I do to take charge of my life, to move from a passive observer to an active participant?
- Am I standing up for myself and clearly expressing my feelings, desires, and aspirations?
- How can I regain my sense of purpose and will to live?
- How can I learn to celebrate and rejoice in my life and its abundant gifts?
- What is most important to me in life, and how can I honor it?
- If I had one last wish, what would it be? Where would I go? Who would I spend my time with? What kind of person would I become?

The Chinese believe that Lung (Metal), Spleen/Pancreas (Earth), and Kidney (Water) deficiencies eventually weaken the *wei chi,* leaving the individual vulnerable to HIV/AIDS. If you are a Metal type, you might ask yourself:

- What can I do to enhance the quality of my life?
- Do I have enough breathing space? If not, what can I do to create it?
- What am I holding on to that I am desperately afraid of losing? Do I really need it? What is the worst possible outcome if I lost it?
- What do I *really* need? What can I not live without?

If you are an Earth type, you might ask:

- How can I allow others to care for me and take care of me?
- What concerns me most about this disease? What am I most worried about?
- How can I set time and space aside for myself?

If you are a Water type, ask yourself these questions:

- Of all the difficulties confronting me, what am I most afraid to face?
- What can I do to restore my faith in my body's ability to heal itself?
- What situations cause me to freeze up? What can I do to create warmth and movement in my life?

A STARTING POINT

Picking and choosing among the many and diverse remedies recommended for HIV/AIDS may seem like an overwhelming task. Where should you begin?

The following supplements, herbal remedies, and healing strategies will give you a solid foundation that you can then build upon. Use the other remedies suggested in this section when and if you need additional support:

1. *Diet:* Follow the dietary suggestions on pages 377 to 379.
2. *Exercise:* Exercise for twenty to thirty minutes every day.
3. *Nutritional supplements:* Take the general formula for Maximum Immunity, with the following changes: *Increase the dosage of vitamin C* to 6,000–10,000 mg. daily, taken in 1,000-mg. doses every hour or two; and *increase beta-carotene* to 200,000 I.U. daily.
4. *Essential fatty acids:* Take both omega-3 fish oils and GLA oils, 1,500–3,000 mg. of each daily.
5. *Thymus extract:* Take two to three 250-mg. tablets twice daily.
6. *Bu Zhong Yi Qi Wan:* Take eight pills three times daily or twelve pills twice daily.
7. *Western herbal formula:* Take a tonic of astragalus, echinacea, licorice, osha root, and dandelion in equal amounts. If osha root is difficult to find, substitute isatis or goldenseal.

*"Alas! The way of healing is so profound.
It is deep as the oceans and boundless as the
skies. How many truly know it?"*

—The Yellow Emperor's Classic of Medicine

APPENDIX I: RESOURCES

HOW TO FIND A PRACTITIONER

To find a practitioner you can trust as an ally in your healing journey, you will need to do your homework. Check the education and certification of practitioners you are considering. Call and ask detailed questions, just as you would interview anyone else you might consider hiring. Ask them how long they have been in practice and what they would do in certain hypothetical situations. Ask for the names of several of their patients who would be willing to talk to you. Above all, trust your intuition. Remember that you are in control; if you aren't impressed with the individual you are interviewing, you have the right to shop around. Many competent and compassionate doctors, acupuncturists, herbalists, and naturopaths are available to assist you.

How to Find a Holistically Oriented Physician

American Holistic Medical Association
4101 Lake Boone Trail, Suite 201
Raleigh, NC 27607
(919) 787- 5181

The AHMA can refer you to a holistically oriented physician near you. They offer a National Referral Directory for $8.

How to Find an Acupuncturist

American Association of Acupuncture and Oriental Medicine (AAAOM)
433 Front Street
Catasauqua, PA 18032-2506
(610) 433-2448

The AAAOM will refer you to a qualified practitioner of acupuncture in your area, and they will provide information on requirements for licensure and practice in your particular state. For a small fee, they will send you a list of qualified practitioners in your area.

National Commission for the Certification of Acupuncturists (NCCA)
1424 16th Street N.W., Suite 105
Washington, DC 20036
(202) 232-1404

The NCCA will provide you with a list of board-certified practitioners in your area.

National Council of Acupuncture Schools and Colleges (NCASC)
P.O. Box 954
Columbia, MD 21044
(301) 997-4888

The NCASC will provide you with a list of accredited acupuncture schools that prepare students for the NCCA exams, which are generally the equivalent of the state licensing exams.

How to Find a Qualified Herbalist

Chinese Herbal Medical Practitioner

A national organization to certify minimum educational requirements for the practice of traditional Chinese medicine was recently established:

National Commission for the Certification of Acupuncturists (NCCA)
1424 16th Street N.W., Suite 105
Washington, DC 20036
(202) 232-1404

The NCCA nationally certifies practitioners of traditional Chinese medicine who have proved their competence by studying at an approved college, practicing for a minimum number of years, and passing a national board examination. Be advised, however, that NCCA certification does not ensure competence. Because NCCA is a new certifying body and many well-respected herbalists may not be NCCA certified, be sure to interview potential practitioners in a discriminating fashion. Ask where they got their training, how long they have been practicing Chinese medicine, and whether they have access to the advice of other experts. Feel free to ask for references and names of other patients they have treated with problems similar to yours.

Western Herbal Practitioner

Although there is no certifying body for the practice of Western herbal medicine, many exceptional colleges are beginning to offer training in this field. Ask your holistically oriented physician, naturopath, acupuncturist, or health food store proprietor for a referral to a good herbal therapist. The England-based School of Medical Herbalism and its U.S. affiliates are among the most renowned training institutions for herbalists. The organizations listed below offer guidelines for finding an herbalist in your area and information on training programs, schools, and resources for buying high-quality herbal products.

American Botanical Council (ABC)
P.O. Box 201660
Austin, TX 78720
(800) 748-2617

The ABC, a nonprofit organization, publishes the excellent *HerbalGram* magazine, provides excellent reference materials, and can direct you to an herbalist in your area.

The Herb Research Foundation
1007 Pearl Street, #200
Boulder, CO 80302
(303) 449-2265

The HRF publishes *HerbalGram* in conjunction with the ABC and can provide abundant information on herbal training programs and seminars in your area. It can also direct you to herbalists or schools in your area to help you to locate a qualified practitioner.

American Herb Association (AHA)
P.O. Box 1673
Nevada City, CA 95959
fax (916) 265-9552

The AHA provides educational material and resources for medical herbalism, which may steer you toward a qualified herbalist or provide information about specific herbs.

How to Find a Naturopath

American Association of Naturopathic Physicians (AANP)
P.O. Box 20386
Seattle, WA 98102
(206) 323-7610

The AANP will send you a list of certified naturopathic physicians in your area; please enclose a SASE when writing to the above address.

BUYING HERBS BY MAIL

The following reputable herb dealers sell good-quality, usually organic herbs, in dried form, tinctures, and capsules. You can order the dried plant material from any of the vendors listed and make good-quality herbal decoctions and infusions yourself. Most of them will send you a catalog on request.

Integral Health Apothecary
3 Paradise Lane
New Paltz, NY 12561
(888) 403-5861 (toll free)

The Integral Health Apothecary is the pharmacy connected with Integral Health Associates, a group practice in New Paltz, New York, whose aim is to treat the "whole person" utilizing various alternative and traditional healing modalities. Nutrition, acupuncture, herbal medicine, homeopathy, psychotherapy, chiropractic, natural vision care, yoga, bodywork, and massage therapy are practiced by experienced health care professionals. At our (Jason Elias and staff) health and wellness center, we have established a pharmacy carrying a complete line of herbal (both Western and Chinese) products and supplements, as well as books and other related products. The following reputable companies offer fresh-dried herbal material for teas and decoctions:

For Western Herbs

Aveena Botanicals
Box 365

West Rockport, ME 04865
(207) 594-0694

Blessed Herbs
Rte. 5, Box 1042
Ava, MO 65608

Green Terrestrial
P.O. Box 41, Rte. 9W
Milton, NY 12547
(914) 795-5238

Herbalist and Alchemist
P.O. Box 458
Bloomsbury, NJ 08804
(908) 689-9020

HerbPharm
P.O. Box 116
Williams, OR 97544
(503) 846-6112

Island Herbs
Waldron Island, WA 98297

Monarda Herbal Apothecary
P.O. Box 505
Rosendale, NY 12472
(914) 658-7044

Sage Mountain Herb Products
P.O. Box 420
East Barre, VT 05649

Trinity Herbs
P.O. Box 199
Bodega, CA 94992

For Chinese Herbs and Patent Remedies

If you live near a Chinatown, you will be able to locate a Chinese herbal shop offering
the patent remedies described in this book. Or you can order Chinese herbs from:

ITM Herb Products
2017 S.E. Hawthorne
Portland, OR 97214
(800) 544-7504

Crane Enterprises
45 Samoset Avenue
RFD #1
Plymouth, MA 02360
(800) 227-4118

NUTRITIONAL SUPPLEMENTS

Vitamin and mineral supplements can be purchased at health foods stores and pharmacies. Quality can vary dramatically, so be sure to ask the advice of a qualified herbalist, holistically trained M.D., naturopath, or health food store proprietor.

Integral Health Apothecary recently expanded their pharmacy to carry reasonably priced vitamins, minerals, and other nutritional supplements as a service to their patients and friends.

Integral Health Apothecary
3 Paradise Lane
New Paltz, NY 12561
(888) 403-5861

FOR MORE INFORMATION:

Allergies, Sinusitis, and Asthma

National Institute for Allergy and Infectious Diseases
Building 31, Room 7A5o
31 Center Drive MSC 2520
Bethesda, MD 20892-2520
(301) 496-5717

Asthma and Allergy Foundation of America
1125 15th Street, N.W., Suite 502
Washington, DC 20005
(202) 466-7643

American Academy of Environmental Medicine
P.O. Box 5001-8001

New Hope, PA 18938
(215) 862-4544

Arthritis and Joint Diseases

National Institute of Arthritis and Musculoskeletal and Skin Diseases
Building 31, Room 4CO5
31 Center Drive MSC 2350
Bethesda, MD 20892
(301) 496-8188

Arthritis Foundation of America
1330 West Peachtree Street
Atlanta, GA 30309
(404) 872-7100

Eczema and Psoriasis

National Eczema Association for Science and Education
1221 S.W. Yamhill, #303
Portland, OR 97205
(503) 228-4430

National Psoriasis Foundation
6600 S.W. 92nd Avenue, Suite 300
Portland, OR 97223-7195
(503) 244-7404
(800) 723-9166

Inflammatory Bowel Disease and Crohn's Disease

Crohn's and Colitis Foundation of America
386 Park Avenue South
New York, N.Y. 10016
(212) 685-3440

Chronic Fatigue Syndrome

CFIDS of America
P.O. Box 220398
Charlotte, NC 28222-0398
(800) 442-3437
(900) 896-2343 (Information Line)

Chronic Fatigue Immune Dysfunction Syndrome Foundation
965 Mission Street, Suite 425
San Francisco, CA 94103
(415) 882-9986

Diabetes and Digestive Problems

National Institute of Diabetes and Digestive and Kidney Diseases
31 Center Drive, Room 9A04
Bethesda, MD 20892
(301) 496-3583

Lupus

Lupus Foundation of America
1300 Piccard Drive, Suite 200
Rockville, MD 20850-4303
(301) 670-9292
(800) 558-0121

Cancer

American Cancer Society
1599 Clifton Road, N.E.
Atlanta, GA 30329
(800) ACS-2345

Center for Advancement in Cancer Education
P.O. Box 48
Wynnewood, PA 19096-0048
(610) 642-4810

HIV/AIDS

AIDS Alternative Health Project
4753 N. Broadway
Chicago, IL 60640
(312) 561-2800

Bastyr University AIDS Research Center
144 N.E. 54th Street

Seattle, WA 98105
(800) 475-0135

WATER FILTERS AND TESTING

We strongly urge you to purchase a water-filtering system for your drinking water and for water used in cooking. Hundreds of U.S. companies manufacture water filters. Differences in quality exist, so be sure to ask around before you purchase a system. Plumbers are often a good source of information, and they can also help you install the more complicated filtering systems.

The following chart is from Elson Haas's book *Staying Healthy with Nutrition* (Celestial Arts, Berkeley, California, 1992):

Water Systems Analysis

Contents	SOURCE		PURIFICATION		
	Tap Water	*Well or Spring*	*Solid Carbon*	*Reverse Osmosis*	*Distillation*
Chlorine	yes	not unless treated	removed	not removed unless carbon used also	removed
Fluoride	if added	natural or if treated	not removed	removed	removed
Bacteria	unlikely	possibly removed	most likely	removed	removed
Parasites	possibly	possibly	removed	removed	removed
Chemicals	likely	likely	removed	removed	possibly*
Basic Minerals	some	likely	not removed	removed	removed
Heavy Metals	possibly	possibly	some removed	removed	removed

Energy Factors

Electricity Used	no	probably	no	no	yes
Wastes Water	no	no	no	yes	some

*Potential volatilization of chlorinated hydrocarbons and other toxic chemicals.

Common Filtration Systems Are:

Activated Carbon Filters

The most common and least expensive type of water filter is available at department stores, hardware stores, and health food stores. These units filter the water mechanically and biomagnetically, removing bacteria, parasites, chlorine, and many chemicals; they are said to filter out all particles larger than 0.04 microns. The filters have to be changed quite often, as there is some fear of recontamination if they are not.

Solid Block and Carbon Block Filters

These filters are not as easy to find, except in specialty shops and through many catalogues; Amway and Multipure manufacture both types. They are more effective than activated charcoal filters: They filter more contaminants and have less danger of recontamination.

The Reverse Osmosis Filter

This filtration system, our personal favorite, employs two or three separate filtering mechanisms: a sediment filter to remove the larger particles, a reverse osmosis membrane, and an activated carbon filter. Reverse osmosis units are more expensive than other filtering systems, but in our opinion they are the superior choice. Filters need to be replaced every year or two.

WHERE TO BUY WILD FISH

Kooskooskie Fish
P.O. Box 1305
Walla Walla, WA 99362
(509) 520-8040

APPENDIX II: MAKING YOUR OWN HERBAL FORMULAS

There's no doubt about it—herbs are expensive. It's easiest to buy a ready-made herbal formula and take it as prescribed, but you will be spending a lot of money. The other choice is to prepare your own herbal formulas, which takes time and some storage space but can be fun; the process itself can become a healing ritual, connecting you to the "root of healing." And of course you will also be saving money. This appendix describes how to prepare your own herbal medicinal formulas, in the form of decoctions, infusions, tinctures, or capsules.

All the herbs presented in this book are considered safe and can easily be prepared at home. You can purchase the herbs in tincture form from a source listed in the Resources section or from your local health food store. (Try to buy herbals labeled organic.) Buy only herbs made by reputable companies; ask a trusted health food store proprietor or health professional for advice on which are trustworthy. In making herbal and supplemental products available to the lay public, we have lost a degree of quality assurance as to the quality and potency of herbal and vitamin products, so "buyer beware" is a good philosophy when purchasing natural herbal products. All of the herbal resources we list sell good dried herbal material, and some also sell good-quality tinctures; call and ask for a catalog.

To make your own decoctions, teas, infusions, tinctures, or capsules, start with good, fresh herbal material. The herbs you buy will be dried, yet their color and texture as well as aroma should be clean and crisp. Good dried herbs should remain similar in color to the fresh plant; they should appear "fresh" and vivid in color, their blossoms or flowers should be bright and colorful, and their roots should also have a rich color.

Inspect the dried herbs to ensure there is no mold, and smell them—they should smell strong and "vital." An herbal store or health food store that sells lots of herbs and has a large turnover will probably have good fresh stock, whereas herbs from a shop with little traffic, where the herbs sit in bottles for months at a time, will quickly lose their "vitality" and effectiveness.

PREPARING A DECOCTION/TEA

A decoction is an herbal remedy made by boiling the hard and woody parts of a plant in order to extract its active principles (those aspects that have the healing effect). Always use stainless steel or ceramic pots to make your herbal brews, as aluminum pots may chemically interact with the herbs. Take the hard and woody parts (root, bark, and twigs), and break them up into small pieces—the smaller the better for extracting the active constituents. To make a decoction, take one ounce of the combined herbal constituents, and place the hard and woody parts into five cups of water. Bring to a boil, and cook at a full boil for ten minutes, or until the five cups of water cook down to four cups. Remove from heat and add the more delicate herbal ingredients, the leaf and flower material; cover and let stand for another ten minutes. Strain the mixture, and enjoy one cup twice daily.

Decoctions will last three to four days in the refrigerator.

PREPARING AN INFUSION

An infusion is made by breaking up the dried plant material (flowers, leaves, whole plant) in a clean cloth; again, use one ounce of herb material per pint of water. Pour the pint of just-boiled water over the dried, bruised herb, and let simmer for 20–30 minutes. Strain the mixture, and drink it hot or cold. Generally, for medicinal purposes, two cups of infusion or decoction is a daily dose.

PREPARING A TINCTURE

Tinctures are generally the best way to use herbs. Alcohol is probably the best medium for extracting the active constituents into the liquid medium; at the same time it preserves the formula for many years, so that its effectiveness remains intact for years rather than days, as in other methods of herbal preparation. A tincture is made by pouring five ounces of alcohol over one ounce of dried herb material or three ounces of fresh herb material. Professional herbal tinctures use very pure and refined grain alcohol (198 proof). To make it at home you can use five ounces of 100 to 120 proof vodka.

Keep the mixture in a sterile, airtight bottle, away from direct light; over time the active constituents of the herbs will be released into the alcohol. In four to six weeks, strain the mixture and press it in cloth to remove the old plant material. Tinctures will last for a minimum of four years.

If you cannot drink alcohol, you might try making tinctures with apple cider vinegar instead of alcohol.

PREPARING CAPSULES

You can buy or make your own capsules by grinding the plant material in a grinder and putting the powder in "00" capsules. Many health food stores carry little capsule-making kits. The advantage is ease of use, but the disadvantage of buying dried herbs is that the shelf life is very limited. If you make capsules yourself, you are assured of freshness if you grind your own herbs, but they should be used within a couple of months from purchase. If you buy dried capsules in a store, look for an expiration date on the label and take it seriously, for old herbs quickly lose their vitality.

APPENDIX III: ACUPRESSURE POINTS

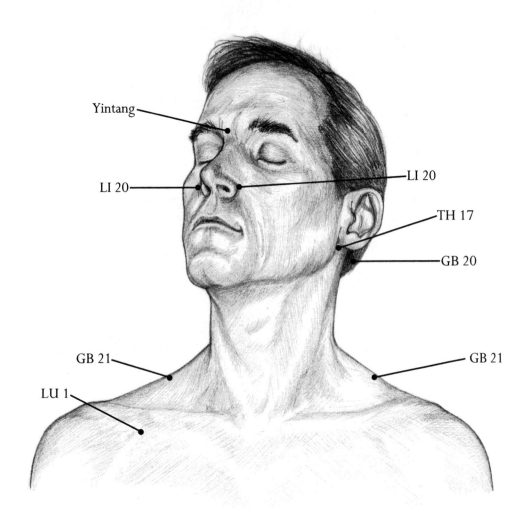

Yintang

LI 20

LI 20

TH 17

GB 20

GB 21

GB 21

LU 1

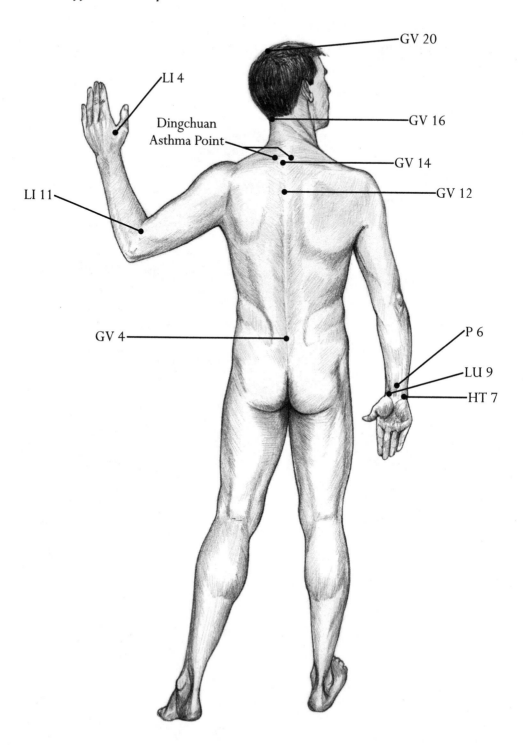

GV 20

LI 4

Dingchuan
Asthma Point

GV 16

GV 14

GV 12

LI 11

GV 4

P 6

LU 9

HT 7

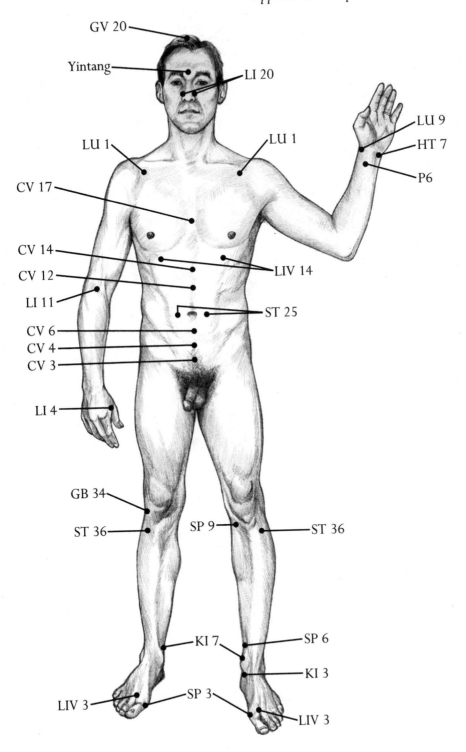

GV 20

Yintang

LI 20

LU 1

LU 1

LU 9

HT 7

P6

CV 17

CV 14

CV 12

LI 11

LIV 14

ST 25

CV 6

CV 4

CV 3

LI 4

GB 34

ST 36

SP 9

ST 36

KI 7

SP 6

KI 3

LIV 3

SP 3

LIV 3

INDEX

acidophilus, 247, 362–63, 380–81

acupoints, 41, 405–7

Conception Vessel *3*, 127, 134, 161, 309–10

Conception Vessel *4*, 385

Conception Vessel *6*, 322

Conception Vessel *12*, 86–87, 336–37

Conception Vessel *14*, 65–66

Conception Vessel *17*, 194, 367

Ding Chuan, 239

Gallbladder *20*, 174

Gallbladder *34*, 294

Governing Vessel *4*, 295

Governing Vessel *12*, 294

Governing Vessel *16*, 174

Heart *7*, 65, 161

Kidney *1*, 128

Kidney *3*, 134–35, 155, 161, 163, 239, 310, 368, 385

Kidney *7*, 322

Kidney *10*, 138

Large Intestine *4*, 158, 206–7, 225, 272, 295

Large Intestine *11*, 295

Large Intestine *20*, 158, 225–26

Liver *3*, 41–42, 149, 152, 157–58, 206, 250, 258, 294, 367–68

Liver *14*, 42

Lung *1*, 111

Lung *9*, 110–11, 163, 194, 239, 309, 322, 368, 385

massaging, 41

meridians, 211–12, 213–14

Pericardium *6*, 152

Spleen *3*, 87, 155, 336

Spleen *6*, 148–49, 272, 336, 385–86

Spleen *9*, 295

Spleen *10*, 272

Stomach *25*, 250, 258

Stomach *36*, 148–49, 250, 258, 295, 386

Triple Burner *17*, 174

Urinary Bladder *40*, 138

Yin Tang, 226

acupoints for specific purposes

allergies, 206–7

arthritis, 294–95

asthma, 239

cancer, 367–68

chronic fatigue syndrome, 322

colds and flus, 194

diabetes, 336–37

Earth types, 86–87

Earth/Water types, 155

eczema and psoriasis, 272

to expel Wind Devil, 174

Fire types, 65–66

HIV/AIDS, 384–86

inflammatory bowel disease, 258

irritable bowel syndrome, 250

lupus, 309–10

Metal types, 110–11

Metal/Water types, 163

Metal/Wood types, 157–58

acupoints for specific purposes (*cont.*)
  sinusitis, 225–26
  warmth, 128
  Water/Fire types, 161
  Water types, 127, 128,
    134–35, 138
  Wood/Earth types,
    148–49
  Wood/Fire types, 152
  Wood types, 41–42
acupuncture
  increasing use of, 214
  moxabustion, 295
  moxa rolls, 135
adult-onset diabetes. *See* diabetes, adult-onset
agrimony, 177
AIDS, xvi, 371–72
  Chinese interpretation,
    341, 376–77
  complementary treat-
    ments, 377–88
  opportunistic infections,
    374–75
  Western interpretation
    and treatment, 342
  See also HIV virus
alcohol, 358
Alexander, F. M., 104
alfalfa, 247
allergic dermatitis, xv
allergies, xv, 196–97
  Chinese interpretation,
    199–200
  complementary treat-
    ments, 200–208
  eczema and, 260–61
  hypoallergenic products,
    274
  Western interpretation
    and treatment, 197–99
  See also food allergies

anemia, 366
anger, 23, 180
Anger exercise, 33
antibiotics, xiii-xiv, 186,
    217–18
antioxidants, 305–6, 360–61
  See also selenium; vita-
    min E
anxiety. *See* worry
armeniaca seed, 236
aromatherapy, 67
  See also fragrances
arthritis, xv
  associated with lupus, 299
  Chinese interpretation,
    286–87
  complementary treat-
    ments, 287–97
  osteo-, 283–84, 285,
    287–88, 293
  rheumatoid, 284-85,
    287–88, 293
  symptoms, 284
  Western interpretation
    and treatment, 284–86
asanas. See yoga exercises
asthma, 228–29
  allergic (atopic), 229
  Chinese interpretation,
    232
  complementary treat-
    ments, 232–41
  exercise-induced, 230
  incidence in children, xv
  secondary, 229
  symptoms, 230
  Western interpretation
    and treatment, 229–31
astragalus, 86, 191, 193,
    204, 321, 363, 364,
    376, 383–84
atopic dermatitis. *See* eczema
atractylodes, 257

autoimmune diseases, 285,
    290, 310
  See also arthritis; lupus
autumn, 101–2, 177
AZT (azidothymidine), 375

back pain, 135
barberry, 161
barley, 177
baths, moisturizing, 273
Ba Xian Chang Shou Wan,
    110
Belly Breath exercise, 80–81
Bender, Sue, 103
Benson, Herbert, 32
Besserman, Perle, 104
beta-carotene, 190, 235,
    246, 305
  effects on cancer, 361
  functions, 267, 319
  immune system effects,
    380
  side effects, 221, 380
betaine hydrochloric acid,
    306
Bi Syndrome, 287
  See also arthritis
bitter foods, 59–60, 67
Bi Yan Pian, 157, 204, 222,
    223
Black Elk, 115–16
Bladder (Chinese view). *See*
    Urinary Bladder
bladder (Western view), 120
Blau, Paul, 301
blood
  abnormalities associated
    with lupus, 299
  Chinese view of, 277–79
  "congealed," 31, 179, 356
  as defense against disease,
    169
  deficient, 279–80

diseases at level of, 280–81

disturbances, 279–80

functions, 278

Heat Devil and, 176

relationship to *chi*, 278–79

Western view of, 277–78

blood sugar disorders, 329

   See also diabetes

body

   connection to mind, xxii, 341–43

   defenses against disease, 169–70, 171, 172, 211–12

bones, 130, 137

boneset, 175, 189

Brand, Paul, 280–81

breast cancer, 361

breathing exercises

   Belly Breath, 80–81

   Calming Breath, 59, 126–27

   for Earth types, 80–81, 88–89

   for Fire types, 58–59

   Invigorating Breath, 126

   for Metal types, 103–4

   for Water types, 126–27

   Whispered Ah, 104

bromelain, 291

bupleurum, 40, 363

burdock, 270–71

Butterfly exercise, 38–39

Bu Zhong Yi Qi Wan, 86, 148, 154, 191, 204, 320, 382

B vitamins. *See* vitamin B

caffeine, 220

Caisse, Renée, 366–67

Calming Breath exercise, 59, 126–27

Cameron, Ewan, 360

Campbell, Joseph, 88, 115

cancer

   breast, 361

   cell types, 350

   Chinese interpretation, 31, 341, 355–56

   complementary treatments, 352–53, 355, 356–71

   incidence, xvi, 349

   Kaposi's sarcoma, 375

   lung, 347–49

   Western interpretation and treatment, 342, 349–55

carcinomas, 350

Casals, Pablo, 345

catnip, 249

cayenne, 177, 179

celery seed, 293

CFS. *See* chronic fatigue syndrome

chamomile, 45, 60, 225, 249

chemotherapy, 354, 361, 362, 364, 366

Cheney, Paul, 314–15

Chen Pu Hu Chien Wan, 291

chi, xxi, 209–10

   disturbances, 215

   functions, 211–13

   meridians, 211–12, 213–14

   relationship to blood, 278–79

   relationship to *wei chi*, 209

   See also wei chi

Chinese herbs

   for AIDS patients, 376

   See also Chinese patent medicines; herbs

Chinese medicine

   as complement to Western medicine, xxii-xxv

defenses against disease, 169–70, 171, 172, 211–12

organs in, 24, 169, 214, 339–44

yielding to illness, 282

See also Five Element System

Chinese patent medicines, 40

   Ba Xian Chang Shou Wan, 110

   Bi Yan Pian, 157, 204, 222, 223

   Bu Zhong Yi Qi Wan, 86, 148, 154, 191, 204, 320, 382

   Chen Pu Hu Chien Wan, 291

   Chuan Shan Jia Qu Shi Qing Du Wan, 270

   Du Huo Jisheng Wan, 291–92

   Gan Mao Ling Pian, 191

   Gejie Ta Bu Wan, 133, 154, 191

   Guan Jie Yan Wan, 292

   He Che Da Zao Wan, 306–7

   Hsiao Yao Wan, 40–41, 148, 151, 157, 204, 223, 363

   Liu Wei Di Huang Wan, 133, 307, 334

   Ping Chuan Pills, 236–37

   Po Chai Pills, 192

   purchasing, 40

   Ren Shen Yang Ying Wan, 382–83

   Restorative Pills, 306–7

   Shen Ling Bai Zhu Pian, 257

   Shen Qi Da Bu Wan, 363–64

Chinese patent medicines
(*cont.*)
   Shih Chuan Ta Bu Wan, 154
   Shou Wu Chih, 133–34, 269
   Shu Kan Wan, 248
   Su Zi Jiang Qi Wan, 237
   Tian Wang Bu Xin Wan, 64–65, 151, 160
   Yeuchung Pills, 334
   Yin Chaio Chieh Tu Pian, 192
   Yunnan Pai Yao, 154
Chinese patent medicines for specific purposes
   allergies, 204–5
   arthritis, 291–92
   asthma, 236–37
   cancer, 363–64
   chronic fatigue syndrome, 320
   colds and flu, 191
   diabetes, 334
   eczema and psoriasis, 269–70
   HIV/AIDS, 382–83
   inflammatory bowel disease, 257
   irritable bowel syndrome, 248
   lupus, 306–7
   sinusitis, 222–23
   Water types, 133–34
cholesterol, 332–33
chromium, 332–33
chronic fatigue syndrome (CFS), 312–13
   Chinese interpretation, 316–17
   complementary treatments, 317–24

Western interpretation and treatment, 313–16
Chu, D., 376
Chuan Shan Jia Qu Shi Qing Du Wan, 270
cinnamon, 179
cleavers, 273
codonopsis root, 363
coenzyme Q-10, 319
coffee, 60
Cold Devil, 173, 178–79, 187, 218–19
   Bi (arthritis), 287, 295
colds, 184–85
   Chinese interpretation, 186–88
   complementary treatments, 188–96
   Western interpretation and treatment, 185–86
colitis, xv
   Chinese interpretation, 254–55
   complementary treatments, 255–59
   symptoms, 253
   Western interpretation and treatment, 253–54
comfrey, 178, 257
complementary medicine, xiv, xxii–xxv
   See also acupoints; diet; herbs; nutritional supplements; *and specific conditions*
Conception Vessel *3*
   acupoint, 127, 134, 161, 309–10
Conception Vessel *4*
   acupoint, 385
Conception Vessel *6*
   acupoint, 322

Conception Vessel *12*
   acupoint, 86–87, 336–37
Conception Vessel *14*
   acupoint, 65–66
Conception Vessel *17*
   acupoint, 194, 367
contact dermatitis, 262, 265–66
Control Cycle, 6, 142, 145
copper, 221
cornsilk, 177
couchgrass, 161
Cousins, Norman, 161, 342
crampbark, 154
Crohn's disease, xv, 251–52
   Chinese interpretation, 254–55
   complementary treatments, 255–59
   symptoms, 253
   Western interpretation and treatment, 252–54
cycles
   Control, 6, 142, 145
   Generation, 5, 141, 142, 145
   Humiliation, 155–56

da chi, 172
Damp Devil, 173, 176–77
   Bi (arthritis), 287, 295
dandelion, 39, 85, 176, 271, 384
dandelion root, 148, 151, 157, 205, 206, 308, 335, 365
degenerative joint disease. *See* arthritis
dermatitis
   allergic, xv
   atopic. *See* eczema
   contact, 262, 265–66

Devils, 172–73
    Cold, 173, 178–79, 187,
        218–19, 287
    Damp, 173, 176–77, 287
    Dry, 173, 177–78
    Heat, 173, 175–76, 187,
        218–19, 287
    involvement in arthritis,
        287
    Wind, 173–75, 187,
        218–19, 287, 376
devil's claw, 293
devil's club, 335
diabetes, adult-onset (Type
    II), xv, 324–25, 326
    complementary treat-
        ments, 329–38
    Western treatment, 327
diabetes
    Chinese interpretation,
        328
    juvenile-onset (Type I),
        326, 329
    Western interpretation
        and treatment, 325–27
Diamond, John, 381
diet
    for arthritis, 287–88
    for asthma, 232–33
    for cancer, 356–59
    for chronic fatigue syn-
        drome, 317–18
    for colds and flu, 188–89
    for diabetics, 329–32
    for Earth types, 81–83
    for Earth/Water types,
        154
    for eczema and psoriasis,
        266–67
    fats, 60–61, 330–31,
        356–57
    fiber, 107, 203, 244–45,
        331, 332, 357–58

for Fire types, 59–61
for HIV/AIDS patients,
    377–79
for inflammatory bowel
    disease, 253, 255–56
for irritable bowel syn-
    drome, 244–46
for lupus, 302–3
for Metal types, 105–7
for Metal/Water types,
    163
for Metal/Wood types,
    157
for sinusitis, 219–20
for Water/Fire types, 160
for Water types, 128–29
for Wood/Earth types, 148
for Wood/Fire types, 151
for Wood types, 33–35
See also foods; nutritional
    supplements
digestive system
    acupoints for, 86–87,
        385–86
    *See also specific organs and
        conditions*
Ding Chuan acupoint, 239
diseases
    chronic, 183, 215,
        344–47
    defenses against, 169–70,
        171, 172, 211–12
    *See also specific diseases and
        conditions*
dong quai, 178, 271
Dossey, Larry, 342
Dry Devil, 173, 177–78
Du Huo Jisheng Wan,
    291–92

ears
    hearing problems, 136
    infections, 188

Earth energy, xviii, 4
    deficient, 77–79, 152–53
    excess, 75–77
    imbalances, 74–79, 337
    organs associated with,
        74
Earth types, 71–74
    acupoints, 86–87
    best time of day, 79
    breathing exercises,
        80–81, 88–89
    color (yellow), 88
    Damp Devil and, 173,
        176–77
    diet, 81–83
    exercise, 83–85
    famous people, 92
    fragrances, 89
    herbs, 85–86
    Indian summer and,
        79–80
    learning to say no, 80
    lifestyle changes, 79–81
    nutritional supplements,
        83
    questions to ask, 90–91
    relationships, 73, 79, 153
    senses, 88–90
    singing, 88–89
    story for, 91
    sweets, 75, 81, 89
    Wood/Earth types,
        146–49
    worry, 173, 181
Earth/Water types, 152–
    55
echinacea, 157, 192–93,
    205, 224, 257, 308–9,
    321, 364, 383
eczema, xvi, 259–60
    allergic, 262
    Chinese interpretation,
        265–66

eczema (*cont.*)
    complementary treat-
        ments, 114, 266–76
    of Metal types, 93–94
    Western interpretation
        and treatment, 260–62
EFA. *See* essential fatty acids
elder flower, 175
elecampane, 109, 110, 157
elements. *See* Earth; Fire;
        Five Element System;
        Metal; Water; Wood
eleutherococcus ginseng, 154
emotions
    anger, 23, 180
    cancer and, 368–70
    chi and, 212
    fear, 173, 182–83, 240
    Five Destructive, 179–83
    grief, 181–82, 207,
        239–40
    joy, 180–81
    role in allergies, 207
    worry, 173, 181
energy. *See chi*
environmental problems,
        xiii–xiv
    indoor pollution, 216–17,
        230, 234
ephedra (*ma huang*), 157,
        179, 205, 206, 223,
        237–38
Epstein-Barr virus. *See*
        chronic fatigue syn-
        drome
essential fatty acids (EFAs),
        256, 381
essiac, 366–67
eucalyptus, 113, 158,
        225
exercise
    asthma induced by, 230
    for Earth types, 83–85

    for Fire types, 62–63
    for Metal types, 108–9
    tai chi, 84, 131, 154,
        288–89
    for Water types, 130–32
    for Wood types, 37–39
    See also yoga exercises
eyes. *See* vision

fasting, 107
fats
    reducing in diet, 60–61,
        330–31, 356–57
    trans-fatty acids (TFAs),
        61, 266
fear, 173, 182–83, 240
Felten, David, xxi–xxii
feverfew, 148
fiber, 203, 244–45, 331,
        357–58
    laxatives, 244–45
    supplements, 107, 332
Fire energy, xvii–xviii, 4
    deficient, 55–56
    excess, 53–55, 158–59
    imbalances, 51–56
    organs associated with,
        51–53
Fire types, 49–51
    acupoints, 65–66
    best time of day, 57
    breathing exercises, 58–59
    color (red), 66
    diet, 59–61
    exercise, 62–63
    famous people, 53, 70
    fragrances, 67
    Heat Devil and, 173, 176
    herbs, 64–65
    joy and, 180–81
    lifestyle changes, 57–59
    nutritional supplements,
        61

    questions to ask, 68–69
    relationships, 58, 68
    senses, 66–68
    story for, 69–70
    stress reduction, 57–59
    summer as best season, 57
    Water/Fire types, 158–61
    Wood/Fire types, 149–52
fish, wild, 317
fish oil, 236, 256
Five Element System, xvii
    in authors' lives, 142–45
    common combinations,
        145–46
    Control Cycle, 6, 142
    description of elements,
        xvii–xviii
    Generation Cycle, 5, 141,
        142, 145
    Humiliation Cycle,
        155–56
    interaction of elements,
        xviii–xix, 4, 141–42
    in personality, 3–5, 6–7,
        141–42
    questionnaire, 9–20
    See also Earth; Fire; Metal;
        Water; Wood
flaxseed oil, 236
flu, 184–85
    Chinese interpretation,
        186–88
    complementary treat-
        ments, 188–96
    shots, 186
    Western interpretation
        and treatment, 185,
        186
food allergies, 196–97
    associated with lupus, 302
    asthma and, 232–33
    Chinese interpretation,
        199–200

common allergens, 106

complementary treatments, 200–208

dairy products, 106

with eczema and psoriasis, 266

inflammatory bowel disease and, 255

irritable bowel syndrome and, 244

Metal types susceptible to, 105–7

symptoms, 105

tests, 233, 244

Western treatment, 199

foods

antibiotics in, xiii–xiv

bitter, 59–60, 67

cooling (*yin*), 59–60

energy derived from, 171

nitrates in, 163, 358, 361

organic, 148

processed, xiii, 200, 357

salty, 128–29, 137

spicy, 113–14

sweet, 75, 81, 89

whole, 201

See also diet; tastes

foot massage, 46

forsythia fruit, 192

fo ti, 178

fragrances

beneficial effects, 44

for Earth types, 89

for Fire types, 67

for Metal types, 113

for Water types, 136–37

for Wood types, 44–45

frankincense, 137

fruits, removing toxic residues, 35

fu organs, 339–40

Gallbladder (Chinese view), 24–25, 340

gallbladder (Western view), 25, 39

Gallbladder *20* acupoint, 174

Gallbladder *34* acupoint, 294

gamma linoleic acid (GLA), 202–3, 256, 269, 290, 306, 319, 362, 381

Gan Mao Ling Pian, 191

gardenia fruit, 176

garlic, 188, 224

oil, 188

supplements, 188

treating colds and flu with, 188, 189, 190

Garrett, Laurie, 373

Gattefossé, René-Maurice, 67

gecko lizards, 133, 191

Gejie Ta Bu Wan, 133, 154, 191

Generation Cycle, 5, 141, 142, 145

gentian, 151, 176

Gersten, Dennis, 33, 135

ginger, 85, 154, 177, 179, 189, 193, 249, 293

foot bath, 128

ginkgo, 136, 238, 335

ginseng, 85, 86, 132, 191, 204, 363

eleutherococcus, 154

Siberian, 320

GLA. *See* gamma linoleic acid

glucosamine sulfate, 291

goat's rue, 335

goldenseal, 193, 206, 224, 321

gout, 293

Governing Vessel *4* acupoint, 295

Governing Vessel *12* acupoint, 294

Governing Vessel *16* acupoint, 174

grapefruit, 188–89

grief, 181–82, 207, 239–40

Guan Jie Yan Wan, 292

guar gum, 332

gu chi, 171

Gurdjieff, George Ivanovitch, 80

Haas, Elson, 35

hawthorn berries, 64, 151, 160

hay fever, 197, 199, 202, 204

See also allergies

head massage, 46–47

hearing

problems, 136

See also sounds

Heart (Chinese view), 51–52, 339–40

circulation of blood, 279

energy created in, 171

Heat and, 173, 175–76

herbs for, 64–65

shen (spirit), 65, 171

heart (Western view), 51, 64

disease, 359

Heart *7* acupoint, 65, 161

Heat Devil, 173, 175–76, 187, 218–19

Bi (arthritis), 287, 295

He Che Da Zao Wan, 306–7

herbs

agrimony, 177

armeniaca seed, 236

astragalus, 86, 191, 193, 204, 321, 363, 364, 376, 383–84

atractylodes, 257

herbs (*cont.*)
  barberry, 161
  barley, 177
  boneset, 175, 189
  bupleurum, 40, 363
  burdock, 270–71
  catnip, 249
  cayenne, 177, 179
  celery seed, 293
  chamomile, 45, 60, 225,
    249
  cinnamon, 179
  cleavers, 273
  codonopsis root, 363
  comfrey, 178, 257
  cornsilk, 177
  couchgrass, 161
  crampbark, 154
  dandelion, 39, 85, 176,
    271, 384
  dandelion root, 148, 151,
    157, 205, 206, 308,
    335, 365
  devil's claw, 293
  devil's club, 335
  dong quai, 178, 271
  echinacea, 157, 192–93,
    205, 224, 257, 308–9,
    321, 364, 383
  elder flower, 175
  elecampane, 109, 110,
    157
  ephedra (*ma huang*), 157,
    179, 205, 206, 223,
    237–38
  essiac, 366–67
  feverfew, 148
  forsythia fruit, 192
  fo ti, 178
  gardenia fruit, 176
  garlic, 188, 189, 190,
    224
  gentian, 151, 176

  ginger, 85, 128, 154, 177,
    179, 189, 193, 249,
    293
  ginkgo, 136, 238, 335
  ginseng, 85, 86, 132, 154,
    191, 204, 320, 363
  goat's rue, 335
  goldenseal, 193, 206, 224,
    321
  hawthorn berries, 64,
    151, 160
  honeysuckle, 176, 192
  isatis, 191, 384
  lavender, 45, 67, 137
  ledebouriella, 175
  lemon balm, 45, 89, 148,
    151, 249
  licorice, 151, 155, 205,
    206, 238, 249, 270,
    293, 308, 366, 384
  licorice root, 157, 193,
    224, 321
  linden flower, 175
  lobelia, 238
  magnolia flower, 204, 222
  marshmallow, 178
  marshmallow root, 249,
    307
  meadowsweet, 154–55
  milk thistle, 39, 148, 321,
    365
  mint, 189
  motherwort, 64, 160
  mullein, 224, 238
  nettles, 308
  oats, 365
  ophiopogon, 110
  osha root, 157, 179, 193,
    205–6, 224, 384
  peony root, 248
  peppermint, 249
  perilla seeds, 237
  polygonum, 134, 269

  poria fungus, 177
  preparing, 401–3
  prunella, 176
  purchasing, 394–96
  red clover, 109, 110, 271,
    365–66
  rehmannia, 334
  rehmannia root, 64–65,
    110, 133, 178
  schizonepeta, 175
  skullcap, 176
  slippery elm, 178, 249
  St. John's wort, 148
  tea, 249
  uva ursi, 161
  vervain, 132, 160–61,
    308
  wild indigo, 321
  wintergreen, 249
  xanthium fruit, 204
  yarrow, 189, 293
  yellow dock, 176, 271,
    366
  See also Chinese patent
    medicines; Western
    herbs
HIV virus, xvi, 371–72
  Chinese interpretation,
    376–77
  complementary treat-
    ments, 377–88
  stages, 374
  transmission, 373–74
  Western interpretation
    and treatment, 372–76
honeysuckle, 176, 192
Hsiao Yao Wan, 40–41, 148,
  151, 157, 204, 223,
  363
Huang Di, xii, xxii, xxv–
  xxvi, 24–25, 339, 341
humidity. *See* Damp Devil
Humiliation Cycle, 155–56

hydrochloric acid, 203, 268, 306
hyperglycemia. *See* diabetes
hypoallergenic products, 274
hypoglycemia, 329, 332

IBS. *See* irritable bowel syndrome
I Ching, 282–83
illness. *See* diseases; *and specific diseases and conditions*
imagery techniques, 135
immune supportive therapy, 354–55
immune system
  benefits of vitamin C, 360
  Chinese concept of, xx–xxii, 341
  herbs for, 364
  Western concept of, xx
  See also autoimmune diseases; HIV virus; *wei chi*
indigo, wild, 321
inflammatory bowel disease (IBD), 251–52
  Chinese interpretation, 254–55
  complementary treatments, 255–59
  Western interpretation and treatment, 252–54
  See also colitis; Crohn's disease
influenza. *See* flu
insulin, 325, 327
interferon, 321, 364
intestines. *See* Large Intestine; Small Intestine
Invigorating Breath exercise, 126
irritable bowel syndrome (IBS), xv, 241–42

Chinese interpretation, 243–44
complementary treatments, 244–51
symptoms, 242
Western interpretation and treatment, 242–43
isatis, 191, 384
itching, relief of, 270, 273

Jacobson, Edmund, 32
jing chi, 119, 171, 172
joy, 180–81
juvenile-onset diabetes (Type I), 326, 329

Kaposi's sarcoma, 375
Kidney (Chinese view), 119–20, 339–40
  acupoints, 127, 134
  Cold Devil and, 173, 178
  deficient energy, 130, 186–87, 228, 316, 355–56
  energy stored in, 171
  herbs for, 64–65, 133
kidney (Western view), 119, 299
Kidney *1* acupoint, 128
Kidney *3* acupoint, 134–35, 155, 161, 163, 239, 310, 368, 385
Kidney *7* acupoint, 322
Kidney *10* acupoint, 138

Lao-tzu, 30, 183–84
Large Intestine (Chinese view), 53, 96–97, 340
large intestine (Western view), 96
Large Intestine *4* acupoint, 158, 206–7, 225, 272, 295

Large Intestine *11* acupoint, 295
Large Intestine *20* acupoint, 158, 225–26
lavender, 45, 67, 137
laxatives, 36, 244–45
ledebouriella, 175
Lemonade, Special, 36, 37
lemon balm, 45, 89, 148, 151, 249
lemons, 45
lemon water, 189
leukemia, 350, 358
licorice, 151, 155, 205, 206, 238, 249, 270, 293, 308, 366, 384
licorice root, 157, 193, 224, 321
Lieh-tzu, 212
linden flower, 175
Lin Yutang, 358
Liu Wei Di Huang Wan, 133, 307, 334
Liver (Chinese view), 339–40
  association with Wood, 24–25
  constrained *chi*, 40, 199, 254, 355, 356
  dietary recommendations, 34–35
  elimination of stress by, 30–33, 243
  functions, 34
  relationship to blood, 279
  Wind and, 173
liver (Western view), 24, 365
  cleansing, 35–36
Liver *3* acupoint, 41–42, 149, 152, 157–58, 206, 250, 258, 294, 367–68

Liver *14* acupoint, 42
lobelia, 238
Lown, Bernard, 342–43
Lung *1* acupoint, 111
Lung *9* acupoint, 110–11,
    163, 194, 239, 309,
    322, 368, 385
lung cancer, 347–49
    See also cancer
Lungs (Chinese view),
    339–40
    allergies related to, 199
    deficient *chi*, 355–56
    Dry Devil and, 173
    functions, 94, 96
    wei chi created in, 172,
        186–87, 214
    See also asthma
lungs (Western view), 96,
    109
lupus, 297
    Chinese interpretation,
        301–2
    complementary treat-
        ments, 302–12
    diagnostic criteria,
        298–300
    incidence, xiv, xv
    Western interpretation
        and treatment,
        298–301

magnesium, 136, 235,
    247–48, 290–91, 319
magnolia flower, 204, 222
ma huang. See ephedra
mantras, 88–89
marshmallow, 178
marshmallow root, 249, 307
massage
    for arthritis, 289
    for Earth types, 90
    for Fire types, 68

for Metal types, 114
self-, 46–47, 138
Swedish, 46, 68, 90
types, 46–47
for Water types, 138
for Wood types, 46
Matsumoto, Kiiko, 222
meadowsweet, 154–55
meditation
    benefits, 32
    for Metal types, 104–5,
        112
    Vipassana, 127
    for Water types, 127
    for Wood types, 32–33
    Zen, 104
meridians, 211–12, 213–14
Metal energy, xviii, 4
    deficient, 99–101
    excess, 97–99, 103, 161
    imbalances, 96–101, 173
    organs associated with,
        96–97
Metal types, 93–96, 104–5
    acupoints, 110–11
    autumn as best season,
        101–2
    best time of day, 101
    breathing exercises,
        103–4
    color (white), 111–12
    diet, 105–7
    Dry Devil and, 173,
        177–78
    exercise, 108–9
    famous people, 116
    food allergies, 105–7
    fragrances, 113
    getting organized, 102–3
    grief, 181–82, 207,
        239–40
    herbs, 109–10
    lifestyle changes, 101–5

massage, 114
meditation, 104–5, 112
nutritional supplements,
    107–8
questions to ask, 114–15
senses, 111–14
spicy foods, 113–14
story for, 115–16
Metal/Water types, 161–64
Metal/Wood types, 155–58
milk thistle, 39, 148, 321,
    365
mind, connection to body
    and health, xxii,
    341–43
minerals
    copper, 221
    vanadium, 333
    See also magnesium; nutri-
        tional supplements;
        zinc
mint, 189
    pepper-, 44–45, 89,
        249
motherwort, 64, 160
moxabustion, 295
moxa rolls, 135
Moyers, Bill, xxi–xxii
mugwort, 135
mullein, 224, 238
mushrooms, 364–65, 384
music, 88–89, 112, 126
myrrh, 137

nettles, 308
nicotine, 359
nitrates and nitrites, 163,
    358, 361
nutritional supplements
    for allergies, 202–3
    for arthritis, 289–91
    for asthma, 234–36
    for cancer, 360–63

for chronic fatigue syndrome, 318–19
for colds and flu, 189–91
for diabetics, 332–34
for Earth types, 83
for eczema and psoriasis, 267–69
for Fire types, 61
for HIV/AIDS, 379–82
for inflammatory bowel disease, 256
for irritable bowel syndrome, 246–48
for lupus, 304–6
for Metal types, 107–8
for sinusitis, 220–22
for Water types, 129–30, 136
for Wood types, 37

oats, 365
olive oil, 266–67
omega-3 fatty acids, 236, 256, 268–69, 289–90, 306, 319, 362
onions, 233
ophiopogon, 110
organs
    Chinese metaphorical view of, 24
    as defense against disease, 169
    diseases at level of, 339–44
    flow of *chi* through, 214
    fu, 339–40
    zang, 339–41
    See also specific organs
osha root, 157, 179, 193, 205–6, 224, 384
osteoarthritis. *See* arthritis
osteoporosis, 130, 137

pain, 280–81
    spiritual, 281–82
Pancreas (Chinese view), 171, 279
Pauling, Linus, 190, 360
peony root, 248
peppermint, 44–45, 89, 249
Pericardium (Chinese view), 51, 52
pericardium (Western view), 52
Pericardium 6 acupoint, 152
perilla seeds, 237
personality, interaction of elements in, xviii–xix, 3–5, 6–7, 141–42
photosensitivity, 303–4
physical therapy, for arthritis, 286, 288
physicians
    Five Failings of, xxv–xxvi
    responsibilities, 341–42, 344
pine oil, 225
Ping Chuan Pills, 236–37
pneumonia, pneumocystic, 374
Po Chai Pills, 192
pollution, xiii–xiv
    indoor, 216–17, 230, 234
polygonum, 134, 269
Porchia, Antonio, 139
poria fungus, 177
protease inhibitors, 375–76
prunella, 176
psoriasis, xvi, 262–64
    Chinese interpretation, 265–66
    complementary treatments, 114, 266–76
    Western interpretation and treatment, 264–65
psychotherapy, 127, 286

pycnogenol, 236, 305–6, 319

Qi Bo, xii, xx–xxi, 45, 51, 81, 113, 120, 341
quercetin, 202, 247, 268
questionnaire, 9–20

radiation therapy, 353, 361, 364, 366
reactive airway disease (RAD). *See* asthma
Reclining Hero (yoga exercise), 84–85
red clover, 109, 110, 271, 365–66
rehmannia, 334
rehmannia root, 64–65, 110, 133, 178
relationships
    of Earth types, 73, 79, 153
    energy created from, 171
    of Fire types, 58, 68
relaxation techniques, 32
Ren Mo, 214
Ren Shen Yang Ying Wan, 382–83
respiratory infections, 109, 205
rheumatoid arthritis. *See* arthritis
Robbins, John, 148

saline nasal spray, 225
salt, 128–29, 137, 160
sarcomas, 350
schizonepeta, 175
seasonal affective disorder (SAD), 128, 159
seasons
    autumn, 101–2, 177
    Indian summer, 79–80

seasons (*cont.*)
spring, 30, 44
summer, 57
winter, 124–25, 128
selenium, 222, 235, 290, 305, 333, 361, 380
senses
vision, 42–44
of Wood types, 42–46
See also fragrances; sounds; tastes; touch
Seven Day Liver Cleanse, 35–36
shark cartilage, 363
shen chi, 171
Shen Ling Bai Zhu Pian, 257
Shen Qi Da Bu Wan, 363–64
Shih Chuan Ta Bu Wan, 154
Shiitake mushrooms, 364–65, 384
Shou Wu Chih, 133–34, 269
Shu Kan Wan, 248
Siberian ginseng, 320
sight. *See* vision
siler tuber, 175
sinus cleanse, 222, 289
sinusitis, chronic, xv, 215–16, 289
Chinese interpretation, 218–19
complementary treatments, 219–27
symptoms, 217
Western interpretation and treatment, 216–18
Skin, as Third Lung, 94, 114
Skin Cap, 272–73
skin disorders. *See* eczema; psoriasis
skullcap, 176

slippery elm, 178, 249
Small Intestine (Chinese view), 53, 340
small intestine (Western view), 53
smell. *See* fragrances
smoking, quitting, 359
Snow, Sheila, 367
sounds
for Earth types, 88–89
for Fire types, 66–67
for Metal types, 112
for Water types, 136
for Wood types, 44
sour tastes, 45, 113–14
Special Lemonade, 36, 37
spicy foods, 113–14
spirituality, 115–16, 212–13, 340
Spleen (Chinese view), 74, 244, 279, 339–40
acupoints for, 86–87
deficient *chi*, 254, 316, 355–56
energy created from food, 171
spleen (Western view), 74
Spleen *3* acupoint, 87, 155, 336
Spleen *6* acupoint, 148–49, 272, 336, 385–86
Spleen *9* acupoint, 295
Spleen *10* acupoint, 272
sports. *See* exercise
spring, 30, 44
Standing Forward Bend (yoga exercise), 131–32
Standing Squat (yoga exercise), 109
Star series (yoga exercise), 63
St. John's wort, 148

Stomach (Chinese view), 74, 340
acupoints for, 86–87
energy created from food, 171
stomach (Western view), 74
Stomach *25* acupoint, 250, 258
Stomach *36* acupoint, 148–49, 250, 258, 295, 386
stress reduction, 246, 358
Fire types, 57–59
Wood types, 30–33
sugar, 220, 330
summer, 57
Indian, 79–80
sunlight, 274, 303–4
Su Zi Jiang Qi Wan, 237
sweet foods, 75, 81, 89
systemic lupus erythematosis. *See* lupus

tai chi, 84, 131, 154, 288–89
tan, 77, 83, 219
Tao, xii
tastes
bitter, 59–60, 67
sour, 45, 113–14
spicy, 113–14
sweet, 75, 81, 89
tea
diaphoretic, 189
green, 60
herbal, 249
Tense and Release exercise, 32
TFAs. *See* trans-fatty acids
thymus gland extract, 381
Tian Wang Bu Xin Wan, 64–65, 151, 160
tinnitus, 136

tongue, 67

touch
Earth types and, 90
Fire types and, 68
Metal types and, 114
Water types and, 137–38
Wood types and, 45–46

toxins
on food, 35
in indoor air, 216–17, 230, 234

trans-fatty acids (TFAs), 61, 266

Triple Burner *17* acupoint, 174

Triple Heater, 52–53, 328, 340

Trombley, Lauran Eugene, 345

ulcerative colitis. *See* colitis

Urinary Bladder *40* acupoint, 138

Urinary Bladder, 120, 134, 340

urinary infections, 160

uva ursi, 161

vaccines, flu, 186

vanadium, 333

vegetables, removing toxic residues, 35

vervain, 132, 160–61, 308

Vipassana, 127

viruses, intestinal, 196
See also flu; HIV virus

vision, 42–44

vitamin A, 190, 202, 221, 235, 361–62

vitamin B, 202, 236, 247, 290, 305, 319, 333, 362, 380

vitamin C
antihistamine function, 202, 220, 234, 318
cancer prevention, 360
for colds, 190
dosage, 220–21, 234–35
functions, 246, 268, 290, 304, 333, 379–80

vitamin E
antioxidant role, 235, 290, 305, 360–61, 380
functions, 202, 221, 247, 333

water
drinking, 81–82, 136–37
filters, 399–400
testing, 35

Water energy, xviii, 4
deficient, 122–24, 149–50, 152, 158–59
excess, 120–22
imbalances, 119–24, 136, 228
sexuality and, 137

Water/Fire types, 158–61

Water types, 117–19
acupoints, 127, 128, 134–35, 138
best time of day, 124
breathing exercises, 126–27
Cold Devil and, 173, 178–79
color (black), 135
commitment to causes, 125–26
diet, 128–29
Earth/Water types, 152–55
exercise, 130–32
famous people, 140
fear, 182–83, 240

fragrances, 136–37
herbs, 132–34
lifestyle changes, 124–28
meditation, 127
Metal/Water types, 161–64
music, 126
nutritional supplements, 129–30, 136
psychotherapy, 127
questions to ask, 138–39
salty foods, 128–29, 137
senses, 135–38
story for, 139–40
winter and, 124–25, 128

wei chi, xxi
attacks by Five Devils, 172–79, 183
as defense against disease, 169, 171, 172, 211–12
emotions and, 183
relationship to *chi*, 209
sources of energy, 171–72, 186–87, 214

Weil, Andrew, 126

Werbach, Melvyn, 268

Western herbs
for allergies, 205–6
for arthritis, 292–94
for asthma, 237–38
for cancer, 364–67
for chronic fatigue syndrome, 320–22
for colds and flu, 189, 192–93
for diabetes, 334–36
for Earth types, 85–86
for eczema and psoriasis, 270–71, 273
for Fire types, 64–65
for HIV/AIDS, 383–84
for inflammatory bowel disease, 257–58

Western herbs (*cont.*)
   inhalations, 225
   for irritable bowel syn-
      drome, 248–50
   for lupus, 307–9
   for Metal types, 109–10
   purchasing, 394–95
   for sinusitis, 223–24
   for Water types, 132
   for Wood types, 39
   See also herbs
wet heating pads, 295
Whispered Ah exercise, 104
white flower oil, 164
Wind, syndrome, 27
Wind Devil, 173–75, 187,
    218–19, 232, 376
   Bi (arthritis), 287, 294
Wind Points, 173–74, 175
winter, 124–25, 178
wintergreen, 249
Wood/Earth types, 146–49
Wood energy, xvii, 4
   deficient, 27–29, 38
   excess, 25–27, 147,
     155–56
   imbalances, 23–29
   organs associated with,
     24–25
Wood/Fire types, 149–52
Wood types, 21–23
   acupoints, 41–42
   anger and, 23, 180

best time of day, 29–30
color (green), 43–44
diet, 33–35
exercise, 37–39
famous people, 48
fragrances, 44–45
Heat Devil and, 176
herbs, 39–40
lifestyle changes, 29–33
Metal/Wood types,
   155–58
nutritional supplements,
   37
questions to ask, 47
senses, 42–46
sour tastes, 45
spring as best season, 30,
   44
story for, 47–48
stress reduction, 30–33
Wind Devil and, 173
worry, 173, 177, 181
Wu Hsing. See Five Element
   System

xanthium fruit, 204

yarrow, 189, 293
yeast infections, 247,
   374–75, 378
yellow dock, 176, 271, 366
*The Yellow Emperors Classic of
   Medicine*, xi–xii, xxv–

xxvi, 24–25, 30, 45,
   51, 57, 102, 120, 125,
   172, 179, 340
Yeuchung Pills, 334
Yin Chaio Chieh Tu Pian,
   192
Yin Tang acupoint, 226
yin and *yang*, xii, 278–79,
   339
yoga exercises
   for arthritis, 288
   Butterfly, 38–39
   for Earth types, 84–85
   for Fire types, 62–63
   for Metal types, 108–9
   Reclining Hero, 84–85
   Standing Forward Bend,
     131–32
   Standing Squat, 109
   Star series, 63
   for Water types, 131–32
   for Wood types, 38–39
   Yoga Mudra, 108–9
Yunnan Pai Yao, 154

zang organs, 339–41
Zen meditation, 104
zinc, 221, 248, 268, 305,
   334, 382
   for colds and flu, 190–
     91
   oxide ointment, 273
   spray, 272–73